MEDICINE, MURDER & MERRIMENT

Medicine, Murder & Merriment

A DOCTOR'S CONFESSIONS

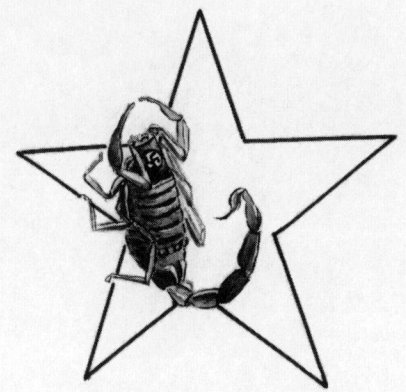

Charles Pole

PENTAGON

0 904288 01 3

Photoset, printed and bound
in Great Britain by
REDWOOD BURN LIMITED
Trowbridge & Esher

With love and gratitude to my wife for her sacrifices and for writing this book (I only dictated it).

With sincere thanks to Morag Campbell, Roy Lenthall, Bob Ryall and Tony Wood for their invaluable help.

With forgiveness to my *old* enemies (I have no new ones).

C.P.

TO THE MEMORY OF
GUSTAV AND LES
MY BEST FRIENDS
WHO LEFT US PREMATURELY

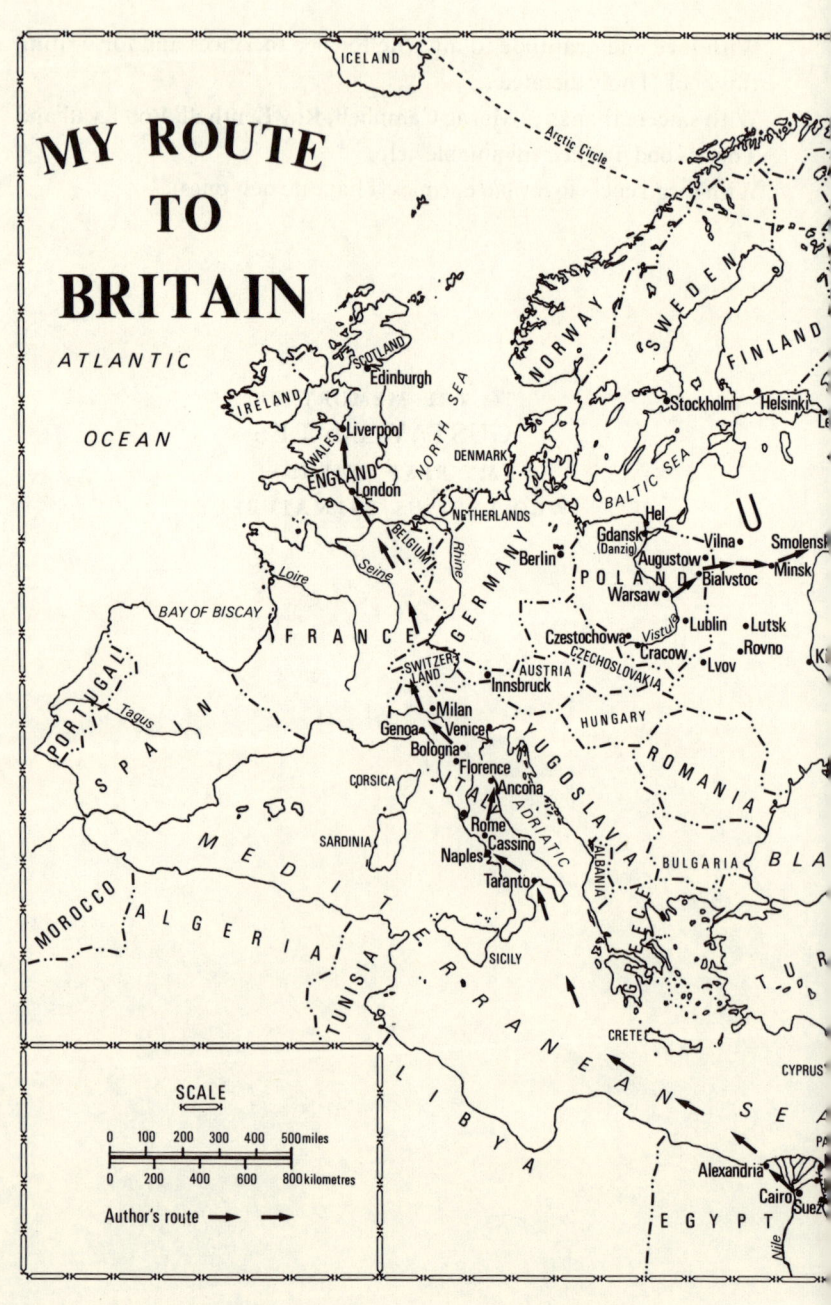

MY ROUTE TO BRITAIN

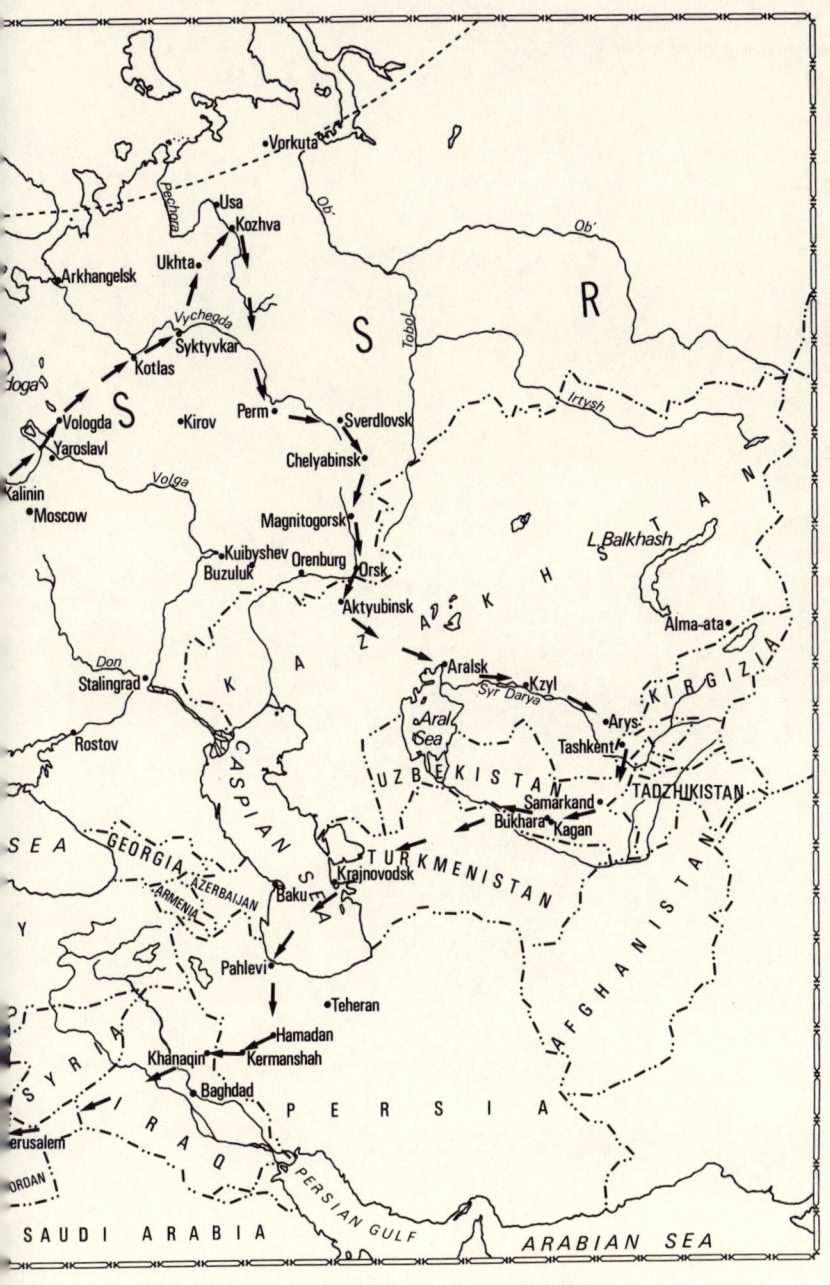

Contents

Illustrations

Preface

I have my moments of frustration, moments of doubt, moments of despair. Such feelings must not be too deep or too long, otherwise there is no possibility of winning.

Martin Luther King

Why have I written this book?

There are many reasons.

Having been swept along by brutal events over which I had no control, I have seen many lands, met many races and lived among people of various tongues, classes and creeds. I have come into contact with remarkable people, people of courage, tenacity of purpose and love for their fellow men, but also with abominable, callous, "human" beings indifferent to the tragedy of others, with selfishness, avarice or self-indulgence written all over their faces. When confronted with humanity their cold hearts became colder still. Fortunately, I found solace and love among animals. Much later, from behind the surgery desk, I was able to observe the intimate behaviour of men more closely and gained access to their lives. Perhaps because of this I am able, by comparison, to appreciate the great features of this country better than many who have lived here longer than the twenty-eight years of my life in Britain. Besides, a doctor who has suffered can identify himself more easily with the patient, and compassion comes to him naturally. I feel I had more reason to write what I have written than an average mortal!

These are my credentials to tell the story. But there is more to it.

We live in eventful times, not only as they were during the years of war but as they are at this very day. Yet, there is a great difference. The war years were turbulent and terrifying. Only afterwards did they become exciting, and the past seems almost insignificant in the light of scientific progress since. I wish to share with the general public my enthusiasm for the incredible advances made in medical knowledge during the last few decades and to let them participate in the thrill of many discoveries, also to put on record the social and moral changes which have occurred. They are not lay readers any more. Thanks to the mass media the public is much more knowledgeable to-day and

1

doctors find it easier to communicate with them; this is rewarding. The gap has been bridged. Yet changes around us are so rapid and so profound that we need all possible help to be able to absorb them. Amazingly, there are a great number of people, especially in the younger set, who have intimate knowledge of a motor-car, motor-cycle, computers and other automatic devices but who know very little about how their own body works. Fortunately, doctors have much to tell, much more than before. They do not wrap their scanty knowledge of yesterday into "pidgin" Latin any more. When they discarded their customary aloofness, they ceased to separate themselves from the rest of their fellow men, their real or potential patients, and delivered modern learning in more comprehensible terms without resorting to mystery and magic. They like to explain to their patients the nature of the disease from which they suffer. Doctors not only became more clever but wiser. It is my hope that the brief account of medical progress reported here will be easily understood and the unfolding of events readable.

This book is, in fact, a continuation of a dialogue I have already had with patients. Until now *they* confessed to me and now *I* confess to them. In this way, I hope, we shall get to know each other better. Patients can see that a doctor is also human — with two sides to the coin. If I complain about a few, it is only to put the record straight — one often hears complaints about doctors, seldom about patients. May I be permitted a gentle reminder that a patient who expects good "bedside" manners from his doctor should display them himself. If I have some desperate things to say, it is because peoples' deeds were outrageous, my words are not. If I am indifferent to religious devotees, it is because I long more for genuine faith than for the promise of the future world. I do not believe people have to be buried before they can be equal and free from worry. I have lived through two wars and hated them. They brought death, destruction, starvation, disastrous epidemics, trench feet, trench fever, gassing, mutilation and the atom-bomb aftermath, with repercussions for life. Efficiency in killing has grown with the passage of time. Not many marshals and generals had been killed or captured; the full impact fell on the "other ranks" and civilian population.

Homage shown to dead heroes should be a warning to those who survived. The greed of the Kaiser and the German desire to have a place in the sun started the First World War, using the assassination of the Arch Duke Franz Ferdinand, heir to the Austrian Throne, as a pretext. Hitler's "great design" for Germany started the Second World

War under yet another pretext – to fight unfaithful Jews and godless Bolsheviks. If I have been biased it is because I cannot conceal my emotions. It is only natural that one hopes for peace and tries to give hope to others, a tangible hope, a hope for cure for the present incurable, brought about by advances in medicine. If I have omitted some gruesome events it was because I chose not to remember them and the canvas was not large enough to embrace everything. I had to pick and choose. If I touched on humour in most unhappy situations I did it in self-defence and expect it to be accepted in this spirit, besides, laughter is the best medicine. If I criticized others I have criticized myself and my countrymen.

This is not an eloquent nostalgic recollection of war-time experiences, even though the persecution turned into adventure. I am not a retired soldier or doctor writing from boredom. I am still in harness. The day when I put my stethoscope away is still far ahead. This is a study of the times I have lived in and of its people, and the flimsy sketch of myself is unavoidable. It is the eventful times which may be of interest to the Reader.

I express my conviction that the world is not in decline and that the ferment we witness is like a purposeful catalyst which helps to shape new forms to come. Science, particularly medicine, shows a continuous progress and brings us more hope and more opportunities. I pause to reflect that the emerging world is like a growing child who needs a great deal of careful planning and adjustment. This should make it possible to live in the exciting and happy future. The reminiscences here are meant to raise the hopes and spirits of the downhearted by showing that even the darkest beginning does not mean a dismal end. Why then despair? I began to write in tears and ended in smiles and laughter, the hope I had lost has returned.

If I have shown compassion towards the Jews, I have done it with the Poles, Russians, women in general, the aged and others, motivated by injustices heaped upon them. I did not lead a personal vendetta against the guilty, all of us have suffered. However, I find it necessary to refresh our memories and to tell the younger generation about our experiences to prevent it ever happening again. Forces by which we were swamped have to be understood to be timely averted. It was a lesson which should not be lost! But this is more of a warning than of a chilling account and aims at inoculating optimism, not hate.

I have discussed life and people. Doctors, I believe, are eminently

3

suited to do it; they are involved in mankind. Surely it is not a coincidence that Friedrich von Schiller, Anton Chekhov, Sir Arthur Conan Doyle, Arthur Schnitzler, Somerset Maugham, Axel Munthe, A.J. Cronin, Albert Schweitzer, Janusz Korczak, Aldo Castellani, Lord Moran and Richard Gordon were all doctors, to mention but a few. Writing has enabled me to put my views across on controversial matters with which modern living is studded. From the reader's point of view, the fictional character of a doctor has been of interest to him for centuries. I imagine reality could be as good as fiction. But I don't expect everyone to agree with all my opinions − it is too much to hope that each reader will see only through my eyes.

My dilemmas posed by war are gone, yet peace, prosperity and progress brought a new one − is it to the patient's good to strip him of all mysteries, to foster his criticism and dispose with the power of suggestion? Should bland truth be told whatever its contents? Due to the insatiable progress in science much of what I write will become obsolete. Yet what I am saying is meant for my contemporaries. Why should I care for posterity, it certainly will not care for me!

Last but not least I wish to show how Britain is seen through the eyes of a stranger adopted by her. The whole world owes a deep gratitude to the British for standing firm against everything Hitler stood for, against his conspiracy of lies and genocide. Britain helped to thwart his plans without sparing sacrifices, thus saving mankind from sinking into the Dark Ages. I admired her people's courage, determination and ability to resist and win. My gratitude is also a personal one. Britain has been like a mother to me and the English language is my adopted mother tongue even though I have never mastered the accent! I have great admiration for her people, among whom I have my best friends. I remember the time their country gave me and my fellow countrymen a helping hand when we were down and out and they in mortal danger. I have no doubt that it was not just an act of self-preservation but one of common humanity and longing for justice. I was uprooted and moved half-way round the world among strangers. It was a grand and forceful tour, perhaps because it was unintended. It came to an end on reaching British shores.

Now I am not a stranger, not even an immigrant any longer. Britain is my country, I belong here. Evidently God was on my side. Perhaps He is our Father and shows benevolence after all. I was wrong to think of Him as a fickle, haphazard Providence! Fickleness was mine and not His. I began to put my trust in God and to look upon Him as our

4

Saviour. Love and forgiveness are his business. He bestowed on us the only religion – it does not know hate and does not need churches, mosques and synagogues, its place is in man's heart. Only man created many versions (like the English language with its many dialects), sometimes uncompromising and with dubious ethics. Religions don't unite the human race, they divide it. The religious enthusiasm which followed the conquests of the Prophet Mohammed and Christian crusades have antagonized people. We have Pagans versus Christians, Moslems versus Hindus, Catholics versus Protestants. Who can tell which is the true church? God has no chosen creeds or nations, nor even people for that matter. Every striving and honest man has a future; a saint has a past.

This is a humble effort executed by one hand, in the knowledge of it being scrutinized by many pairs of eyes, preceded by this statement of my intent.

1
Childhood

You can take a boy out of the country but you can't
take the country out of a boy.
Arthur Baer

Indeed, I tremble for my country when I reflect that God
is just.
Thomas Jefferson

Czestochowa is a Polish town renowned for its textile industry and the
fortified monastery on Jasna Gora.* In my youth it had 100,000 inhabitants. The monastery, perched on a hill and surrounded by thick
walls, was successfully defended by fanatical monks under the Prior
Kordecki from the invader King Gustav Adolph of Sweden. The Swedish army was led by General Mueller. The year was 1655 and the
siege lasted from November 18 until December 12. The enemy outnumbered the defenders almost by twenty to one.** In 1702 the monastery withstood yet another Swedish invasion, and, in 1809 resisted
an attack from the Austrians. The monks and Holy picture of the
Virgin Mary of Czestochowa, reputed to be responsible for many
miracles, have never been forgotten by the Polish nation. Famous visitors from abroad including the French Marshal Foch were conducted
with pride to the monastery. It was with similar pleasure that I showed
it to the major of the French Military Mission in Poland, who had recently married my cousin, when he came to visit "my" town in 1921.

Not everything, however, was holy on Jasna Gora. A few years
before the First World War, a prior named Macoch fell in love with a
nun and removed the precious stones, mostly rubies, from the Holy
picture giving them to his beloved. When this was eventually discovered, the infatuated monk was defrocked and the name Macoch
was used as a curse for a long time after.

I am writing about this "Holy Town" not because of my religious
convictions, but because I was born there in August 1910 and lived in
it for the next eighteen years. The year of my birth Agnes Baden-

* Mountain of Light.
** 230 defenders repelled the 4,000 strong enemy.

6

Powell and her brother Sir Robert founded the Girl Guides Movement and Peyton Rous discovered the first tumour-inducing virus.* One may say that one of these happenings was a non-event.

It was on my third birthday when my parents took me to a fête saying that it had all been arranged especially for me. I listened with delight to a band and watched, full of curiosity, a sack race, an egg-and-spoon race and a balloon man. I felt very important yet annoyed seeing other children getting balloons which should have been mine!

For a full four years I was able to live peacefully in "my" town, then World War I broke out. I saw the last Kazakhs leaving the town in a hurry and soon after the Germans marched in. I was just four years old, and fascinated by the sight of endless heavy boots raising dust from the trembling soil. I saw the goose-step for the first time. They were all boots, only boots . . . One of the soldiers gave me a bar of chocolate – how nice they are – I thought. It was not long before my fascination changed to fear. I remember seeing a man chained between big horses which carried puffed-up, arrogant, fierce looking, overfed soldiers wearing spiked helmets and spurs. They spurred their horses and the unfortunate man was dragged by the leaping animals. Brutes! Soon our house was requisitioned and we had to live and sleep in one room, the kitchen being taken over by the army cook; mother was allowed to use it only when the soldiers had satisfied their appetites. One morning an officer heard me crying. He rushed to my mother rattling his sabre and yelling: "Silence that bastard at once or I will chop his curly head off!" I was petrified. Some time later the same officer ordered my mother's bed to be taken away, and that at the time when she was confined to it after an accident; he found the bed to be more comfortable than his own.

The following summer we spent in Kociezowy, a village some forty miles north of our town. Here I saw Austrian soldiers for the first time. Their uniforms intrigued me. Had I not had the past unpleasant experience, I would have enjoyed this pantomime.

The years were flying by crowded with events, the Russian Revolution and German defeat among them.

Soon I was eight and helping my parents to decorate our balcony with pots of flowers and to hang a colourful carpet from the balustrade – we were celebrating the independence of Poland. New buff uniforms appeared and I admired the smartness of the officers and their high

---

* He successfully transmitted a cell-free filtration from sarcoma of one chicken to another, which led to the link between viruses and cancer.

7

shiny boots. I also liked the blue uniforms of the police. In no time we were asked to part with all our brass, copper and leather goods for a good cause. For the next twenty years the men in uniform were our masters, the clergy being second in command, and we believed in their strength, their honesty and their patriotism.

We lived in comparative peace. People, mostly peasants, were flocking to the monastery from afar on organized pilgrimages, crawling on their knees for the last few hundred metres, crossing themselves frequently, kissing the earth, some in tears and praying for a miracle. The shuffling of hundreds and hundreds of feet and the monotonous singing of "Aaave Mariiia" reached our school. They then wandered in the monastery grounds as in a trance amid the Fourteen Stations of the Cross, only to kneel for hours on the stony ground, chanting or in prayer before the bejewelled picture of the Virgin Mary of Czestochowa, and pursuing unhygienic rituals such as kissing Holy objects and the like, common among most religions. Barefooted, in patched but clean dresses to look their best, they admired the ornate attire of the bishop who celebrated Mass and gaped with reverent amazement at the immense treasures displayed in the vault, after paying an entrance fee. I always understood that Christianity aims at equality of worldly goods . . . They greeted each other with "Praised be Jesus Christ" which was answered by "For the centuries of centuries, Amen". On leaving the monastery the worshippers were instantly surrounded by vendors who were selling various trinkets and "holy pictures". These "sacred" objects were later finding pride of place in their poor homes, and so some people found peace, some prosperity, while others were deprived of both.

In 1921 our town witnessed a pogrom in which several Jews were killed, among them a feldsher* named Nasanowicz, who appeared in the street during the riots answering a mercy call from a hospital, although he was warned of the danger to himself.

This did not appear to worry people who were used to years of turbulence. The creation of Sovereign Poland brought dispute over the Russian/Polish frontiers and culminated in fighting. In 1920 Warsaw was saved by a hair's breadth from advancing Soviet armies under the command of General Budenny. Skorupka, a fanatic priest, threw himself in front of the counter-attacking Polish troops brandishing a cross and was killed; he stirred anger in those who were following him. The

* Assistant surgeon.

8

Polish nation calls it a "miracle upon Vistula"* It was a miracle also for my uncle. A dental surgeon in the Polish Army, he was awarded the "Cross of Valour". He told me his story. When out riding through the woods near Warsaw in the company of two cavalry officers, they suddenly heard Russian voices; his two companions spurred their horses and got away. My uncle, still on his horse, was petrified and glued to the spot. His mare's rein slackened. The foreign voices became louder and louder, and soon five armed Russian infantrymen appeared surrounding the frightened horseman and demanding to be taken prisoners, they had had enough of the fighting. My uncle who by now had regained his composure, led the "prisoners" to the camp to be greeted by cheers and clapping from his amazed fellow officers. The Russians, however, caught up with him after their entry into Poland in September 1939, he was arrested and perished in captivity.

After its rebirth the country showed many signs of unrest. The first President of newly independent Poland, Professor Narutowicz, left Switzerland and his teaching post but was soon assassinated in the country of his birth by one of his subjects. Rivalry existed between the legions of General Haller and that of Marshal Pilsudski. Intrigues, squabbles, recrimination and personal issues were many. 150,000 citizens emigrated each year, mostly to the United States of America, and this remained the pattern of this struggling country for a long time. There was no place in this new Poland for Ignacy Paderewski – a great pianist, patriot and humanitarian – who was its Prime Minister for only a brief period. His stay in Poland brought him worry, misunderstandings and unhappiness. And yet Professor Robert Lord, a member of the American Delegation to the Peace Conference in Paris, said of him: "He founded the first government of the new state that was accepted by everyone at home and recognized by all the powers . . . He successfully held the country together during the first and most trying year of its existence . . . He gained a great many things for Poland that a statesman who was less trusted could never have secured . . . He did what no other Pole could have done."

Paderewski brought to realization the hope of his grandfather Professor Nowicki of the University at Vilna whose dream of freedom resulted in exile to Siberia for him and his family. Paderewski's mother was born in Siberia. My memory of these times is the meeting of General Weygand, the head of the French Military Mission. On a collection day for the Red Cross I noticed the General accompanied by

* Warsaw's river.

9

others, in their impressive uniforms, entering the park. Excitedly, I rushed towards them holding my collection box and gabbling: "Monsieur le général c'est pour la Croix Rouge, s'il vous plait" (I had recently started to take lessons in French from Madame Zarembska, the widow of the Polish painter). General Weygand bent down and on tiptoe I pinned the paper flag on to his tunic but with some difficulty owing to its thickness. He smiled and said something in French I could not understand; his gold braided cap and dark clipped moustache became imprinted in my mind.

I was spellbound when taken to the circus for the first time by my mother and found the clowns intriguing. I tried to catch everything they uttered and picked up a strange word. Turning to my mother I asked: "What does prostitute mean?". Ma pretended not to hear so I asked again and again, louder and louder. People began to look at us, some were smiling. My mother's face became redder and redder. Suddenly she gripped my hand and led me to the exit. I pondered for a long time after why little boys can not pose questions to their elders.

I was now twelve years old and my first flickering doubts about the infallibility of the police, the military and the clergy* who could not save the President, the feldsher Nasanowicz and many others, began to form.

The country had not yet recovered from its war wounds. There was a great deal of poverty and hunger, and the American Relief Organization distributed extra food for us children. I enjoyed waiting in the queue and have never objected to it since!

On April 1, 1923, my grandfather, then eighty-nine and still extremely agile, came to me full of excitement brandishing a newspaper. On the front page, in large print, was: "The Tsar Nicholas II is alive and is marching with his loyal troops on Moscow". He immediately went to his chest where he kept thousands of worthless roubles and the same evening I heard him playing The Radetzky March on his decrepit violin for the first time in many months. My parents and I were unable to convince him that it was a Fool's Day hoax and he kept returning to his chest. For my grandpa The Tsar was alive, but it was wishful thinking. He did not believe that the Tsar and his family were assassinated at Ekaterinburg (now Sverdlovsk) on the eastern slopes of the Urals on July 16, 1918.

My school years were peaceful enough, part of them spent amongst animals as keeper of the school zoo. I fed them each morning and when

* Poland had a privileged state religion which was Catholicism.

they heard me coming the zoo was in an uproar. The lion roared, the bear grunted, the wolf howled, but the noisiest of them all were the monkeys. I particularly liked a monkey named "Daisy" who displayed many human traits − attachment to her mate, vanity, jealousy, temper, hate, deceit . . . I sometimes thought the reverse was true, that the people were apeing my Daisy . . . Some do! They chatter like monkeys and display animal behaviour. They prey upon others, scavenge, steal, fight, grunt, breed . . . They can be as false as a cat, as thick-skinned as a rhinoceros and as obstinate as a mule . . . They can shed crocodile tears . . . They have similar sexual urges, though do not confine themselves to seasons. Like animals they can be killers of their own species and of others. Like animals they display various instincts and show some good, even admirable trends. Some are as brave as lions, strong as oxen, busy as bees, wise as owls and gentle as lambs. This kinship is more obvious among the animal loving British. There is an uncanny bond between them, one need only look at a zoological keeper, a police dog handler or a pigeon fancier.

Many animals serve man in various ways and even risk their lives for him, be it medical research, or amusement such as bull fighting, steeplechasing or hunting. They might possess considerable intelligence. Sea-lions have been trained to retrieve lost objects from the sea bed at depths of 500 feet. They quickly adapt to training; captured wild, sea-lions will submit to a harness within two to three weeks. Dolphins − intelligent, playful, able to dive to 1,000 feet − have a good inter-relationship with humans and are known to communicate among themselves. A three-year-old chimpanzee at the Emory University in Atlanta has been taught to read and write with the help of a computer. She makes her requests by pushing the right combination of buttons and sentences must begin with the word "please" (many humans would benefit from such a schooling!). I admire animal wisdom − they spurn alcohol, tobacco and gambling!

Animals share with man the same diseases − rabies, tuberculosis, diabetes, nephritis, ringworm, scabies, trichinosis, brucellosis, psittacosis, toxoplasmosis − furthermore − slipped disc, hernia, cleft lip and palate . . . After all, man is a civilized, or not-so-civilized animal. When a fox managed to escape from our zoo, the chickens kept by the school administrator began to disappear. As it turned out the beast was not responsible, it was the janitor . . . How apt is the saying: "Cats and monkeys, monkeys and cats − all human life is there." It is a well known fact that a cat's behavioural response to drugs is more like that of man than of any other laboratory animal. Nature shows humour – a pig is the animal most akin to the human organism and out of the whole animal kingdom pork insulin is the nearest to his own.

At the beginning of term, when the weather was still warm, I let my pet monkey, Daisy, out to play in the school's vast garden. Sitting in the shade of a chestnut tree, I often experienced a direct hit by chestnuts thrown at me with full force by the monkey. Looking up I caught her grinning with another chestnut in her paw ready to aim at me again. Some times I rode my bicycle in the school grounds with Daisy on my shoulder, one of her paws holding tight to a tuft of my hair pulling fiercely at each bend and giving a squeak. Once I took her on a lead to a local grocer. As soon as Daisy spotted an open sack full of flour in front of her, the mischievous creature turned the place into a busy mill, emptying the sack in no time.

I got very attached to my zoo population. I was not afraid of any of them and they were not afraid of me. To the visitors I pointed out that they had nothing to fear, after all these were only animals. As far as I know, Noah was not alarmed to be amongst his animal travelling companions with whom he had spent fifty-four days in his Ark. It made me sad when the skunk died, and reminded me of the grief I experienced walking behind the coffin of my school friend who died of typhoid. Our school band led the procession and played Chopin's "Funeral March."

I remember another bleak day on which my mongrel dog disappeared. The town was employing a "flayer" to catch and destroy stray dogs should no one claim them within a week. My first thought was of him and so I went on a bicycle to the flayer's kennels, three miles out of town. My deduction was right! I saw my dog jumping and barking with joy and excitement behind bars. After the happy reunion I rode home with him running behind me. At one point I was stopped by a passer-by who admonished me for being unkind to my pet. "I have rescued it from the clutches of death, we are rushing home", I shouted triumphantly.

Two sights made me feel particularly uncomfortable – a patient with an infectious disease on the way to hospital in a two-wheeled cart, well hooded with a canvas, pushed through the streets by a hospital attendant, and that of a priest in a horse-driven cab on his way to administer the last sacrament to a dying person. The priest's server, sitting next to the cabman, was ringing a small bell and the passers-by stopped and knelt in prayer for the departing soul.

I was fortunate in having art lessons from the outstanding painter

12

Zak, a good friend of my parents. He soon settled in his right milieu – Paris – where he was happy in spite of frequently being hungry. When he died in poverty, of a heart attack, his wife, who proved to be a good business woman, opened a successful exhibition of her husband's paintings. Zak was at last recognized, his family became prosperous.

When I was a sixth former, I developed an interest in cycle racing and this is how I got my first medals!

Like most boys I enjoyed pranks. The geography teacher, a petite spinster wearing high heeled shoes in an attempt to correct nature, was on our "wanted list". On one occasion we spread glue on the classroom floor at the entrance and the poor thing got stuck to it, falling out of her shoes. Another time we hung a pair of trousers over the blackboard and the geography teacher, suspecting someone was not decently dressed, was afraid to come in. As it happened the trousers belonged to her favourite pupil, a meticulous twerp who was in the habit of changing his trousers whilst at school so as not to lose the crease in his better pair. I sometimes think that my neglect of geography was the reason for my long travels I had to make later on! When one of my aunts arrived to visit my parents, I was spurred to action. I disliked her intensely – she never smiled, looked austere, was strict with me, and did not once bring me a present! So I raised the back legs of the sofa, on which she always slept, with my geography atlas and other books. Not suspecting anything, the silly old fuss-pot rolled off the sofa on to the floor three times during the night. The next morning my aunt declared she would be leaving as the sofa was very uncomfortable. I pretended to be sorry to hear it . . .

One summer's day, when I was thirteen years old, I went with my mother and another aunt on a holiday to the mountain resort of Zakopane in the south, in the high Tatra, which is as spectacular as the Alps. She was an entirely different kind of person – gentle, kind and considerate, who never forgot my birthday. Several years before, when she arrived late, bringing my favourite sweets – chocolate buttons covered with poppy seeds – I was already in bed, and my aunt, presuming me to be asleep, put them under my pillow. As soon as she left I tucked into them, with the result that even now I cannot look at this particular brand!

On the way we visited Cracow – a mediaeval city which was the capital of Poland for 300 years up to 1596. We saw the impressive castle of the Polish kings picturesquely situated on Vavel Hill by the Vistula river, and I was intrigued by the big bell "Zygmunt" cast from enemy cannons captured in the 16th century. I liked the market square with the Drapers Hall, originally 13th century merchant stalls which still serve as a bazaar, the old streets with burghers mansions, the city walls with bastions and dungeons, the church spire from which a bugle call is played every hour (it has a break in the melody in memory of the trumpeter who was struck by a Tartar's* arrow while sounding his instrument). In later years I have often returned there in memory, reminded of Cracow by the publicity of its citizen – graphologist Raphael Scheermann. By studying one's handwriting he was able to reveal man's innermost secrets. He was sought after by courts of justice and medical men in difficult cases, and people from all over the world consulted him. Scheermann influenced the fate of many. The ancient** Jagiellonian University was also very much in the news. It took its name from the dynasty which reigned at the close of the middle ages and ended in 1526 with the slaying of the last ruler by the Turks.

Next day we visited a salt mine thirteen kilometres from the town dating from the 11th century and still in operation. I admired its underground passages and the chapel hewn in salt and decorated with salt carvings. When in Zakopane we made a trip to the famous beauty spot of "Eye of the Sea" (Morskie Oko). My mother hired a highlander who took us there in a horse driven cab. He was wearing a colourfully embroidered white wool jacket and tightly fitting trousers to match, with a belt studded with brass tacks. He had a hat of black felt with a band of white shells, and an eagle's feather. We reached the "Eye of the Sea" – the vanished glacier – now a lake with pine trees skirting it, and my mother paid the highlander for the trip on the understanding that he would wait to take us back after our visit to "Black Lake", 100 yards higher, which we set out to explore on foot. Paying him was a mistake. During our not-too-long absence he spent the money on drink and was in a condition which a police surgeon would describe as "unfit to drive". We took the high road winding its way down along the precipice back to Zakopane. The highlander was urging the horse, clicking his tongue and shouting encouragement, the cab pushing on to the poor animal's hind quarters. We were all frightened, except our man who was enjoying himself singing and swaying. His strong hiccups added to our discomfort. A spectacular descent at breakneck speed. Both ladies were standing on the side of the cab away from the precipice preparing to jump clear – the panoramic trip

* Tartar raiders destroyed the wooden buildings of the town by setting them on fire.
** Founded in 1364.

14

changed into a nightmare. In this unhappy situation I climbed to the front seat next to the driver, pulled the reins out of his hands and managed to bring the cab to a standstill. The highlander, half gone, was helped down from his seat by the three of us and was now sitting in a sorry state on the ground. I took his hat to the nearest stream, filled it with water and then poured it over him. I repeated this performance several times before he could mount his cab again, but by now all was well. I was proclaimed the hero of the day by the ladies.

My parents were strict but kind, and provided me with regular pocket money which I liked to spend on seeing silent films with my friends. My favourite film actor was Eddie Polo, a fabulous horseman and adventurer whose films were serialized, each part ending at the most crucial moment to the sound of "Light Cavalry", in breathtaking tempo, performed by a first class twenty-strong symphony orchestra. I waited impatiently for the next week's follow up and discussed the possible outcome with the other boys. It was therefore a great punishment every time my parents withdrew my pocket money for misbehaviour.

About that time a sixteen-year-old girl, a violinist in Spoliansky's orchestra, was hiding her still undiscovered legs when playing in Berlin cinemas. Her name was Marlene Dietrich who shot to fame after appearing in the film "The Blue Angel" which I saw in Vienna in 1929.

We held regular concerts at school, in one of which an unknown singer Jan Kiepura took part. We admired his beautiful strong voice, and he promised to sing for us again, but it was not to be. Jan Kiepura went to Germany soon after and became a widely-known film star overnight. Our other favourite was a strong man Breitbart. He had the face of a Greek god and an exquisite physique. Breitbart was a showman extraordinary. We watched him in a huge arena standing in a chariot drawn by two pairs of magnificent horses and holding a ring with harness attached to it between his teeth, this way forming a link between the horses and the chariot. He broke iron bars and heavy chains with ease. It was with horror and daze that we learned of Breitbart's death. He died in his early thirties from blood poisoning due to a slight injury from a broken chain. There was nothing the doctors could do for it in those days.

In February 1922 a fascinating hobby began to spread all over the world. The Eiffel Tower station in France began to broadcast regular programmes. In May of the same year the British Broadcasting Corporation had its début, and about the same time the United States of

America claimed some 750,000 enthusiastic amateurs pursuing the new craze. In 1923, a school pal of mine made a wooden box and, following instructions from a magazine, installed a mass of wires in it – a wireless receiving set. I was invited to the demonstration and with immense curiosity listened through one earphone, the other being used by his mother. Suddenly she exclaimed, "I can hear the Warsaw trams!". It was only interference on the air . . .

I developed a liking for Polish literature encouraged by my teacher, the daughter of a doctor and philosopher – Bieganski. Befittingly my school was named after the venerated Polish writer Sienkiewicz,* the author of "Quo Vadis." I was also interested in life and living creatures. Mechanical things appealed to me only from a utility point of view. I was more interested in Darwin than Edison. I watched with great curiosity Dr. Roszkowski examining my urine by adding reagents to a test tube and holding it over the flame of a spirit lamp. He was the son-in-law of Dr. Bieganski and himself a much sought after physician. I learned later that he described a useful method of detecting dilatation of the aortic arch by percussion. Those were the days of practising medical *art* without the availability of sophisticated ancillary methods. For several years before leaving school I knew what I wanted to be. My hero was the feldsher Nasanowicz, and I longed to save the life of another Breitbart. I would be a doctor!

* Sienkiewicz received the Nobel Prize for literature in 1905.

2
Student in Vienna and Berlin

A man should be just cultured enough to be able to look with
suspicion upon culture.   *Samuel Butler*

In 1929 I was able to enroll at the Vienna University. The twelve
months spent there were happy ones. I admired the beautiful
Kaerntner Ring, Graben and its buildings, the busy Mariahilfer
Strasse, the Palace of Schoenbrunn where the Hapsburgs reigned supreme, the University, the Burgtheater and other theatres, the coffee
houses, the slow tempo, and above all the humour, friendliness and
hospitality of these easy-going people. They were German speaking,
but the language was somewhat mellow, melodious, more of a Welsh
quality. One saw many strolling people, only a few looking busi-
nesslike. Soldiers were scarce, some armed with briefcases on the way
to the University. Austria had a very small army after the war. Once
Professor Pick came half-an-hour late for his lecture and said with a
twinkle in his eye to the amused audience that he was prevented from
crossing the street in time by a long column of marching troops. Everyone laughed knowing that this was not true, but by now I had lost my
interest in uniforms.

My command of German was not very good. I remember asking a
passer-by if he knew of a film worth seeing. No doubt he noticed my
accent. "Of course", he said with a smile, "I will direct you". I thanked
him and thought he was going my way. It took us ten minutes to reach
the picture house, where my companion departed in a hurry, saying
casually, "I have an appointment you know and it is in quite the opposite direction!" He left me dumbfounded. On another occasion I
entered a shop asking if I might use their telephone. "Certainly you
may Sir", said a woman with a smile, "but can you!"

The Vienna of 1929 had numerous coffee houses which were a
second home to many people. The Viennese referred to them as their
own and spent the best part of the day in their favourite one. Here
everyone knew everyone by first names, an unobtrusive waiter would
bring black coffee and a glass of water on a silver tray, and if not called
again, would leave the customer playing cards or dominoes unmolested
in the warmth, thus saving fuel in the guest's own home.

17

The war impoverished a great many people. Half of the population lived by letting rooms to students. I lived in one, sparsely furnished, but expensive, near the Anatomy Building. When I moved in my landlady pointed out, with some pride, that the house was free from bugs, a rarity in Vienna. I shared a room with another student by the name of Willy. Unfortunately, Willy was in love with a girl called Mitzi. We had an understanding that on special occasions I would leave the room at his disposal and would be warned by a red towel hanging from our window. As time went by, the red "flag" was flying more and more frequently and I had to join the other Viennese in finding my "own" coffee house.

Students dominated the life of the city. A great many arrived from foreign lands and the biggest welcome was afforded by the University authorities to people from the territories once ruled by the Hapsburgs' Empire — the Hungarians, the Rumanians, the Czechs, the Jugoslavs and Poles from Galicia.

As a student I was able to be a "claquer" — a clapper in a theatre — without pay, but with free access which enabled me to satisfy my urge for the theatre. Poor me, I could not even afford to pay for the cloakroom, but was now in a position to frequent the splendid opera and playhouses. I enjoyed Pickaver and Jeritza, Leo Slezak, Hans Moser, Alexander Moissi, Hans Jaray and many many others.

During the day I attended various lectures and tried to learn as much as possible of the whole concept of medicine. Vienna then had many luminaries of the profession like Professor Neumann, the ear, nose and throat specialist whose skill was sought by the crowned and famous including the Duke of Windsor; Professor Chwostek and Professor Wenkebach — the medical specialists; Professor Wangemann, the eye specialist; Professor Wagner von Jauregg* — the man who gave hope to those demented by syphilis by infecting them with malaria, and many more. The lecture halls displayed portraits of their famous predecessors — Auenbrugger — the inventor of percussion, Semmelweis — the pioneer of antiseptics in obstetrics, Skoda — a physician, Zuckerkandl — an anatomist, Rokitansky — a pathologist, Billroth — "the father of visceral surgery", Politzer — an otologist, Kaposi** — a dermatologist, Wertheim — a gynaecologist . . . Professor Chwostek was an anti-feminist who barred female students from his lectures. I saw

* His able successor was Professor Poetzl.

** He was Moritz Kohn, a Hungarian Jew, who found life easier after changing his name to Kaposi.

him interrupt his discourse – he pointed at a casual woman visitor saying "*What* is this!" The poor stranger blushed at this trying experience.

I visited Allgemeines Krankenhaus (The University Hospital), Steinhof Asylum – a town in itself with a population of nearly 2,000 and its own hospital, chapel, theatre and workshops. I frequented the lectures of Professor Poetzl, a disciple of Freud, and of course I was a regular attender of lectures in anatomy by Professor Tandler. Professor Tandler was an excellent teacher and speaker; his books on anatomy, each volume weighing some six pounds, were translated into many languages. We found his lectures most intriguing and tried to catch every word he said. Once, a student of small stature, in the front row next to me, sat on two volumes of the Professor's Anatomy, but this was noticed by Professor Tandler who stopped his lecture, pointed his thick finger at my blushing neighbour and pronounced gravely – "My dear young man, you will never learn anatomy that way!".

They were happy days, but slowly the clouds began to gather. There were two lecture halls in the Anatomy Building where at the time Professor Tandler was delivering his lecture on the ground floor, Professor Hochstaetter was holding his in the room above. Professor Hochstaetter was an older man and a poor speaker. His audience consisted of students who boycotted Professor Tandler – a Jew. It soon came to clashes between both factions of students when they met face on when leaving the building after the lectures. I witnessed these happenings on several occasions. I was disenchanted – they were not the gay, light-hearted and learned people I had hoped for – the nationalism and anti-Semitism of the budding intelligentsia horrified me. I looked at the Danube, but instead of the blue river I saw muddy water. I instinctively thought how unkind Vienna was to Franz Schubert. His first and only public concert took place there in March 1828. Eight months later he died leaving the Unfinished Symphony, unable to fulfill all the possibilities of his genius. He struggled throughout his life and died wretchedly poor at the age of thirty-one. This happened when Vienna was the musical capital of the world. I decided to leave this city for a happier place . . . Berlin, where my aunt lived. The year was 1930.

I found the life in Berlin and the people very different; their language was harsh and clipped, their manners less pleasing, their humour unsophisticated, even coarse, but they were an industrious people, punctual in their habits, thorough and well organized.

19

To join the medical faculty I had to pass the examination in Prussian history, but at last I was a medical student of the Kaiser Wilhelm University in Berlin, with its wonderful libraries, the famous teaching hospital "Charite" and household names like August Bier, Ferdinand Sauerbruch – surgeons, Professor Bergmann – medical specialist, Professor Planck – a Nobel prize winner in physics. Their list was a long one. They followed such eminent medical men as Meckel, Romberg, Waldeyer, Helmholtz, Virchow, Koch, Kocher, Ehrlich, Gaffky, Loeffler, Behring, Wasserman . . . I was industrious in the dissecting room, where I learned not only the intricacies of the human body, but also to smoke and tell jokes. I found time for other activities too. Once I listened to Albert Einstein and his exposition of the Theory of Relativity. He was speaking to a lay audience in simple terms everyone understood, giving numerous examples from life and daily happenings; listening to him the whole subject appeared to be so obvious. He was a man of small stature, with a large head, bushy greying hair, impressive dark eyes, mild voice, quiet manners and an engaging smile. I heard a young Indian philosopher, Krishna Murti – good looking, fond of fast cars – telling his listeners about meditation. I did not find his exposé particularly useful in my later years of imprisonment, and after my release there was no time for meditation anyway.

I visited some theatres. Berlin of 1930 and 1931 was a lively city. The entertainment world was dominated by Emil Jannings, Hans Albers, Gustav Froelich, Willy Fritsch, Richard Tauber, Magda Schneider, Marlene Dietrich, Martha Eggert who married Jan Kiepura, the baker's son with a golden voice, and the clown Grogg. I could not see all of them, besides, there were no hired applauders in Berlin. I noticed with interest that Berlin had a "Warsaw Bridge", that some Germans bore Polish names like that of von Bronikowski, a biographer of Frederick the Great, Heine and Wagner, that of von Drigalski, a Berlin bacteriologist, or of Kempinski, the well known wine merchant and restauranteur, and that they had a slang word "dali dali" meaning "hurry up" and taken from the Polish language. I remembered my visit in 1927 to Danzig (Gdansk in Polish) and Zoppot (now Sopot), a seaside town on the Baltic Sea in the then so called "Corridor", seeing the German and Polish communities living in apparent harmony. I know of a German pianist of international repute, Egon Petri, who settled in the Polish mountain resort of Zakopane in 1925 and lived happily there until 1940 when he fled from the Nazis to the United States.

It took me some time to realize that the life in this large German city

20

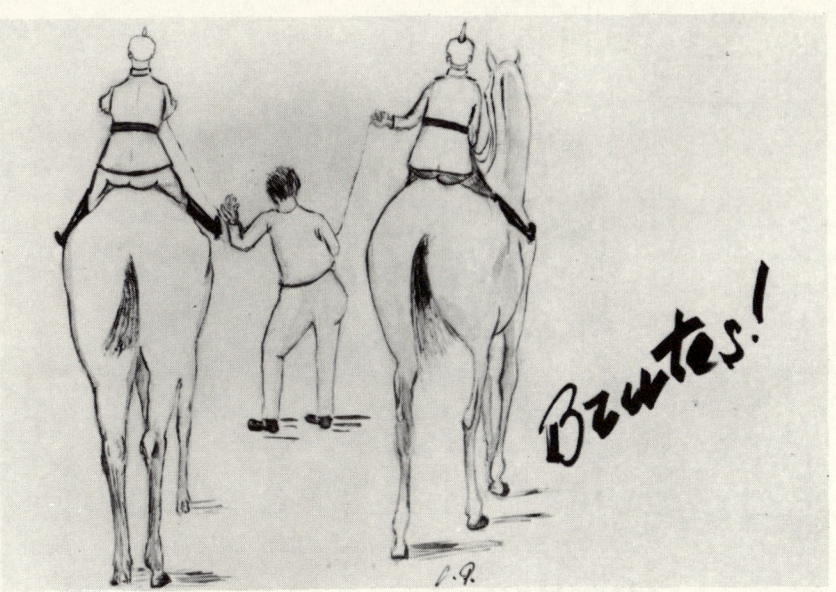

Czestochowa under German occupation, 1914

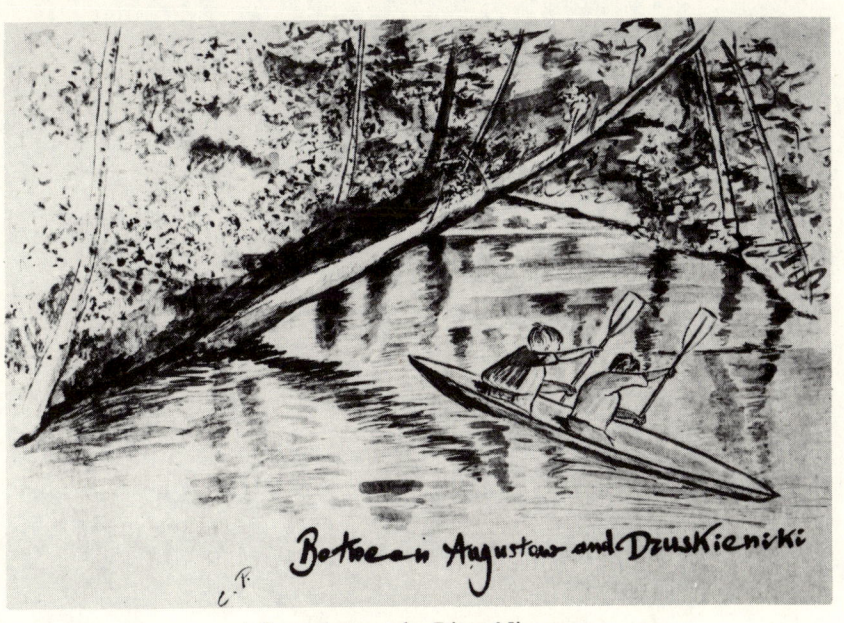

Canoeing on the River Niemen

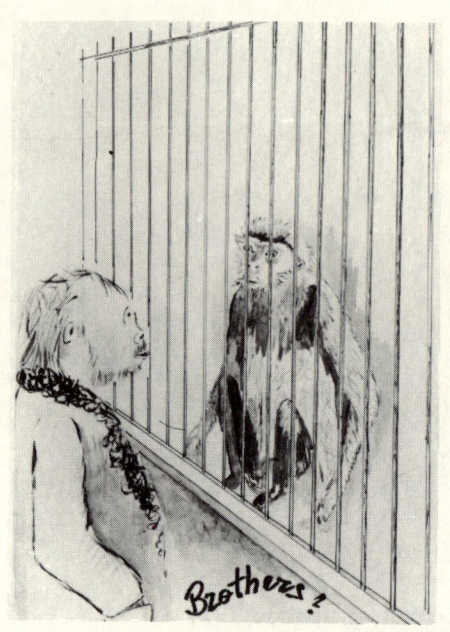

Brothers!

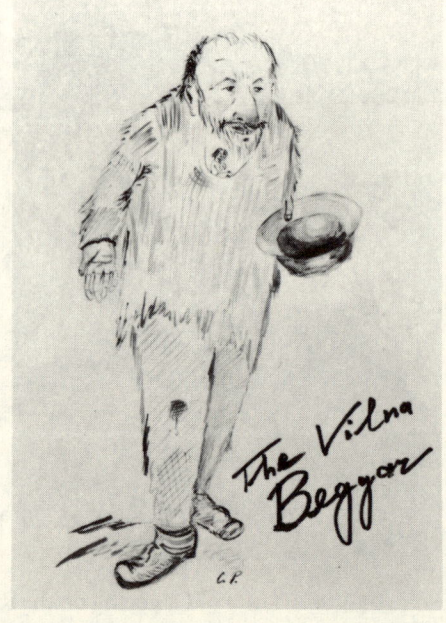

The Vilna Beggar

was not the paradise I had dreamt of — far from it! When my infatuation began to wane, I noticed the hungry faces of the unemployed with placards on their shoulders offering themselves for any available job, prostitutes parading in great numbers on the fashionable Kurfuerstendamm in high red leather boots — their trade mark — the right atmosphere for Bertolt Brecht's cynical humour, "Threepenny Opera", and "Mac the Knife". I read an advertisement in a paper about lessons in bridge. When I rang the bell at the given address, the woman who answered the door just smiled — it was a brothel.

3

Berlin under Hitler

> I hate mankind, for I think myself one of the best of them, and I
> know how bad I am.
> *Samuel Johnson*

The post-war German Republic was in turmoil. Before the end of 1930
some six million were jobless. The discontented people, many of whom
had lost their life savings during the worst inflation of 1923*, encouraged by Communists and their strong party under the leadership of
Ernst Torgler and Ernst Thaelmann, gathered at angry mass meetings
in various parts of the city. The Nazis were trying to disrupt these
meetings, but at first had little success. However, the rowdies were able
to break up some rallies of the Social Democrats – then the ruling
party. Cinema performances of "All Quiet on the Western Front",
based on the successful novel by the pacifist Erich Maria Remarque,
were sabotaged by various means which included the planting of
hoards of white mice and rats by Nazi thugs into the picture houses. I
was there in the midst of screaming women as the rodents ran loose
amongst the stricken audience. The Nazi uniform was looked upon
with disdain – only a very few brown shirts were seen in the streets.
Hitler, with his feeble attempt to overthrow the government on
November 8, 1923 and the unsuccessful writer of "Mein Kampf"
first published in 1925, was mentioned only as a joke. This soon
changed when on April 10, 1932, polling for the Presidency took place;
Hitler was standing against Hindenburg. On the eve of polling day we
heard that Hindenburg, now 85 years old, had died of a heart attack. It
turned out to be a Nazi hoax, but this unscrupulous lie did not help
Hitler to win the election.

Yet the Nazis were more and more in evidence, provoking anti-
Semitic disturbances. On January 30, 1933, Adolf Hitler became
Chancellor and the National Socialist Movement was on the march.
People rushed to buy papers. I remember seeing a photograph of Hitler
in the centre of the new Cabinet on the front page of a newspaper. The

* Shortly before the end of inflation a restaurant dinner cost ten to twenty billion
marks.

22

photograph was purposely of very poor quality with the caption: "This is how the new Cabinet of Germany looks, more comments are forbidden by the Censor". It was the last vestige of freedom papers were able to enjoy.

In the "Kabaret der Komiker" a comedian, Werner Finck, brought five little pigs on the stage, calling them by the first names of the top Nazis. "Hermann, come here", he ordered, beckoning a piglet, "and you Josef, and you Rudolf, and you Julius and you A . . . .", stopping at the first letter and pointing at the remaining animal with a shake of his head and the explanation: "I will not go to prison for this pig". But these were only glimpses of freedom soon to be denied the whole of Germany. In a short time Finck found himself in a concentration camp.

The streets were getting more and more crowded with Nazis in uniform. Jewish shops were battered and one witnessed Jews being molested in the street, even spat upon. "The Chosen People" were not allowed into train compartments and had to stand in the corridors, and were often forcibly removed from trains and the Underground. Signs – "Jews not admitted", "Jews out", "Jews must perish" appeared. Goebbels was more subtle, announcing that he would treat Jews like flowers . . . he would deprive them of water and they would die. Nazi columns were marching through the streets to the accompaniment of brass bands, the beat of the drums or the sound of a tambourine. They were all "Germanic Men", "The Masters", even if they came from the slums of the Moabit quarter of Berlin. Professor Sauerbruch had a long lost battle defying the dismissal of his first assistant, a Jew. Professor Lipmann, a gynaecologist, author of a renowned Atlas and the man who in 1929 introduced subdued colours in his operating theatre instead of the conventional white so as not to strain the surgeons' eyes, had to relinquish his university post, and so had Professor Rona, an authority in chemistry and a Hungarian Jew. Mendelssohn's music was banned despite his conversion to Christianity in early childhood.

Persecution had only just begun. The Nuremburger laws depriving Jews of citizenship and forbidding mixed marriages* had yet to come, but the offspring of such marriages, Richard Tauber was one,** were told that they were Jews. For the present, however, the full impact of

* Hitler distorted the idea of hereditary improvement of men and animals by selective breeding advanced by Sir Francis Galton in the later part of the 19th century (eugenics).
** The same happened to the famous Austrian conductor Josef Krips whose father was once Jewish.

23

the Nazi rule was stalled; Hitler had his eye on foreign visitors who came to Germany for the Olympics of 1936 and successfully deceived the world about his militant intentions. The seventeen-year-old future British war hero, Leonard Cheshire, sensed no danger when he visited Berlin in 1935, and this in spite of staying quite a long time with a German Admiral and his family.

The Hitler Youth were very active, spending most of their time away from home on indoctrination and marching. My landlady looked with pride at her teenage son parading in a brown shirt with swastika* and high black boots.

Once I was sitting in a park engrossed in reading when a man tapped me on the shoulder and motioned that I should rise — young Nazis were passing us singing the Horst Wessel** song, Hitler's Official Anthem. These youngsters, proud of their uniform, carrying collection boxes, enjoyed extorting money from passers-by who were afraid to ignore them. They did not confine themselves to the streets but tried to force their way into private homes with the Nazi salute. In University buildings Jews were forced to sit in the last rows. It became routine that the leader of the local Nazi group addressed the audience before the lectures. There were no clashes similar to those in Vienna, both communities ignored each other, except for a peculiar breed of militant "Couleur" students (I would prefer to call them Koller students, "Koller" means frenzy in German), with their strange caps, high boots and facial scars from duelling. Some people began to realize the gravity of the situation, few expressed their doubts, fewer still raised their voices faintly in protest. One who took a firm stand was Carl von Ossietzky. A journalist, editor of Weltbuehne and author, he repudiated militarism and championed democracy. When the Nazis came to power, he was arrested and disappeared into the dungeons. In November 1936 Ossietzky was awarded the Nobel peace prize when an inmate of a Nazi concentration camp. Hitler, in fury, forbade him to accept it. At the same time he issued an order that any German subject who might be offered such a prize in the future must also decline it.***
Several writers left the country, among them Thomas Mann and Erich

*Once an ancient religious symbol; it was adopted by the Nazis as their official emblem.

** Horst Wessel, who composed this song, was killed in a fight with the Communists in 1930 when still in his twenties.

*** In 1939, in accordance with the instructions of the German Government, Gerhard Domagk — the discoverer of "Prontosil", a forerunner of sulphanilamide — declined the Nobel prize for physiology and medicine.

Maria Remarque, but other liberally minded people, for instance the scientist Professor Oskar Vogt, stayed on. Yet concentration camps were no secret to anyone; a well known clergyman, Pastor Niemoeller, was interned for seven years. A joke circulated in great secrecy about a man whose cat had kittens, one being a Socialist, the other five National Socialists. When asked about the kittens the next day, he said: "There are five Socialists and one National Socialist, the kittens have now opened their eyes!" Even the Jews were able to joke, telling about the boy who when asked by his teacher what he'd like to be if his father were Adolf Hitler, answered shyly, "Please Sir, may I be an orphan?". The "Good Day" greeting was abandoned by the German people in the realization that there wasn't to be one. "Heil Hitler!" was the only greeting.

As an alien I was able to leave Germany and return to my own country and studies, finding life quiet for a time.

I returned to Berlin in 1938 for a fleeting visit to see my aunt. By then life was considerably more dismal. In the restaurants, I frequented, I noticed people whispering and looking around furtively. Once a month a one-pot-dish was served – a thick soup, the only food allowed in any restaurant for the price of a full meal. This applied to private dwellings also; the money saved then being collected for Nazi funds in the guise of the "Winter-help" ostensibly for the poor. The same thing happened with the collection for the delivery of "Volkswagens" – a deferred promise – which, to my knowledge, has not been fulfilled. These were some of the measures which enabled Germany to rearm.

My aunt who escaped the Russian revolution introduced me to her friends – prominent Russian intellectuals, like the chief librarian of the last Tsar. They were émigrés who formed a large colony in Berlin – pathetic figures shabbily dressed, near starving, and cut off from the rest of the community owing to a poor command of the German language. Such existence frightened me and I told my aunt that I hope never to be an émigré. She sadly smiled. I will always remember this smile and the gentle acceptance of her fate – like many of her friends, she perished.

I paid a visit to an old Aryan friend, a lawyer married to an attractive Jewess who had recently borne him a child. I found him in distress, as he had been given an ultimatum to divorce his wife or be sent to a concentration camp.

I visited an "exhibition" where the photographs of Albert Einstein,

Heinrich Heine, Stefan Zweig, Lion Feuchtwangler, Siegmund Freud, Ludwig Zamenhof, Hermann and Bernhardt Zondek, Richard Tauber, Otto Klemperer, Bruno Walter, Charlie Chaplin and others of considerable intellectual attainments were shown under the heading: "These are the people we have had to endure." I noticed a notable omission, that of another Jew — Paul Ehrlich — the discoverer of Salvarsan; the Nazis preferred him to syphilis.

One dark evening, overpowered by curiosity, I watched a mediaeval scene in a large square lit by torches — a burning effigy of a Jew suspended over an enormous pile of books blazing fiercely. Over a loudspeaker I heard the piercing voice of Goebbells condemning Jews for all the wrongs in the world. When his voice ceased, thousands of Germans joined in singing the Horst Wessel song, their arms raised in the Hitler salute. After the singing, the formidable frightening shouting "Sieg Heil! Sieg Heil! Sieg Heil!" echoed round the square. It was sorcery and had to be seen to be believed. I was too dumbfounded to be frightened, and "decent people" were saying "We do not approve the methods, but we whole-heartedly agree with Hitler's aim." They strutted around in brown and black uniforms and found it necessary to replace the customary salutation "Greet God" ("Grüss Gott") with "Heil Hitler" whose violent language stirred the German masses, now convinced that who was not a German was "Untermensch" (subhuman). Hitler offered them leadership, relieved them of war obligations, and was now saving them from unemployment and Communism which were gaining ascendancy; they believed he was rescuing them from chaos. Leading industrialists, among whom were the descendants of Alfred Krupp and the Chairman of I. G. Farben — Karl Duisberg, looked upon Hitler as their own protector. They conformed to the slogan "Fuehrer befiel, wir folgen" (Fuehrer command and we follow you) which was heard all over Germany.

In 1936 Hitler undertook a successful military action in the Rhineland without repercussions. In March 1938, a few weeks before my visit to Berlin, the German army entered Vienna. I had to go to the German Consulate in Warsaw to obtain a visa and heard a German official asking a client what his nationality was. "Austrian", he answered. "So", muttered the clerk, "you are in fact a German." Hitler had been preparing for the annexation of Austria from the day he took power. In October 1933 the Nazis made an unsuccessful attempt on the life of the Austrian Chancellor Dolfuss who was opposed to them,*

* Among other measures, Dolfuss banned the use of Nazi uniforms.

and they succeeded in assassinating him on July 25, 1934. His determination to maintain Austria's independence brought him into conflict with Nazi interests.

Professor August Bier, like many others who looked on and pretended not to notice what they didn't wish to see, lent his name to Hitler's propaganda and was a signatory to several of the Fuehrer's manifestos. He must have had second thoughts in later years as he devoted them to the study of harmony in nature.

It was with relief that my short visit to hellish Germany came to an end and I was happy with the thought that I was parting from the Germans for ever. Alas, how wrong I was!

4

Vilna

> The first half of life consists of the capacity to enjoy without the
> chance; the last half consists of the chance without the capacity.
>
> *Mark Twain*

I went back to my medical studies at the Stefan Batory* University in
Vilna. I passed the necessary entrance examination, and sat for the
subjects of the first two years study for the second time. Vilna was once
the capital of Lithuania reunited with Poland by its strong man, Marshal Pilsudski, in 1920. It was a lively city, dominated by students,
where several cultures blended into a unique intellectual atmosphere.
This place embraced Poles, Lithuanians, Latvians, White Ruthanians
and Jews with their various cultures, languages and press. A number
of intellectual homes were in the habit of inviting students for the
evening to hold interesting discussions. Professor Rose, the neurologist, at the piano, Professor Jakowicki and Professor Michejda, the
surgeons, at his side, were helping the medical students to prepare a
puppet show featuring the luminaries of our medical faculty. The
atmosphere, even in difficult situations, was always cordial. Once at a
students' meeting, a Communist speaker was praising the achievements of Soviet Russia only to be gently reminded by the smiling Professor Jakowicki that there was no need to protect it, it being a big
enough country to defend itself . . . I remember seeing the ageing Professor Senkowski,** the Head of the chemistry department, puffing
and out of breath after negotiating two flights of stairs with the help of
his twenty-year-old usher, asking him with concern if this exercise had
tired the young man . . .

I recollect the day I won a lottery after buying a ticket at a charity
function a few weeks earlier. A blissful feeling took charge of me. The
win amounted to one hundred zlotys on which one could live for a few
weeks. It conveniently happened towards the end of the month when

* Stefan Batory – the name of a Polish King in the 14th century, and of the luxury
liner which made headlines in the world press after the last war, during which it was
temporarily converted into a troop-ship.

** His assistant was Osman Achmatowicz who later became a professor at the
Warsaw University, Under Secretary of State and a member of the Polish Academy of
Science.

my money was running out. I called on a girl-student inviting her for a meal at a first class restaurant. At last I was in a position to entertain, taking full advantage of it. I ordered the best the establishment could offer. We were in the middle of the second course, gulping wine and laughing, when my face froze. The girl watched in amazement my half open mouth which I was unable to close for a moment. I had just realized I shared the lottery ticket with four of my colleagues, only twenty zlotys would be mine. In fact it was less than that, I forgot the tax. When the money arrived it just covered the restaurant bill I incurred by my impetuosity.

I was fond of the twisting alleys and of the cobbled streets which echoed the hollow sound of horses' hooves. I was fond too of the surrounding hills where I often pursued gentle skiing, and of the people – not prosperous, but friendly. For little money I could enjoy a ride in a cab which had large inflated tyres to cushion the jolting and noise of the cobbled stones. In the winter I could drive a sleigh, wrapped in a fur rug, to the sound of horse bells. The jolly, informative cabmen were always ready to talk about the beauty, history and secrets of their lovely city, or just to gossip. They reminded me of the Viennese Fiaker; they were of a similar breed. Even the beggars had a local flavour, were more sophisticated and professional than their colleagues in other cities, and were also better performers. Each day, returning home from lectures, I was confronted with one of these colourful gentlemen stubbornly holding on to his beat – unshaven, his high complexion revealing an alcoholic, his bare chest displaying a tattoo of a decorative maiden, his patched trousers smeared with grease, his face contorted with misery, his clawlike hand outstretched, his voice somehow aggressive. A friend, a constant companion of mine, had great compassion for this individual – he would grip my arm whispering, "Give something to this poor fellow." It was always me who had to part with the money. No wonder I tired of this and one day, hearing from the beggar that he had not eaten in two days, I remarked sarcastically, "You must force yourself." The next day he accosted me again saying, "I am hungry, governor." "It is a good sign, you must be getting better", I muttered wearily. He was not surprised or annoyed at my reaction, realising by now that I would not give way to his plea. I already noticed some hopelessness in his tone, his ebullient cockiness gone; this was my last encounter with him, I decided to change the route.

It was a serene life – the lectures, the social events, even the examinations gave me a thrill. I often studied with a friend who had a room above me where we lodged and when he wished to contact me he just knocked on the floor. He had a nice voice and liked to sing at the slightest provocation. I missed his singing when I didn't hear it for several days. My deduction was correct – my friend had failed an examination. A week after we met again, we studied, we passed, only to prepare for yet another "ordeal." My friend was failed by Professor Pelczar, a stringent examiner and our youngest and most able scientist. Professor Pelczar held a Chair of Pathology and was a keen researcher in cancer, with important works to his credit. When the Germans occupied Vilna, he was one of the first prominent citizens taken hostage, and was shot soon after; a dedicated scientist and not involved in politics, he was only thirty-seven years of age. In 1942, in similar circumstances, they shot the renown Polish novelist Boy-Zelenski.

Such reprisals were not exactly Hitler's invention; when Lenin was seriously wounded by an assassin in August 1918, 500 distinguished citizens of the old régime were summarily shot. After Kirov's murder on December 1, 1934, numerous people in high positions were liquidated and Soviet Russia trembled to its foundations (of 71 members of the Central Committee of the Party only 16 survived, more than 7,000 Communists were shot and tens of thousands of innocent citizens tossed into the labour camps). Stalin's tomb should have the inscription found on Tamerlan's sarcophgus, "Were I alive today, mankind would tremble". It would be appropriate to mention here, that Professor Jakowicki was arrested by the Russians when they entered Vilna in September 1939 and died in one of their prisons after deportation.

When the vacations came, I spent them on Lake Narocz, four kilometres in length, not far from Vilna. In the past I canoed on the River Niemen, its tributaries and canals which link numerous lakes, exploring the thick wooded area between Augustov and Druskieniki. For weeks on end, my friend and I lived on the canoe doing our own cooking, visiting remote hamlets, sleeping in barns. Days passed without hearing human voices, only the singing of the birds in the trees and the splashing of the paddle. The stillness of the water and the green reflection of the trees bending over nature's mirror, their branches intertwined like embracing sisters, had a divine quality. Nature is God and God is nature, I echoed my favourite poet Slowacki.* And I remembered how the great composer Beethoven expressed his communion

* Polish romantic poet of the early 19th century.

30

with nature. "I love trees better than man. Almighty God! In the woods I am happy – I am happy in the woods where each tree speaks of Thee – O, my God, what splendour! In the forests, on the hills, there is peace – peace in which to serve Thee."

It was a beautiful warm evening when we were invited by the scouts camping near the river, to their jamboree. We sat cross-legged in a large circle around a blazing camp fire singing traditional songs, the sun sinking in the West, twilight descending, eyes fixed on the glowing embers, ears catching the cracking of the burning branches and the tolling of a distant church bell when the singing stopped. Not a breeze, not the slightest rustle, the twittering of the birds ceased – they had gone to rest for the night. Only the smell of the pines from the nearby forest remained. We were mesmerized by this other-worldliness. All sense of time seemed to slip away. At intervals a sudden eruption of the camp fire and the warmth which came from it brought us out of the trance. When the bugle sounded, we rose to our feet, the flag with Polish National Colours was lowered from the mast, and we saluted. Thus ended another perfect day. It was truly heaven. Back at home, I read a story of a vagabond "Lampion kisses girls and birches" again and again, reliving those happy times.

However, everything was not rosy. Two medical students in my term joined the International Brigade which fought in the Spanish Civil War against General Franco and they both perished. A university colleague of mine was taken to a forced labour camp in Bereza Kartuska without a trial, where he found, apart from Communists, respectable politicians who did not toe the line dictated by the government.

A honeymoon period had developed between Poland and Germany. Many German tourists were visiting Vilna and one heard more and more of what was going on in Germany. Nationalistic student factions began to boycott Jews. Soon Jewish students were forced to sit on the left-hand side of lecture halls, separated from the rest – "the bench ghettos". Even the daughter of Professor Rose, a Jew, was segregated during her father's lectures; no one knew or cared what was going on in the mind of this high spirited man who once pronounced that he was a Western European and not a ghetto Jew, but during one of his lectures he collapsed and died of a heart attack in the presence of his tormented daughter. He had many qualities; apart from being a warm human being, an accomplished pianist and an excellent teacher, he was also a prominent neurologist and researcher who advanced the knowledge of "cytoarchitectonic" of the brain. When Pilsudski, "the strong Marshal", died, Professor Rose was entrusted with the examination of his brain by the politically minded colonels. I do not know what the Professor was asked to look for, but it was never revealed.

Shortly before Rose's death our University conferred an honorary degree on Oskar Vogt, a German neuro-pathologist; it was an impressive ceremony. This distinction was brought about by the efforts of Professor Rose himself who had worked with Professor Vogt in the past in harmony. Vogt, an authority in his field, was the first to describe bilateral spastic paralysis and a syndrome of spasmodic outbursts of laughing and crying with slow movements of the hands and feet, both due to a brain lesion and named after him. The Russians entrusted Vogt with the morphological study of Lenin's brain which he undertook in 1925 with his wife Cecile at his institute in Berlin. The brain showed extensive softening caused by cerebral sclerosis in a man who died at the age of 54, but no clue could be found for Lenin's great intelligence. I would imagine that he overtaxed his brain. The atmosphere at the time of Professor Rose's death was electric and non-Jewish students boycotted his funeral, although the professorial body was fully represented. He was taken to the cemetery on a hearse which was only used for Catholics and from which the cross had been removed, so as not to draw too much attention.

The Chair in Neurology at our faculty was dogged by bad luck. Before Professor Rose, it was occupied by Professor Wladyczko – a kindly man, a keen specialist and lecturer. When he became ill he consulted Professor Bergmann in Berlin, introducing himself as a patient of Professor Wladyczko, and asked for a full report to be sent to his doctor, in fact, to himself. The diagnosis came – cancer of the stomach; he knew what it meant, and so hanged himself the same day.

The National Radical Party, formed in 1937, proclaimed a full Nazi programme and outbid its predecessor – the anti-Semitic National Democratic Party. Creation of the Union of Young Poland with the same aim followed. It was not long before Jewish shops were molested, windows broken – the picture so well known to me reappeared. Once I had to ask my way of an elderly Jew. He was suspicious and I noticed his frightened look. "Why ask me?", he said, anxiously shaking his head, "There are other people in the street . . ." "Oh! not again", I found myself muttering. Thank God the happenings here were nothing like those in Germany, where there was nothing to thank God for. Fortunately I was preoccupied with my examinations and lectures.

I vividly remember an operation and the professor's commentary on a schoolgirl of seventeen, beautiful but drained of blood due to a profuse haemorrhage into her abdomen, caused through rupture of the tube in the early stage of a pregnancy no one suspected. Seeing her brought into the theatre in shock and on the verge of death left on me a lasting impression which influenced my stand in the raging controversy over "the Pill" in later years. Watching for the first time a Caesarean section, a delivery through an incision in the abdominal wall and the womb, was also imprinted indelibly on my memory – I saw and heard a baby coming into the world this unusual way – just as Julius Caesar allegedly arrived over 2,000 years ago.

When I was a student intern in the Obstetric Department, a heavily-built woman, apparently in the last stages of pregnancy, was brought in, groaning with pain. Hurriedly I ordered her to the Delivery Room and the Consultant who looked in told me to sit beside her and to call him when contractions became frequent. I sat near her studying the manual on confinement, preparing for the event. Soon the woman quietened down. I was with her for a few hours, able to finish the relevant chapters, but nothing happened. The Obstetrician arrived, surprised at not hearing from me, and after examination I was informed that she should be sent home as she still had two more months to go . . . It was her first pregnancy and the last chance. The woman was forty-one and full of expectation – wishful thinking had got the better of her. I was teased afterwards by my colleagues who named me "the delivery man of a woman with the one and only pain". I also remember the first case of gonorrhoea I saw in a young woman. She was reluctant to be examined by the gynaecologist in front of students and claimed to be a virgin. "A virgin, my foot!", he said, shaking his head in disbelief. "Open your legs", he shouted, and this she did meekly.

I admired the first surgical assistant for his skill. It was only later that I heard he was an alcoholic who drank spirits in front of a mirror (for company!) before operating, to steady his hands.

An unusual event caused a stir in the university. An able assistant, singled out for professorship, was accused of indecent assault by a young and attractive female patient who showed paranoic features. The woman occupied a private single room in the University Hospital and on one occasion, when the assistant visited her on his round unescorted, she became aggressive and he had to restrain her. No one believed in the patient's accusation, but a doctor's reputation must be untarnished, and so the unfortunate man had to relinquish his post.

At last I passed the final examination and was soon proudly holding my Diploma. In my Hippocratic Oath I promised "to obey the rules of the profession, to work for the good of my patients and never to do harm to anyone, to preserve the purity of life and my art and to keep secret", but I found the request "*never* to reveal" impossible to follow. After all, this pledge, admittedly of the highest order, is some 2,400 years old and in variance with to-day's standards.

5
War!

We should live and learn, but by the time we've learned, it
is too late to live.   *Carolyn Wells*

As a newly invested M.B., Ch.B., I boarded a train for Warsaw, where
my parents now lived. Warsaw with over one million inhabitants was a
much larger city and here the ferment was less noticeable. On the surface the city was full of life and gaiety. In the cabaret "Cyrulik" the
comedians Dymsza and Krukowski reigned supreme. Their audiences
found the song "Dan-zig-zig, bum-zig-zig" amusing. The year was
1939.

For some time Germany played a cat and mouse game with Poland.
In the beginning, tourism to and fro was encouraged and skiing and
other joint sporting events were welcomed by the two nations. Goering
visited Poland, ostensibly to hunt bison, a disappearing species in the
Forest of Bialowieza;* this was not his first visit, he had previously
accepted the Prince Radziwill's hospitality. The encouraged mouse
showed its tiny claws. Polish rulers, all military men known as "The
Colonels Régime" who once spoke for colonies, were now boasting
strength and waged a war of nerves with the Czechoslovaks taking
Tesin** by force. Only one minister*** showed practical sense busying
himself by building the much needed public lavatories all over the
country. His not-so-practical colleagues removed him from his post.
Soon the cat changed its tactics. Hitler was now demanding Danzig
and the Corridor, and radios were transmitting the hysterical speeches
of the Nazi Gaulieter of Danzig – Foerster. Ribbentrop arrived in
Warsaw to repeat his master's demands. Warsaw remained calm. We
were kept in ignorance by our rulers; no evacuation of women and
children took place.

We thought that Germany was making empty threats and we
believed in our own strength – had not the Polish armies crushed the

* The Forest of Bialowieza covers an area of 782 square miles and is a Nature
Reserve.

** Tesin had 80,000 Poles and 250,000 Czechs.

*** Slawoj-Skladkowski.

Teutonic Knights in the Battle of Gruenwald 539 years ago, had they not invaded Russian territory and occupied Moscow 200 years later? No wonder the singer Jan Kiepura, standing on the roof of his car in a bellicose pose, was delivering defiant speeches.

I carried on with my daily routine as so many others did. Most of my days were spent in the Czyste Municipal Hospital where even the poorest people had the best attention from a team of excellent doctors. The large tubercular ward was the hospital's Cinderella. Here, patients spitting blood, some dying with frightful haemorrhages, were kept out of sight. I was unable to help. No cure for tuberculosis was yet in sight. Open air treatment in the Swiss Sanatoria for the rich and in the nearby Otwock (pronounced Otvotsk) for the less rich, brought some comfort to these patients, but seldom a cure. Frederick Chopin died of this affliction at the age of 39, Carl von Weber at 40,* Louis Braille – French inventor of the standard alphabet for the blind – in his 43rd year and Alexander Moissi at the peak of his acting career. Consumption killed the novelist Charlotte Brontë when she was 39 and the same fate met her mother, brother and four sisters. Tuberculosis was just as rampant among doctors. One such victim was William Withering, M.D. (Edinburgh), who introduced foxglove – the source of digitalis – in the treatment of a failing heart. In modern times they would have been saved for humanity for many more years. Early this century a tuberculous illness interrupted for twelve years the successful career of the Italian actress Eleonora Duse. Even an opera was preoccupied with this disease – the heroine of "Traviata" – a young girl, Violetta, was portrayed as dying of consumption. To-day it is an almost forgotten illness.

In the hospital for infectious diseases patients with typhoid were dying from intestinal perforation or suffering from effects of horse serum, the only treatment available at that time. In the children's annexe the poor wretches were lying with tubes in their throats choking from diphtheria. The staff of this hospital consisted mainly of Sisters of Charity who had divided loyalties – patients and the chapel; I witnessed a similar situation many years after the war – in Eire.

I dreamt that one day I would be able to go to London or Edinburgh for postgraduate studies. British scientists like Harvey, Sydenham, Willis, and a host of others had an international reputation. Besides, I have always been curious about Greenwich to which our time referred.

* Weber died in London, but galloping consumption did not prevent him from completing his last opera "Oberon". He threw all his remaining strength into this work, which miraculously was not affected by his mortal illness.

Each evening I arrived home by tram, was greeted by my parents, enjoyed a meal together, and spent the rest of the evening chatting, reading or listening to the radio. It seems so ordinary, not worth mentioning, but looking back after more than 30 years it means a great deal. My parents were professional people. Father was an easy going, friendly, hard-working man who liked to take to the flute when threatened with an argument. Mother was more vivacious, a driving force; they had many friends and no enemies. I was their only child and we were very united. Then came September 3* and we had to part, as it happened, for ever.

I left Warsaw to join the Military Hospital No. 10 in Przemysl. I kissed my parents with a brave smile saying, "I'll be back in a few weeks", and left home hurriedly, afraid to look back. A day before I saw placards plastered all over Warsaw depicting our planes and cannons in great numbers. They impressed some people and many were confident of the outcome in the knowledge of the British** and French support.

We used to hear that "Great Britain may lose 99 battles but will win the 100th". People stored food, collected gas masks and blacked out their windows. Poland's strong man, Marshal Pilsudski, had been dead for some time – a great many Poles wept at his funeral, a premonition of terrible things to come. Following the teachings of the German historian Treitschke which once influenced the Kaiser, Hitler conceived a visionary scheme based on a divinely appointed mission and biological necessity for war. He was helped by Nietzche's concept of "Supermen".

On August 23, Hitler announced, "I am now fifty years old. I prefer a war now to when I am 55". This time he was as good as his word. The Germans attacked Poland on September 1. They had been preparing for it meticulously, sending spies and saboteurs, engaging "Volksdeutsche". A few days before the war broke out, I saw some saboteurs captured by Polish people being led away through the streets of Warsaw. For months mysterious fires broke out all over Warsaw; the main railway station was not spared. The "Fifth Column" was at work. I also saw the capture of two young German airmen who had parachuted after their plane was hit on the first day of the war; they were very arrogant imagining themselves to be the master race. Tem-

* The general mobilization was delayed until the last moment to appease Hitler.

** The Anglo-Polish Pact of mutual assistance was signed on 25 August 1939.

pers were running high long before Hitler struck. Once, when leaving the tram on the journey home from hospital, I called out to Mary, a travelling companion and colleague of mine, "Give my love to Adolf", meaning her husband. I noticed my blunder when all the passengers turned their eyes on me, looking disgusted.

The motorized German armies and their heavy guns crossed the Polish frontier at several points supported by Guderion tanks, while fighter planes – the Stukas and the bombers – roared overhead. The noise of the planes and the blast of the bombs was terrific and destruction found everywhere. The natural frontier barrier of the Tatra Mountains in the south did not stop the invader. Attacking troops were lead by German skiers who had competed in the previous championships in Poland. The Polish forces put up resistance as best they could. Bayonet charges took place, the cavalry – brandishing their lances and sabres against the guns – attacked tanks and dragged the crews out, but this was futile and carnage was inevitable. This gallant self-destructive resistance had no hope of stopping the Germans from blasting their way into the heart of Poland.

On August 22, the German people heard Hitler say, "I keep my Skull and Cross-bones Formations ready to kill, without mercy or pity, men, women and children of Polish origin and those who speak Polish. That is the only way for us to get the living space we need". He loved hate and spread it. In those difficult days Adrian de Wiart, the head of the British Military Mission which was sent to Poland in the earlier years, fought with the Polish people.

It was just twenty years since Germany, defeated in World War I, signed the treaty of Versailles. Inspired by the U.S.A. President Wilson, an idealist, the treaty began with the covenant of the League of Nations aimed at prevention of future wars. Barely three years later Mussolini and his Fascists marched on Rome and the following year Hitler attempted a "coup d'état" at Munich. There was still hope – in 1926 Germany was admitted to the League of Nations and her Chancellor Stresemann won the Nobel prize for peace, but in 1935 Mussolini attacked Abyssinia and did not hesitate to use poison gas. A year later the German troops occupied the Rhineland. Experiences of World War I were by now forgotten and the stage set for World War II.

On the evening of September 3, mobilization papers in my pocket, I boarded a tram which took me through a blacked-out city to the railway station. Here I pushed my way through heavy crowds and reached the open wagon of a goods train, the last to leave Warsaw.

During a short stay in Otwock, ladies from the White Cross offered us hot tea, sandwiches and cigarettes – this was my last decent meal for some time. Later on I saw railway stations and various buildings in ruins, some still smouldering. The sun was shining as if nothing had happened. Suddenly screaming Stukas appeared, diving towards the train to the accompaniment of machine gun rattle. Several bombs shattered the earth. The attack destroyed the engine and killed some people. A mother cried hysterically at the sight of her dead son. The train journey was at its end.

With a colleague who was on the way to join the same military hospital as myself, we collected some potatoes from the fields and made a fire with twigs. Now our wandering on foot had really started and we headed east, away from the Germans, the distant roar of guns, their angry flashes and the red flames in the darkness of night constantly behind us.

Just as we were reaching Garvolin, we witnessed an air attack and threw ourselves into a nearby ditch at the sound of sirens. A mother with a child was in front of us. Suddenly the child waved a handkerchief towards the diving planes, babbling with delight. The frightened mother snatched the "white flag" and pressed the child against the ground. We heard a tremendous bang and the earth shook around us. I experienced a hit and anxiously felt my back, but it was only a clod of earth. Four metres away the bomb had left a large crater. I am alive! Unhurt! I start to believe in fate; I am not frightened any more. With smiles on our faces and covered with dust we marched through Garvolin, which was full of destruction and partly burned out. Dazed people pottered among the ruins trying to salvage possessions which had withstood the attack. We headed for Lublin. Along the road were many dead and passers-by were covering them with branches full of leaves; some were saying prayers. In the fields horses, cows, even pigs were lying shot, a target for the trigger-happy German flyers. For them it was just an exercise.

We found that Lublin's suburb had been destroyed by bombs and chose Lutsk, further away from the Germans. We slept in barns or fields, sometimes in bombed out trains, and once in a dilapidated Synagogue. We lived on potatoes and turnips from the fields, and if lucky, on bread from a sympathetic peasant.

On several occasions we, two young doctors, attempted to obtain a night's lodging in houses of medical men; these people were fortunate to be living in their own houses with their families around them and

39

were too damned comfortable to commiserate with us. We met with polite refusals and excuses all the way. But we did find shelter in the homes of a shoemaker, ill with tuberculosis, and of a hawker, whose house was full of bed bugs. I learned at first hand, there is no shame in being poor, but it can be a blasted nuisance.

En route to Lutsk we came across an abandoned train with army supplies. Hungry people fought to get into the carriages which were full of canned food, coffee and biscuits. A lot of food was wasted through being trampled on.

Days of marching on a half-empty stomach tired me out. It was now an effort to carry a neat suitcase my mother had lovingly packed with some cutlery, brushes, underwear and other necessities. When I spotted some soldiers in a horse-driven cart plodding along, I asked if they would relieve me of my load for a short while. This request was willingly met and I began to walk alongside holding on to the cart for support. Suddenly the driver whipped up the horses and away they galloped their mocking laughter echoing behind. My last possessions disappeared. I felt like crying but did not dare to show any weakness to my companion. After all, losing faith in others, we both depended on mutual courage.

We entered Lutsk on the evening of September 17, our feet swollen from the long walk. The familiar uniforms of the army and the police disappeared, we learned the Russians had crossed into Poland. A few hours earlier we had stopped a policeman riding a bicycle and asked the way to Lutsk; he shrugged his shoulders and said: "Go home, Poland is finished." We had no idea what was going on and to hear such a pronouncement from the "law" was a great shock to us.

The entering Soviet troops went out of their way to show friendliness. They said they came as brothers anxious to protect the Ukrainians and Byelorussians, to defend the peasants and workers against capitalists, and to restore peace and order. They called it liberation. In fact the partition of Poland, the fourth* in its history, was taking place with the help of the Germans** who had been penetrating it since the 11th century. The Russians reached the demarcation line along the rivers Narev, Vistula and San, and took 180,000 Polish prisoners on the way. This happened in spite of a Non-Aggression Pact signed by

* First partition 1772, Second 1793, the Third 1795 (the extinction of Polish independence).

** The Russian–German Treaty of 23 August 1939 decided on the present partition of Poland.

Poland and the Soviet Union in 1932, and a 10 year Pact of Non-Aggression with Germany in 1934. The cause of this was primarily the unfortunate geography – a virile nation sandwiched between two powers. Many centuries earlier Poland was menaced by Tartars in the east and south and by Teutonic Knights in the west.

The Russians met hardly any opposition from the Poles; few believed their propaganda, many lost heart. Two days before the arrival of the Russian troops the Polish Government crossed the frontier into Rumania leaving behind the struggling nation. We were left in the lurch. Yet the fight against the Germans went on. The battle of Bzura was fought west of the Vistula River, other engagements took place, the last one near Kock on October 5th. Warsaw had resisted, Modlin, the fortress, did not capitulate until September 30, the defence of the Hel peninsula on the Baltic coast lasted until October 2. All this was in vain, the speed of the "Blitzkrieg" prevented any intervention from outside. Poland had lost 200,000 men. The whole nation showed courage and magnificent spirit which the enemy was unable to break. Some continued guerilla warfare, others were waiting for a second chance to fight; two Polish submarines, "Orzel" (Eagle) and "Wilk" (Wolf), escaped from the Baltic – after all – insurrection was a Polish tradition. But, as usual, it was the ordinary people who suffered most.

In Lutsk I spent days queuing in good company for a bowl of soup and a piece of bread. With me was the popular cabaret artist Lavinski, the head of my department in Warsaw Hospital – Dr. Kobryner, the renowned Warsaw surgeon – Dr. Goldstein and other well known figures, all of them refugees like myself. A few days after my arrival there I was introduced to a well-to-do local family and asked to see their son who had suddenly become ill. I diagnosed acute appendicitis and contacted Dr. Goldstein, who was given facilities in the local hospital, half empty, with only a skeleton staff. I assisted Dr. Goldstein in the operation and was given thirty zlotys by the grateful parents. I was very pleased with myself – after all this was my very first private patient!

I purchased a Russian dictionary. The similarity between Polish and Russian is at times a drawback. In many instances the same word has one meaning in one language, and a completely different meaning in the other. I heard a Russian complimenting a Polish girl on her . . . crowing, meaning her singing, and he was pondering why she was not flattered. I was able to live in the hospital for a while. One evening rather late, when I was already in bed, a Soviet sister arrived, looked into my single room and taking me for a patient enquired about my trouble. Not wishing to inconvenience the administrator of the hospital, I said evasively, "It is my pauperitas and the lack of locum (place), sine pecunia,* you know." She did not know, but was sympathetic and said "I hope you will be better soon". Alas, she was very wrong! Not to embarrass the administrator I left the hospital the next day and wandered aimlessly through the streets of Lutsk. I saw the "Politruks", the official Soviet propagandists, trying to draw the attention of the disinterested passers-by. Here and there Russian soldiers talked to the local people and shared their rations with them. They tried to buy watches which were scarce in Soviet Russia, and looked for prostitutes, banned in their country. The town was full of red banners with printed slogans, portraits of the Politbureau** and the ubiquitous pictures of Stalin. A tribune was erected in the centre of the Square, on it was a lifesize picture of the Russian dictator with a child in his arms, surrounded by small boys and girls with happy faces, garlands of poppies on their heads, bunches of flowers in their hands. They were scattering petals at Stalin's feet. It was a striking picture, in glaring colours. A column of Russians was approaching, singing. The song stopped abruptly; changing to goose-step, heads turned towards the tribune, they saluted the picture. Josif Vissarionovich Djugashvilli, alias Stalin, son of a Georgian peasant shoemaker, was a cult for them, his name uttered in a whisper. They called him "The beloved Leader", "The Great Teacher", "The Father of the Nation". They grieved when he died, and preferred to think that all wrong-doings were not his but caused by his wicked lieutenants who deceived him. The atheist rule played havoc with family life. The Russian people, deprived of liberties and reduced to a status of forgotten orphans, looked for moral authority. They therefore welcomed the fatherly "godlike" image of their master whom they identified with "Mother Russia". In fact, Stalin was a most monstrous figure – merciless, without restraint, intoxicated by limitless power. When he spoke of "enemies of the people", "the will of the masses" and "dictatorship of the proletariat", he meant his own enemies, his own will and his own dictatorship.

In a nearby street I saw a queue of people. They were not seeking bread, but standing in front of a prison enquiring about their relatives. The first arrests took place. Further down I noticed troops in their

* Pauperitas – Latin for poverty. Sine pecunia – without money.
** Politbureau – a policy making body of the Central Committee, which in turn governs the Communist Party.

familiar Polish uniforms, unarmed, surrounded by Soviet soldiers, rifles in their hands, bayonets fixed. Several days passed. I heard that Warsaw, with my parents still there, had fallen into German hands after twenty-six days of heroic resistance. A colleague who tried to reach his wife, who had been left behind, was drowned in the River Bug. A well known neurologist hanged himself. In the streets Soviet soldiers were chanting "I don't know a more happy country than ours". Slogans were shouted through powerful loudspeakers and "Long Live" cries followed me everywhere as if people worried about someone who was very ill! It was a demented sight.

The wet autumn descended. I was near breaking-point. I wished to escape from all the noise, propaganda and the rain, to find a quiet, warm corner, to talk to someone. I noticed a shapely figure in a door-way. She smiled at me and I smiled back. As I came near to her she whispered: "I only take roubles". I passed her by, and when I looked back I saw her motioning two young Russian soldiers who followed her eagerly to the house.

To live I had to apply to the Soviet Administration for a job. I became a hygiene inspector. In this capacity I had to visit numerous houses and on one occasion I asked casually why an elderly lady stayed in bed. I was told she had developed a stomach upset the previous day, and her daughter, hearing that I was a doctor, asked me to look at her mother. I did, diagnosed an acute intestinal obstruction, and rushed her to hospital. My job was not as dull as it first seemed after all, but my salary was not worth the shoes I was wearing out, an item which was hard to come by.

I decided, like many more refugees, to head westward to be nearer Warsaw and my parents. For a short time I worked at the St. Roch Hospital in Bialystok, attending to the confinements of the wives of Russian officers. They complained that no one hurried in our country. If they were in Russia their babies would be born much quicker . . . The surgical ward was full of casualties. The winter of 1939/40 was unusually severe* and to cross the German/Russian demarcation line was an ordeal. A great number of casualties did not reach the hospital; some died peacefully from exposure, overcome by utter exhaustion and sleep. One who did reach the hospital, a boy of nineteen, was stopped by a Russian sentry when crossing the border and held until relief arrived. He was too tired to stand, and so he sat in the snow, watched by the sentry. He was brought to the hospital with severe frostbite of

* The Thames froze for the first time since 1814.

43

the buttocks which caused erosion of the large blood vessels. He was bleeding heavily and since there was no way to stop it he soon died. The walls of the waiting room were decorated with large placards depicting smiling faces and figures, figures, figures – a measure of happiness.

Refugee doctors were not particularly welcomed at the hospital; the medical staff who previously worked there were now returning.

My next stop was a clinic near Bialystok serving several villages. There was a great shortage of drugs and, remembering times when camomile was used against inflammation and the healing properties of eucalyptus, liquorice, valeriana, garlic, peppermint, poppies and the like, I turned to herbs. Do we not owe many important drugs like quinine, belladonna, rauwolfia, digitalis, senna, to the plants! Ergotamine, used for the treatment of migraine, and ergometrine, an obstetric drug, are the alkaloids of a small fungus known as ergot which grows on rye. Pliny the Elder, a contemporary of Jesus, wrote several books on medical botany and the Romans claimed their armies needed no doctors if they had sufficient herbs. And so, with the help of a well informed farmer, I stocked my medical chest with various plants and, remembering my lessons in pharmacology, set to preparing various infusions.

I had no means, however, to attack germs. It is true that Domagk of Germany had been using sulphanilamides against them very successfully since 1935, but the drug was very scarce. Bearing in mind my hospital experience, I was taking 10 to 20 millilitres of blood from the patient's vein, immediately injecting it into his buttock, or simply introducing sterilized milk* the same way, to raise the patient's temperature, thus aiding nature in its fight against bacteria.

It was a quiet place in which to live, away from the noise of the town and the restless crowds. I found myself surrounded by humble, grateful people. I needed them as much as they needed me. I witnessed an epidemic of meningococcal meningitis rife among children, a few cases of tetanus, attended to confinements, accidents and daily ailments. Patients came from afar, women dressed in their best, carrying brand new shoes so as not to wear them out. They brought their problems to me, asking for advice and requesting medicines. Once I was approached for a pint of castor oil. "Are you that bad?", I asked with surprise. "Oh no", said the woman cheerfully, "I am taking it for my cow". I imagine she cared for the animal as much as for her own baby – after all a cow produces milk and drinks only water, a baby does just

* The action of a foreign protein on the body.

the opposite!

The summer came and I was delighted with the place. Patients brought various gifts for me – pork, butter, eggs, honey, fruit, and on one occasion some homespun linen – the patient must have noticed that my suit was wearing out! I took the precious linen to the village tailor and was soon parading in a white jacket and trousers which reflected the bright sunshine. It was too heavenly to last.

A few months earlier I was interviewed by an N.K.V.D.* man and had to tell him about my medical studies abroad and about my parents living in Warsaw. I was offered a Russian passport but declined. Polish people were encouraged to obtain Russian citizenship and work in the Soviet Republics. A school pal of mine, who was good at Latin, obtained a post as a lecturer at the Tashkent University. I heard a story about a Pole who, on departing for Russia, promised to let his friends know what life was like there. They arranged that he would send his photograph which would show him smoking a cigarette should conditions in Russia not prove to be up to his expectations; they soon received it; he puffed three cigarettes simultaneously . . .

I then received a telephone call from the same N.K.V.D. official, who had already interviewed me, asking me to come to his office. He was very polite, and before saying goodbye he commented, "Please do not inconvenience yourself, doctor, there is no hurry, come when you can". It did not sound like a summons, but I had my misgivings. One heard of frequent arrests. The date was June 20, 1940 . . . At the beginning the N.K.V.D. concentrated on the Polish police, judiciary, members of the administration and communal organizations, later, on the Socialists, members of the "BUNT",** on prominent communists labelled as Marxist-deviationists and writers, evidently not liking independent thinking, and then on non-political people – engineers, architects, lawyers, doctors, dentists, teachers and the clergy. They were pruning the Polish intelligentsia. The arrests were usually made at night, surreptitiously; people disappeared mysteriously, without anyone's knowledge.

With this in mind, I burnt two books of André Gide – a Nobel prize winner and a French communist whose journey to Russia in 1936

* N.K.V.D. The notorious State Security Organization, with its own armed force and wide powers. This body was so unpopular that it had to change its name frequently. Originally the "CZEKA", set up in 1917 to combat counter revolution, renamed GPU in 1922, OGPU in 1924, and KGB today – the descendants of the old Tsarist OCHRANA.

** BUNT – The Jewish Socialist Party. Its two prominent members, Ehrlich and Alter, were shot a few years later.

sobered his enthusiasm – and a book on history showing a photograph of the early Soviet Government headed by Lenin and Trotsky, with Trotsky's name underneath. A few weeks previously I had a Russian visitor who was horrified to see this photograph and warned me that possession of such a book would brand me as a Trotskyist and would cost me my freedom. I noticed that he had a distorted knowledge of world history which was based on "A Concise History of Communism", widely circulated in the U.S.S.R.

The next day I appeared before the "law" wearing my summer suit. Outwardly composed, I felt my heart beating and my head thumping. A man behind a desk, with a picture of Stalin on the wall, asked me to sit down. He offered me a cigarette, enquired my name, then went for papers already filled in during my first interview. He was interested to know who paid for my studies in Germany, and when I said, "my parents", he shook his head in disbelief.* Suddenly his face changed, the smile disappeared, he got up to search me. He found a few Polish coins on me and to prove the point he threw them on the floor and stamped on them contemptuously, shouting, "You must know that Poland is finished. From now on there will be only roubles and kopecks." He pressed a button and a soldier by the name of Vanya appeared. I was told he would escort me to another office.

For several minutes we walked through the streets in blazing sunshine, Vanya wheeling his bicycle and I acknowledging greetings from passers-by who knew me. We turned into a side street, and, when we approached a disused factory, Vanya carefully leaned his bicycle against the wall, opened a side door and without any warning caught me by the scruff of the neck and pushed me inside, locking the door behind me.

With the turn of the key I became a prisoner.

* In Soviet Russia the State pays for education.

6
Prisoner

A reasonable amount of fleas is good for a dog; it keeps him from
brooding over being a dog.   *Edward Westcott*

Over the clang of the key I heard voices: "Who is it this time!" When
my eyes got used to the semi-darkness, I found myself in a cell about 3
by 4 metres with a small barred window high up, the place already
crammed with eight poor wretches like myself. I recognized some of
them – a lawyer, a dentist, a teacher. The place was full of stench and I
soon had a headache and felt nauseated. Any attempt to get near the
window was thwarted by others, afraid of being deprived of what little
air there was. Some of the inmates were sitting, and some were lying on
the concrete floor. One could hardly move due to lack of space. We had
to take turns in stretching our legs.

Twice a day a soldier, a Tartar, brought us a bowl of skilly – half
cold and tasteless – once a day a hunk of sour black bread, and we tried
to make this last as long as possible. We were only let out once each
day, the guard on our heels, and had to urinate in a corner of our cell;
the captors must have thought that with us they arrested all of our
body functions as well. Each day was the same. Soon none of us had
enough strength to move and we were lying like fish without water,
breathing heavily, our mouths open, our lips and tongues bone dry. We
were kept alive by a fellow prisoner, a petty thief, con-man and a braggart. The conditions were familiar to him, he was in his element. The
man was a marvellous story teller and we listened to his narratives
from early morning till late at night. He must have been at the top of
his profession!

On the second night I was taken for interrogation. It was 2.a.m.
Half asleep, I dragged myself along, the soldier beside me. Some minutes later I appeared in front of a young Security Officer whom I had
not seen before. A strong light hurt my eyes and I was soon wide
awake. On the desk I saw a file with my name on it. The officer asked
me abruptly the same questions as his predecessor and I gave him the
same answers; he banged on the desk in annoyance and ordered me
back to my cell. All my fellow prisoners were also interrogated long

47

after midnight.

On the fifth day the door of the cell burst open and our soldier appeared jangling his bunch of keys, this time without soup, bellowing, "Bring your things along". I have heard this command several times since.

An army lorry took us to a detention camp near Bialystok. The place was surrounded by barbed wire and held 2,000 people. Here I recognised a watchmaker from Warsaw who had lost a leg in his childhood. He told me his story. A German officer left a watch with him for repair. The following day a soldier walked into his shop, noticed the watch and took it, leaving some money behind. The watchmaker tried in vain to explain, tears in his eyes, that the watch was not for sale. "Don't lie, you Jew", he heard, the door slammed, and this was the last he saw of the soldier and the officer's watch. Distressed and frightened, the watchmaker boarded a train and left Warsaw for the border. On the way he was thrown out of the train and had to walk on crutches until he reached the German/Russian Zone. There the Russians "took care" of him. After the fall of Poland, the Germans did not lose any time with indoctrination – a travelling exhibition called "The Jewish Contagion" toured its towns for several years.

They did not confine themselves to indoctrination alone; in Czestochowa, the town where I was born, they committed mass murders and executions on Poles and Jews as early as September 1939. They soon used gas-vans at Chelmno – less time consuming than death marches.

We slept on the bare ground, in barracks built for tanks some time ago. For a while water was a luxury and none of us was able to wash. Then the rainy weather arrived in drenching, cascading torrents, and the sky remained black for many days. Through the roof of loosely joined planks water poured in on us. By now the comradeship began to wane; it was every man for himself and the struggle to keep alive was first priority. The detainees grooved small channels to deflect water from themselves to their neighbour and no one cared to warn his fellow men of imminent search any more. We were hungry, thirsty, bearded, dirty, lousy, and without sleep. During the night we leaned against each other for a few hours, at times water dripping on the ground from the wet garments, eyes closed, our consciousness suspended from exhaustion, unable to lie on the ground for pools of water.

We were still in Poland. Sometimes someone would throw a parcel of food over the barbed wire, but before it could reach us the sentry would trample on it until it was destroyed. Many got dysentery. There were no proper latrines, no screening; we squatted in a line over long narrow ditches which we had to dig ourselves, our bare bottoms facing the sentry. I would have revelled in this gesture for as long as possible but for the flies which were fiercely attacking the exposed flesh. Soon the ditches assumed the Soviet national colour. No paper was available. We used Russian currency instead as a defiant gesture and knowing full well that the money would be taken from us anyway. People often fainted. The few Russian nurses there doused them with water giving an aspirin – the only drug available. Lice were everywhere, each one of us scratched mercilessly, and it was a consolation to see the sentry doing the same. I watched a soldier on duty taking off his shirt to catch the beasts and smoking strong tobacco rolled into a cigarette from a scrap of paper. Lice have a strong instinct of preservation and it was extremely difficult to find all their hiding places to defeat this enemy. It did not dishearten our guards who were commenting philosophically, "One must get used to such things or perish". Anyway, scratching was the only pleasure left to us all, and so handy. It was the itch-scratch-itch merry-go-round. Doctors call it "pediculosis," a term for yet another medical condition, but for the Russians it was a mode of life.

After a few weeks of this existence, deportations started. We counted it as a blessing. Nothing worse could happen to us, we thought . . .

One day N.K.V.D. officials called my name, shaved my head but not my beard and photographed me in full face and in profile with a four figure number plate on my chest. When I had a chance to glance at my photograph I could not recognise myself and thought I looked like a hardened criminal with a five year sentence passed on me – I must have been psychic! They took my finger prints, ordered me to undress and to queue with others. A search in a standing and half sitting position followed. Shivering all over, teeth chattering from the cold, I followed the orders, "Open your mouth!" "Spread your legs!" Someone peered into my anus. He was looking for hidden treasure, I suppose. I wondered what would happen next. To cheer myself up I thought of an old tale – an Austrian medical officer, serving under the Kaiser Franz Josef, was only interested in two ailments when conducting the daily sick parade – inflamed tonsils and haemorrhoids, his finger the only means of inspection. Wishing to be popular among the soldiers, he encouraged them to voice their requests before the sick parade and so a soldier stepped forward and, standing to attention, recited, "May I be examined first, Sir, I only have a touch of tonsilitis."

"Get dressed", came the order at last, and we did as fast as we could. We now sat on our bundles waiting for the next command, "Bring your things along!" Which things? – my name should be Adam, Adam without Paradise, I mean. I heard people saying, "The first man must have been created on Soviet territory – Adam had no clothes, no shoes, and was reported as living in Paradise." But then, I never believed in Paradise.

One night, stealthily, under cover of darkness, they took us through side roads to a train waiting in a disused place, away from the town. We were marched, six in a row, surrounded by guards with rifles at the ready who warned, "One step to the right or left and you will be shot." It was the exact replica of a picture by the well-known Polish painter Artur Grottger depicting the deportations to Tsar's Russia 100 years ago, the picture I saw in my schooldays. A prisoner in my row started to cry and a guard slapped his face, "Shut your gob, you son of a bitch." His cry turned to a muffled sob. We stopped at last. In front of us, in the full glare of lights, was a goods train, so long that its end was not in sight. The wagons were of the type usually used for carrying cattle. Watched by armed soldiers, we were told to squat in front of the train and had to wait to be herded into the wagons, forty into each one. Once we were inside they were bolted by iron bars. It took me quite a while to get used to the semi-darkness; very little light was coming through small barred windows, high up, on each side of the wagon. There was a hole in the floor which we had to use in full view of each other for our urgent needs. In front of every "carriage" stood a soldier on guard.

Each evening we had a count and recount. "All over to the other half" was shouted, and forty people were herded together like cattle. It did not pay to hesitate – a dawdler was sure to be kicked by the guard's heavy boot. Several times during the night we were awakened by stamping on the roof – a routine check to prevent escape. At night the train was in a blaze of lights – at the back of each wagon was a powerful reflector in operation. The train remained stationary for two days and we were without food and drink until a few hours before we moved off, when delicious Astrachan herrings and a bucket of water were brought in, but no bread. During our stay we banged in despair on the door, shouting "Bread", "Wa-ter, Wa-ter, Wa-ter". The guards responded by hammering the door with their rifle butts and yelling, "Shut up Polish swine". Those who attempted to put their hands through the barred window, in the hope that someone would give them a little bread, were poked by the guard's bayonet. I would have liked to have had a long stomach capable of extension, such as a snake, which could then take a fortnight to digest a meal and free me from eating for months, and also a fang with which to defend myself . . .

Suddenly there was a jolt, and we started to move, heading east. Most of the precious water in the bucket spilled on to the floor, splashing some people squatting nearby and on to our bundles; we were nearly all in tears. No more water was given to us until the next day; our lips were parched, our throats dry after the Astrachan herrings.

We soon learned that the best way to travel was in a squatting position owing to the constant jolting. From time to time one would climb on another's shoulder to obtain a quick look at the Polish meadows and pastures slipping behind. I saw a dog heading westwards. Lucky dog! I thought.

The next day we noticed unmistakably Russian faces, plump and rosy, the women in headscarves, the many bearded men in caps, wearing blouses belted at the waist, their baggy trousers tucked in high boots.

The landscape had not changed very much, the people had. We were in the Union of Soviet "Socialist" Republics, in short, the U.S.S.R. Our status as detainees changed into a more significant one – deportees.

The train came to a halt. The Russian people looked at the goods train with its escort of armed men with curiosity. Someone spat high up into our window, "Polish lords, damned capitalists!" A glazier from Nalewki,* who was in the same wagon as myself, straightened up – he was visibly honoured by the remark. Unhappily, we did not lose the status of the "Wandering Jew."

We moved on again, leaving behind the sound of an accordian and laughter. On the ninth day we reached the deportation point at Kotlas, with its many watchtowers and sentries. The place looked like a human zoo. By the barbed wire fence, watching our arrival, were various races and nationalities – Turkmen, Jews, Azerbaijani, Armenians, Georgians, Tartars, Kazahks, Kalmuks, Yakuts, Uzbeks, Tajiks, Karakalpaks, Bashkirs, Chinese, Samoyeds, Europeans . . . They talked in Russian, Ukrainian, Byelorussian, Lithuanian, Polish, German, Yiddish and various oriental languages; Russians account for just over half the population of the Soviet Union. They had various occupations – lawyers, doctors, teachers, Russian military men dis-

* A poor Jewish quarter of Warsaw.

51

honourably discharged but still in uniforms stripped of insignia, land-owners, priests, thieves and spives. Unbearable tumult. Utter confusion. Pandemonium. Someone was yelling "Scum!" "Sod!" "Swine!" "Bastard!" "Shit!", another was pick-pocketing, someone else was forcibly taking the shoes off another man's feet, people were screaming at each other, a number of them came to blows, whistles pierced the air, a shot rang out from a watchtower, a guard was searching for watches . . . Humanity was at its lowest ebb.

On the fourth day of this hell we were marshalled into barges which took us on the river Vychegda – a large, dull, lifeless stretch of water. The next day we were transferred into open trucks, only to be marched the last forty kilometres on the point of exhaustion, carrying our bundles. Twice I was tempted to abandon my bundle and twice my instinct of preservation told me to hang on to it. Whoever stopped was immediately shouted at – "Get moving", and kicked by the guards. Our escort bellowed: "Faster! Faster!" but we ignored them, hardly being able to trudge.

On the way we saw Polish prisoners of war, still in their uniforms, building a railway; with what little strength I had left, I waved to them and they waved back. It cheered me up and gave me strength; not everyone was a stranger here after all.

At last we arrived in Labour Camp Number 12. The Russian word for a labour camp is "lager", a word which none of us will ever be able to forget. There I was allowed to work in an infirmary. I was treating dawdlers and desperate people who preferred to cut off their fingers, to poison themselves by drinking strong infusions of tobacco, or to become blind by self-administration of obnoxious powders, rather than to work. People who had contracted syphilis a long time ago queued for injections of Neosalvarsan and Bismuth. Some were incredibly tattooed. I remember the French called syphilis "The Russian disease" and the Russians – the "French disease". A great number suffered from frostbite. One of them, whom I knew before the war, told me he was awakened by the N.K.V.D. men in the middle of the night, not allowed to collect his shoes from another room, and taken away in slippers and deported. His frostbitten feet were wrapped in dirty rags held by string. It was not courage which stopped him from shedding tears, only deficiency of vitamin A!*

On arrival at the camp I was still wearing the linen suit made by the village tailor. The temperature was near freezing.

* In vitamin A deficiency the eye is deprived of lacrimal fluid.

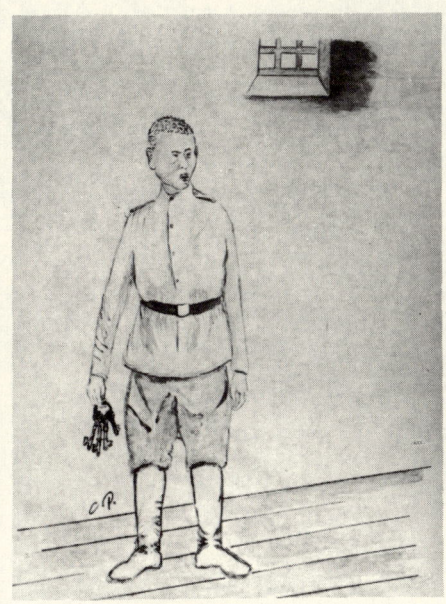

A Tartar Jailer

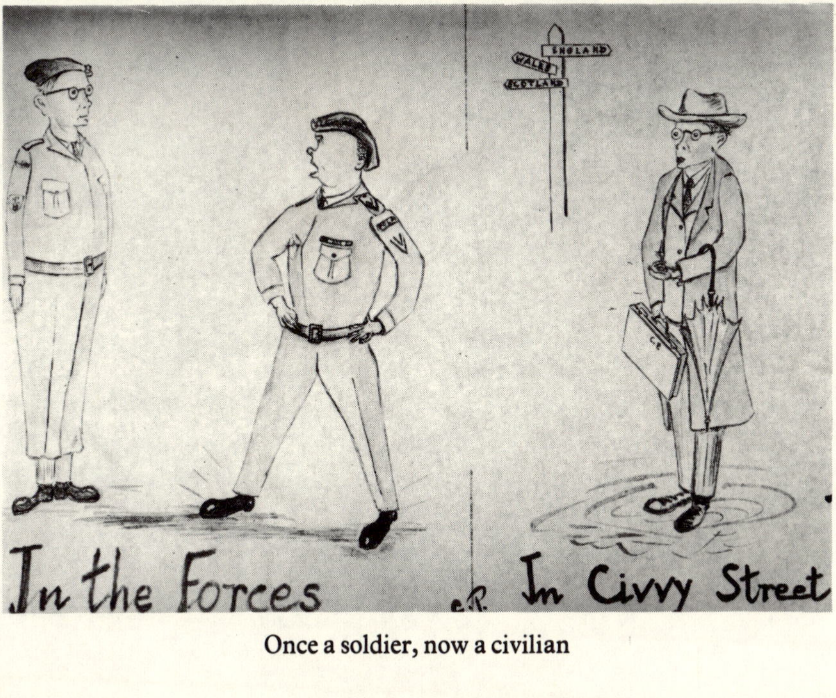

In the Forces   In Civvy Street

Once a soldier, now a civilian

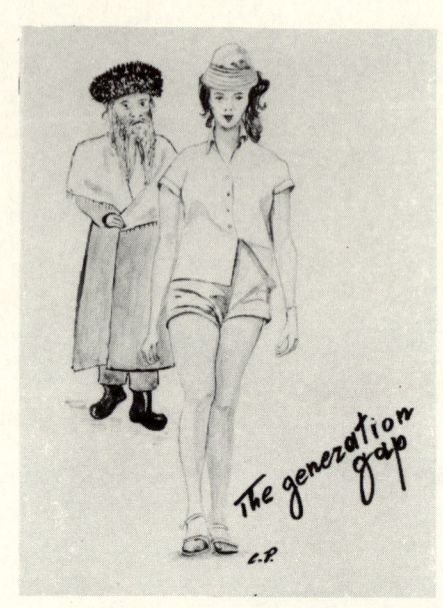

The generation gap

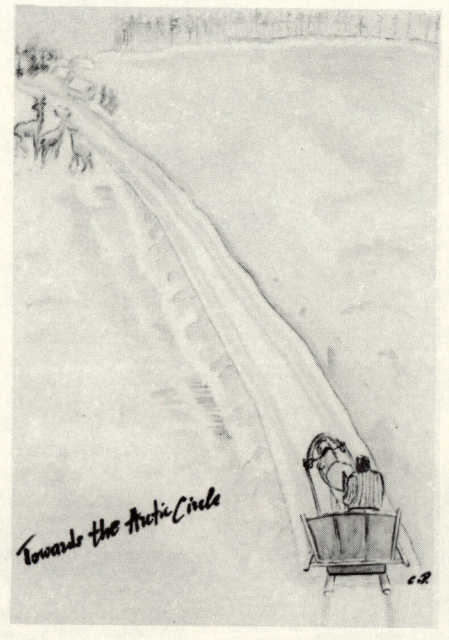

Towards the Arctic Circle

Women were difficult to treat – cases of tuberculosis, severe hysteria, absence of menses caused by emaciation, and again determined dawdlers – a woman with a large benign tumour of the womb pretending to be pregnant, who had been moved from camp to camp "unfit for work" for the last sixteen months, women simulating to be continuously unwell with the help of lipsticks . . . Many of my patients were singers, dancers, past dignitaries, thieves or prostitutes. This camp knew the father of the executed head of the N.K.V.D. – Yagoda. The old man was able to survive his son, but not for long. The Soviet Constitution declares that the father is not responsible for his son nor the son for his father; old Yagoda was sentenced on his own merit – on suspicion of espionage – a guilty man unless he could prove his innocence. It was a vivid example of Soviet perfidy.

The Constitution presented by Stalin to the Congress and adopted on December 5, 1936, laid down that all citizens have equal rights. It also guaranteed freedom of speech, press, assembly and demonstrations.* December 5, is celebrated as Constitution Day. And yet in 1948 Shukhevich, a boy of fourteen, was sentenced to ten years imprisonment because his father was one of the leaders of the Ukrainian nationalist movement; in 1958, on the day of his release, a further ten years was added . . . There were numerous examples of this kind. The heads of the State Security were not immune and did not last for long. First was Dzerzhinsky, then Menzhinsky, Yagoda, Yezhow, Beria. The prevalent complaint of both sexes in the camp was blindness, which affected people from dusk till dawn owing to lack of fats and vegetables. Cod liver oil remedies this, nevertheless, I saw two people who lost their sight in the final stages of night blindness. No wonder Igor, a former school teacher, now a prisoner in Camp Number 12, was keen to be a latrine attendant – a job which gave him an extra ration of a quarter of a litre of milk, a bare cup, a day. When his fellow men were escorted to work some way outside the camp, each morning before dawn, he was able to remain behind; therefore it was not surprising that many prisoners tried to snatch his job. Two more "posts" were coveted in the camp – the keeper of the delousing station and the attendant of the steam bath; besides them, the cook and the administration the only people left in the camp during the long working day were a few sick men looking after the empty barracks – the barrack orderlies.

The delousing station was the pride of the Russians who were saying

* Articles 123 and 125.

53

"It is proof of our culture". They were also saying "We are the only country which puts people into prison for swearing in public". I was told earlier of a salesman at "GUM", Moscow's departmental store, who brought out endless bales of material for a woman's selection, but still she could not make up her mind. Finally, his face flushed in anger, he muttered, "Please wait," adding in a raised voice, "and I will go to hell!" . . . so saving himself from prison. "You mustn't" is the Russian battle cry for culture, but there are many "mustn'ts" there – one mustn't be outspoken, choose one's work, friends or dress, read or write freely . . . The word "individual" is out, replaced by "collective". The Russian people are collectively educated, indoctrinated, employed, entertained and condemned, and they plan, eat, play, sleep and confess collectively. The non-conformists are the enemies of "culture". Hell and damnation, they call it culture and fancy themselves to be the centre of it but, in fact, their culture is drab and brings indifference, resignation and unhappiness. Like "Mustn't", there are many "Musts". One must obey, vote, suffer . . . Compulsion replaced compassion.

The steam bath, similar to the Turkish bath, is an old Russian institution. I took one on a cold dark evening and had a feeling of entering heaven. A small hut, built entirely of logs, with a wooden floor, had a large oven made of stone, the top of which had holes covered by sizeable stones. The oven with its stones was brought to intense heat by burning wood a short time before our arrival. I stripped naked in the ante-room, entered the heavenly bathroom, dark, except for a flickering glow from the oven, laid down on the bench along the wall, resting and sweating profusely. After a while I lazily left the bench, picked up a wooden vessel full of water and dragged myself towards the oven, not too close and slightly to one side. I threw water on to the stones, enjoying the dense clouds of rising steam. At last I lifted another wooden vessel full of water, poured it over myself, dried with a towel, dressed quickly and left the place reborn. It was my first real bath since my imprisonment and it was a success. I made a point of getting acquainted with the intricacies of the Russian steam bath and I followed its rules scrupulously. A fortnight previously a prisoner died from severe and extensive burns because he went too near the oven after throwing water on to the hot stones.

Not far from the camp was a hospital for the personnel and the previous deportees who had settled in the region after completing their sentences. The doctors there had a lot to contend with. When an epidemic of gastro-enteritis was raging among the infants, causing high mortality due to the poor condition of the nursing mothers and the lack of facilities and drugs, the doctor in charge was arrested. Therefore it was with trepidation that I answered an urgent call for a doctor needed in the camp, in the absence of the obstetrician, for a woman who was in difficulties during labour. "Hurry up doctor", said the soldier escorting me. It was the first time since my arrest that the "authority" had called me that.

I found the woman already many hours in labour without much progress, and the foetus with signs of distress. She was well built and the neck of the womb was fully dilated. I could feel the head of the baby, but her contractions were poor. There was every indication to apply forceps except one – I had never applied forceps before! I had watched this procedure many times in the past and it did not look too difficult. I took a snap decision to use the blasted things. I had nothing to lose, I was already a prisoner anyway!

With another doctor pouring ether on the woman's face I managed to deliver the baby alive! It was a relief for everyone concerned. I remember a story told by our Professor of Gynaecology about an assistant who was deputizing for his professor at a difficult delivery. Everything went wrong. The young man had to perform trepanation* to save the mother. His patient died during this procedure. The distraught father committed suicide . . . The doctor had three deaths on his hands! Some time after, the same assistant-obstetrician found himself confronted with yet another similar situation, but this time he reported cheerfully to his superior, "Sir, I was able to rescue the poor father"!

The father of the baby I delivered, an N.K.V.D. officer, had good reason to be grateful, and so he took me by lorry to a shop in Syktyvkar – a town some distance away from our camp. It was not 4.p.m. when we arrived, but it was already dark, with stars shining in a cloudless sky. When a nice, elderly salesman learned that I had come from the labour camp he gave me a razor, the thing I wanted most. "Poor you", he said, "you are here for good; believe me, I know." I heard later that the deportees, who returned home after completing their sentence, were usually brought back to the far north on trumped-up charges.

I did not enjoy my razor for long. Two days later I was thoroughly searched; two N.K.V.D. men looked everywhere – their hands fumbling in my pockets, my mattress and my pillow. The rummaging

* Trepanation. An obsolete procedure to destroy the embryo in the womb.

55

ended with the taking of a few roubles and my razor. The whole place was left in a shambles. A few days passed and I was informed that I would be leaving the camp as no sentence was ever passed on me. A free man? Was I hell! "Bring your things along", the order echoed again. An open lorry took me to the station where five other detainees, all doctors, were assembled. No one was able to tell us our destination. We were taken to a nearby bathhouse where we had a hot bath, a change of linen and were issued with fufaikas* and padded trousers. After that I felt my spirits rise. Someone in authority asked us if we wished to make any requests. My colleagues, much older than I, were silent and downhearted. The question put me on my guard. I now suspected a long journey to the North, so I asked for valenki,** a Russian cap with earflaps, and mittens. To my surprise I got them, together with two pieces of linen for wrapping the feet inside my boots. The thermometer registered 30°C below zero. We were ordered to board a train and found ourselves in yet another goods wagon, this time with a little iron stove inside. We soon got to know each other – one Austrian, one German and three Russians.

We moved with a jolt and listened to the monotonous rattling of the wheels. We were heading north! One of the Russians, silent and visibly depressed, suddenly gripped his chest, his face contorted with pain. We looked at him with compassion, all of us doctors, not able to help, this time not because of lack of knowledge. Thank God his attack passed quickly, but I really should not use that expression. After three days of travel in "luxury" – the complete goods wagon for only six people – we reached Kozhva. For the first time we left our wagon without an escort.

* Fufaika. A quilted coat.
** Valenki. High felt boots.

7

Doctoring in Russian Labour Camps

Russia is a riddle wrapped in a mystery inside an enigma.
Winston Churchill

We watched with amazement soldiers unloading carcasses of meat from the train – a long forgotten sight. We soon learned that we and the carcasses were to be despatched to the prison hospital near Kozhva, by order of Beria's* office, because of the high mortality among prisoners from pellagra. The hospital had 600 patients, the majority in the late stages of the disease. They looked like skeletons, their eyes sunken, their skin almost transparent, dry and creased, extremely pale. They were all emaciated, had no strength to move an arm or even utter a word, only their dry lips quivering. They were incontinent, with watery motions like dishwater, a great number with swellings all over the body. Some had hallucinations and delusions, some a severe squint. The thermometer's mercury did not rise above 34°C. This was pellagra in its most florid form. They arrived in hospital too late and the most skilful handling could not save them. Despite this there were several arrests of hospital doctors. The unfortunate patients suffered because of prolonged deprivation – green vegetables, meat, milk, and milky products were denied them for a very long time. When they became tired and irritable, were unable to sleep and complained of sore tongues, bright red in colour, and of dyspepsia, no one took any notice. The bread ration was cut to 300 grams a day, the only other food being skilly. "He who does not work, does not eat", was the camp's ruling to preserve the image of the "Worker's state". The poor wretches stopped caring, they lost their appetites anyway. When they looked like skeletons, unable to raise themselves from the bunk, they were rushed to hospital. The other illness was scurvy, owing to lack of fresh fruit and vegetables. This caused not just bleeding gums and falling teeth, but large painful haemorrhages into the joints and muscles making them bedridden, even causing death. Scurvy was a potential hazard for all of us, therefore I was glad to learn that eating the shoots of dried peas, which I cultivated by placing the pea on muslin over a glass of water,

* Beria. Head of N.K.V.D. executed after Stalin's death.

57

provided me with the vitamins I was lacking in my food; sipping "hvoya" prepared from needles of fir trees was another counter-measure. To have the full quota of vitamins, I also made a habit of taking cod liver oil on a piece of bread each day. This way I escaped night blindness.

The doctors in this hospital were partly free people and partly under sentence. The free people kept apart, addressed each other as citizens or comrades and seldom acknowledged greetings from the rest. They must have thought we were infected with the plague!

The doctor who was on duty the previous night reported a "quiet state of affairs". "Only seven patients have died." Among the dead was a prisoner by the name of Sergejev. He succumbed to a brain abscess and blood poisoning. There were no facilities to treat his diseased mastoid bone.

I was glad to learn that I was in transit, my final destination being 250 kilometres away. I was told that a horse drawn sledge was waiting for me. My instructions were to follow the track until I reached the main infirmary of the region and to look after the precious horse well. "You will find food already in the sledge and do not forget to grease your face." Full of thrill and expectation, not scared of the unknown, I said a cheerful "Hello" to my companion – the horse – who lifted his head wearily. The poor animal looked as if he was nearing the end of a ten year sentence. He started to paw the ground, eager as I was to leave the place. I had a feeling the horse was as disenchanted and famished as myself. I found the sledge full of hay, with only bare necessities for myself – a few tins of reindeer meat, one of marmalade, black bread already cut, a few sweets, a tin opener, billycan, spirit stove, a container with methylated spirit, a box of matches (incidentally, an item which was difficult to come by), also a thermometer but, unfortunately, no dark glasses.

And off we set, the horse and I, working our way through the only track available, mostly on the ice of the frozen Pechora River, strong enough to bear our not too heavy bodies, in one direction – North, exploring the vast land of Komi, A.S.S.R. and getting nearer and nearer the Arctic Circle. The journey took six days. It was a cold enterprise! Time and time again I halted to give the horse a rest, to warm myself by flailing my arms against my body, stamping my feet, running around the sledge, putting my chilled hands under the horse's belly. It was also feeding time for both of us. When I had warmed myself sufficiently to ease the stiffness of my hands, I took some hay out of the sledge and gave it to my friend, then opened a tin of meat and melted some snow over my spirit stove.

Both refreshed, we plodded on again. The warning "Grease your face" was always with me, the temperature nearing minus 40°C. It was like a white desert – a plateau covered with snow as far as the eye could see. There was nothing in the way apart from our breath vapourizing as each of us exhaled. The air was pure and I felt its vibration, a clear sky with a weak sun, perfect visibility, not the slightest breeze; the stillness was uncanny. The dead silence was only broken by the crunching sound of the horse's hooves, or my felt boots treading in the thick snow. The constant reflection of it tired my eyes causing moisture which rapidly turned into icicles.

Once I ran into a snowstorm and in no time we were covered heavily with a blanket of snow. The storm soon died out, but for a while the going was difficult. Suddenly, I saw two sledges in the distance moving swiftly across the plain, pulled by reindeers. What a novelty! It was getting darker, the day and our labours were coming to an end for the present. We had covered some fifty kilometres in the course of the day. Luckily for us we were nearing a settlement consisting of log houses, not too late to find a place to stop. This region was sparsely populated and the villages were very few and far between. I found the people primitive, illiterate, poor but hospitable. They were Samoyeds – well developed but short in stature, with oblique Mongolian eyes. They dressed in skins, lived mainly by hunting and fishing, and kept reindeer which provided them with transport, food and clothing. I was told they believed in ghosts, in the wandering of the Soul that was able to enter into the bodies of other men and animals, and cherished superstitions. (In this context it is worth mentioning a Polish belief that at Midnight on Christmas Eve animals can speak with human voices.) Their god Ukko or Nim, the chief spirit, was supposed to be influenced like other spirits by the spells of shamans – virtually sorcerers – who work cures, etc. by magic, bringing themselves to a frenzy. It is possible that Samoyeds are the descendants of the Mongolian expeditionary forces led to the North by Ghenghiz Khan in the 13th century. They prepared kumiss from mares' milk and used this for libations, as quoted by E.D. Phillips in "The Mongols".

The female population dominated each settlement, many of their men being taken away to labour camps. I will continue to refer to these camps as "labour camps" throughout the book, but the term "prison camps" would be more appropriate. The illiteracy of the Samoyeds saved them from political discrimination; most of them got only short sentences, two or three years – for sabotage, not being able to deliver the amount of products required from them, or for incompetence and other trivialities.

Samoyeds have their own language and only a few spoke Russian. The word "Abu" occurred again and again in their conversation and, intrigued, I asked the meaning of it. I was told it is the equivalent of the Russian "Nietu" – "not available".

When, much later, I found myself in the Uzbek Soviet Republic, the first word I learned was "Yok" – "Nietu" in that language, but then it was wartime.

I slept among the Samoyeds for five nights and found that lice were in greater strength than I had ever experienced before. This may have been because the Russian civilization and its delousing stations had not reached them! I witnessed their own battles against this invader – a mother of a teenage daughter was killing lice and nits galore in the girl's hair by constantly crushing the beasts and their eggs with the flat of a knife after a meticulous search. She did it in a matter-of-fact fashion, not in the least embarrassed by my presence. The task completed, she cut a portion of black bread with the same knife, inviting me to share it with them. Both mother and daughter looked pale and famished; they were fending for themselves in the absence of the deported head of the household. Such a gesture of sacrifice could not be ignored. I, a man in a fufaika, a prisoner in the far North, tried by miming to explain, I was not hungry . . . I showed my goodwill though by accepting "Kipietok",* and offered the girl a sweet wrapped in paper. The poor creature did not know what to do with it; she had never seen a sweet before.

I departed next morning leaving a tin of meat, which I opened for them, to show my gratitude. I kept going. On the way I saw a herd of wild reindeers but no man in sight and soon heard the sound of their hooves as they raced away.

At last, on the sixth day, tired but in good spirits, I reached my destination. I noticed that my thermometer had frozen** and from now on only one filled with alcohol was any use. I enjoyed the trip and I honestly think it was worth while. I had learned that much more about life.

I was now steps away from the Arctic Circle and some two hundred kilometres from the Arctic Ocean. Winter was long and severe, the

* Kipietok – Hot water for drinking.
** Mercury freezes at 39° centigrade below zero.

temperature reaching 50°C below zero. The days were as bleak as the nights, an anaemic-looking sun appearing very briefly,* only lasting blizzards breaking the monotony. According to the camp ruling, prisoners should be excused from work when the temperature dropped to 40°C below zero, but the overseers and the rest of the administration, keen on maintaining the output, often tampered with the thermometer displayed outside the guard-house.

In the spring I watched huge blocks of unthawed ice floating on the river with its strong current, but not for long; the Pechora was frozen solid nine months out of twelve. The short Spring and Summer had many sunny days and for several weeks the nights were as bright as the days; I had to cover my windows with blankets to enable me to sleep. These were the white nights of the Arctic. The warmest months were July and August, with frequent mists and heavy showers. During this time nature was coming to life. I enjoyed the hum of various insects but not the whine of angry mosquitoes. Swarms attacked us fiercely, making our life hell. I had to protect my face with a net and to wear gloves when out of doors; a few people developed malaria. To guard the living quarters against the mosquitoes we burned rags at our doors. We were in a tundra district, swampy and full of moss as water cannot filtrate through the perennially deep frozen earth; an ideal breeding ground for the newest enemy.

There were no latrines. We had to take positions in the tundra, pants lowered in a flash, without any chance of meditation, unless one was prepared to take the consequences! I had to treat several patients after they communed with nature. The labour camps were scattered around in the vicinity of taiga-forest. Prisoners were marched into it, in parties, each morning at 5 o'clock, when still dark, for tree felling. They had to work hard until late in the evening, a good eleven hours, under the eyes of the overseer and armed guards, to earn their meagre rations. At roll-call I had to hold a sick parade and see them off. They arrived back into the zone long after darkness had descended, only to stand in the frost in front of the guard-house where they were counted and searched; it could take hours. After a frugal meal, followed by a mug of hot water, they laid their weary bodies packed together on the hard planks of the barrack bunks.

Only men were in these camps, most of them inexperienced in this kind of work, and accidents happened to which I was called quite often. Attractive jobs like overseer, "educational" officer, cook and ad-

* During the winter months the sun does not rise above the horizon.

ministrative posts were only given to criminals, who were the trusted people.

The felled trees were sawn into large logs and assembled into piles to await transport. There was no railway near, so the timber was floated down the Pechora during the few months navigation was possible. The virgin forests were of great value to Russia; the mass deportations to these areas provided the necessary labour otherwise impossible to recruit on a voluntary basis. We were pioneers by force! Komi, A.S.S.R. is a vast region and the labour camps were tucked away from the eyes of the Komi people already scattered over this territory.

I made some journeys in this area but I never came across the Komi inhabitants. On one occasion I was ordered to see patients in a labour camp, some forty kilometres away. I was given yet another horse, in a much worse condition than the first. He had something wrong with one leg and was limping slightly. I was most uncomfortable as I did not get a saddle. Twice we sank deeply into marshy ground; nevertheless, I was glad of the exercise. No wonder that on my return to the infirmary after the two days trip I had a succession of troublesome boils in most unsightly places. It showed I was not the best of horsemen!

By now I was used to living and working among prisoners. When I first arrived at the infirmary, my superior — "the Citizen" Yegorov — asked me what my offence was and what was the sentence. It struck me then that I had never been tried or sentenced, although it was ten months since my arrest.

The infirmary was a wooden building. There was a very large room with sixty beds close together and two small rooms adjacent to it, one of them being the medical inspection room with dispensary. This had to be kept locked when not in use. The people who were running the camp and had easy access to the infirmary were picked from criminals ("urkas"), usually hard drinkers. I caught them drinking Valeriana, "gastric drops" and other medicines, in short, they drank anything which smelt of spirit. I had to treat one of them for chemical burns of the mouth and throat, the label "Aromatic Spirit of Ammonia" led to his blunder. Such was the "élite". I found that the great majority of patients suffered from advanced pellagra, scurvy, malnutrition with generalized swelling. There were also two cases of open pulmonary tuberculosis, a man with a shot gun wound, and one malingerer whose determination brought him suffering. For months he pretended he had lost his leg. He had it tightly bandaged in a fully bent position to his thigh, never attempting to straighten it; when it was discovered, he already had an irreversible contraction.

It was not long before I had an argument with my superior.

A patient in his thirties, big and swarthy, was admitted to the infirmary because of paralysis of his legs and dog bites. He gave a history of a sudden stiffness of his lower limbs when in the camp, which prevented him from joining the working party. The camp authorities considered him to be a malingerer and let loose ferocious dogs on him. The shock aggravated his condition and he became paralyzed.

My superior, a free man who was the medical administrator of the camps in the region, was convinced that the camp authorities were right. "I can smell a malingerer for miles", he said. He poured a few drops of boiling water on the patient's leg, causing blistering, and pricked the man with a needle, not getting the slightest response. "This man is from Baku,* he is a fakir," my superior pronounced without examining him. I showed that the man had abnormal reflexes and drew attention to the peculiar articulation of his speech, "Without any doubt he is a wheel-chair case", I declared; he was not convinced, but left me to deal with the patient.

In one of the adjacent rooms I had the two patients in advanced stages of tuberculosis, kept in isolation. They were toxic, flushed, feverish, sweating profusely, emaciated and too weak to walk. I was powerless; there was no known drug which could help them. I wished to build them up with food but they could not eat.

Two cows were allocated to the infirmary. In charge of them was a youngish, fair haired, blue eyed woman, the only one of her species there. When she first spoke to me she was on her best behaviour, but on hearing her swearing incessantly at the guard without running out of foul language and seeing her spitting in his face, I guessed what her crime was. She unmistakably belonged to the most international and oldest profession known under various names − courtesan, moll, geisha, wanton, slut or "fallen woman". But to be more precise people speak of a street-walker, harlot, call-girl, prostitute and plain whore. I only then realized how rich and picturesque the Russian language is. It confirmed my previous admiration of the able and concise descriptions in it, like the word "Sumashedshe", for instance, which means a madman and translates "He who went off his mind", or the expression "Soul pinching music". I once heard a Russian philosophying: "One can't make rude noises higher than one's buttocks, neither can one

* A port on the Caspian Sea.

jump above one's penis, but there is no harm in trying." No wonder the Russians are not interested in Latin but prefer a living language instead!

Some patients did improve in the infirmary – we had better food, vitamins and a few drugs. One of them, a Polish Jew, was admitted in a state of exhaustion, covered with horrible boils from head to foot. When he started to improve he made himself useful by helping to wash the patients, taking temperatures and delivering drugs to individual beds.

His name was Leib. After a few months with me, Leib had red rosy cheeks, healthy skin and ten pounds added to his weight. I helped a few more by keeping them as long as possible and writing in the hospital records additional diagnosis – kidney stone? gall stones? peptic ulcer? angina? . . . Sometimes I had a social visit from the Administration of the nearby camps – they enjoyed our food and liked to talk about the victuals of the past . . . . "I remember" was said with sentimental sadness many, many times. In this way I made the acquaintance of an interesting Russian man. Distinguished looking, with silver hair and moustache, highly intelligent and widely read, he once was a factory manager with a degree in mathematics and Russian literature. He was sentenced for misappropriation of funds and was now a planner in one of the camps. He introduced me to Pushkin and Lermontov and advanced my knowledge in the Russian language. This proved very useful when I took a job as a Pathologist in our infirmary on the transfer of another doctor. At last I had a safe job and no one could accuse me of a wrong diagnosis or of harming a patient.

It was a ruling that all people who died in a hospital had to have a post-mortem and an assistant surgeon was helping me with this task. He was a quiet, unassuming person who struck me as a man of intelligence and knowledge. He also knew Latin, a rarity among lower medical personnel in Russia.

After a few months, when we knew each other better, he confided in me that he was in fact a fully qualified doctor. "I concealed my Diploma, it was only a burden to me. I now do a doctor's work, I eat the same as you and do not bear any responsibility."

With his help I was able not only to carry out post-mortem examinations, but to write lengthy reports, in Russian of course! I found most striking changes in the human bodies – smooth atrophic lining of the large intestine with ulcerated walls, fatty degeneration of the liver, spleen reduced to the size of a fig, gall bladder creased, half empty, with transparent liquid of lemon colour. One case concerned a man who became ill suddenly when in a working party engaged on floating timber. He had had to sit for hours near the river waiting for the party to be taken back to camp. He could not march quickly enough for the guards who were anxious to get home. He was pushed and struck several times. On arrival he was pale and feeble. They took him to a steam bath-house where they poured cold then hot water alternately over him until his colour returned. He brought up some blood, but this was due to rough handling, they thought. It took three more days before the camp orderly decided to send the man to the infirmary. The patient was soon dead. He was only twenty-five years of age. I found his right lower and mid lobes as solid as an ox-heart, and many bruises. He died of pneumonia which could have been prevented. I reported the incident to the Medical Administration of the Region. I received no acknowledgement. Human life was cheap. "Russia has a great many people," in fact 220 million, we were told.

Post mortem examinations on people who met a violent death were carried out by a forensic expert specially sent for. However, during the summer thaw when huge blocks of ice were rushing down the stream of the Pechora river, we were cut off from the mainland for several weeks. Consequently, I was ordered to carry out a post-mortem on a twenty-year old shot by a sentry. I found the bullet in his brain. Its entry was near the lumbar spine and it came out between the shoulder-blades, finding its second entry in the back of the head. The sentry claimed that the prisoner tried to escape and did not stop when challenged. How could he when he was in a stooping position? Anyway, where would he run to – to the tundra? to the swampy forest to die of starvation? and what would be waiting for him at home? All prisoners knew, no one wanted them there after several years of deportation; it would be impossible to get a job, one would live in fear of denunciation and further deportation; they were suspects, and old friends were afraid to have contact with them. I knew of cases where wives turned against husbands having settled to a new life with a new man. No wonder many prisoners preferred to remain in the place of deportation after completing their sentences. Stalin was arrested five times by the Tsarist police and each time managed to escape, like many of his associates. Obviously the old régime was more lenient, or less efficient than his.

I had yet another forensic post-mortem examination. A body was brought in from a punishment cell of the camp – the name itself raised

65

fear among the prisoners. The guards had to overpower and bind by rope the doomed men before they could drive them away like bullocks to the slaughter house. The punishment cell was small, dark and cold. The prisoner, who was now dead, had been put on a starvation diet consisting of 200 grams of bread a day and water.* The post-mortem examination revealed only extreme wasting in an otherwise healthy individual. I saw this place and once watched a prisoner stumbling and swaying when coming out of it, with eyes half closed against the light.

The first camp Commandant I met was a charming person, and so was his wife. Both were good looking, tall, dressed in sheepskin coats and mink caps. They enquired about my work, my patients and myself. They spoke softly and listened attentively, obviously interested in the people around them. The couple arrived a month before me; I got the impression they had held an important post in the past and that the transfer to this camp was not a promotion.

Two months later they left. I was told they had been arrested. To be a camp commandant was an insecure post. During my stay in the infirmary there were three of them in succession. I was rather unlucky with the second one. He consulted me because of an abscess in the most delicate area of his bottom, necessitating surgical intervention. In preparation I cleaned the skin with iodine, the only disinfectant available. Two days after, he saw me again. He was in great discomfort and visibly annoyed, his skin grossly inflamed and blistered, no doubt because of his sensitivity to iodine. "You hoped to finish me off", he remarked. "It is against the Hippocratic Oath", I said. The communist hierarchy did not believe one could have high principles. In January 1953, nine prominent physicians were arrested on Stalin's orders and charged with attempts to poison members of the Presidium who were their patients. Two were beaten to death, and only the timely end of Stalin saved the others.

Iodides in those days were the most used remedy — for disinfection, goitre, tonsilitis, bronchitis, asthma, circulatory affections, to promote the secretion of urine, for treatment of lead and mercury poisoning, syphilis, inflamed lymphatic nodes and testicles, rheumatism, sciatica, muscular pains, shingles, cataracts, radiography, against various parasites . . . The list was endless, in spite of the great hazards of such a remedy which sometimes resulted in death. We had mixtures, solutions, paints, liniments, ointments, powders, vapours, injections,

* Prisoners who went to work during the day, returning to the punishment cell for the night, had their bread ration increased to 300 grams.

66

but times have changed and it is not used any more.

The last Commandant was the opposite of the first one, to put it mildly. One day, fourteen months after my imprisonment, he summoned me to his office and in a harsh booming voice read out the sentence of five years, passed on me by the Soviet Supreme Court *in absentia*, without any pretence of a trial, as a "socially harmful element"; they eventually found the article of the penal code which would suit my case. My status changed again, I was no longer a detainee, I was now a prisoner in my own right – under sentence. Justice, which came to a halt a long time ago, was being taken over by the law. It did not upset me unduly for it was like yet another pantomime, too ridiculous even to be angry. Anyway, I was convinced that everything would come right in the end – my thirty-one years helped me in my optimism. The majority had much longer sentences and they referred to one of five years scornfully as a child's sentence. The Commandant, a short fat man with high cheek bones and small pig-like eyes, his voice raised to a crescendo, told me what a lucky man I was and how lenient the Court had been with me. His arrogant behaviour showed me unmistakenly how much this little bumptious man was enjoying his power.

When he had finished, I departed without a word – I had none for his behaviour and the trumped up charge. I was dismayed, but perhaps I should have shown good manners by thanking him . . . after all, to me he was nothing more than a faceless nonentity. I went back to the infirmary and the books I was able to get hold of. The modern Russian literature which I read was full of human misery, drabness and hopelessness – the heroes finding death in battle, drowning in floods, or killing themselves; not once did I come across a book even remotely resembling "Lampion kisses girls and birches". In medical books I often found authors' names blocked out – "Trotskyists" no doubt.

8
Crossing the Urals and reaching the army

A yawn is a silent shout.
Gilbert Keith Chesterton

On the world's arena, Russia took possession of Bessarabia and Northern Bukovina* in June 1940 and of the 3 Baltic states – Lithuania, Latvia and Estonia – two months later; officially these countries were "admitted" to the Soviet Union just as I would be admitted but for my refusal to accept the Russian passport offered to me. The United States and Britain had never recognised the incorporation of the Baltic States into the Soviet Union.

On June 22, 1941, Hitler's armies poured into Russia and barely four months later they were just sixty-four kilometres from Moscow, forcing the Soviet ministries to be evacuated to Kuibyshev. On November 21, Rostov – the gateway to the Caucasus – was captured. On December 2 a reconnaissance battalion penetrated to a Moscow suburb. A few months earlier, on July 30, 1941, an Agreement was signed by Stalin and the Polish General Sikorski proclaiming general amnesty for Polish people, and on August 14 it was decided to form a Polish Army on Russian soil, both in consequence of a Russian Treaty with Great Britain concluded a little earlier. I found it of great interest that in May, 1940, Britain saved Allied troops retreating from Dunkirk.

I knew nothing about these swiftly moving events being "in retreat" since June 1940. The first intimation of this news came over the loudspeaker installed in the camp. I heard that the Russians and the Poles were now friends and allies and that we would be released, and sure enough I was soon called to the Camp Commandant's office. He, trying to be nice, his voice cloying in its affability, asked me to sit down. "You will soon be free", he said, "We can offer you an attractive job in the region", and he proceeded to paint a rosy picture of my future under his wing. I was still smarting from our first encounter, I was

* Bessarabia and Northern Bukovina are now known as Moldavian Soviet Socialist Republic.

68

not interested anyway. "I wish to join the Polish Army", I told him with determination. The mask dropped off his face. "You will be sorry", he barked through clenched teeth, rising from his chair and shrugging his shoulders. Before I left, he told me angrily that I was lucky to be released. I learned from this tactless little ferret that the Medical Administration resented my forensic reports. He was informed by a medical orderly whom he had "planted" in the infirmary without raising my suspicions, of my activities and disparaging remarks. He finished, saying, "We would have doubled your sentence but for the amnesty". He got on my nerves. I stormed out full of contempt and had difficulty in restraining myself from shouting "To hell with you!"

Before I left, I said goodbye to a few people in the Administration. With their help I got spare linen, a towel, several tins of meat and marmalade, and also dried fruit. I put my treasures neatly into the small wooden case with which I was provided and waited until an army lorry could take me to the N.K.V.D. Quarters in Kaninnos. Here I found a crowd of prisoners who had been waiting for several weeks to be called out, some among them pretending to be Poles, but it was not easy to deceive the N.K.V.D.

I came across one man by the name of Samuel Rosenbaum who was a genuine Polish citizen; his relatives abroad, hearing of his arrest, got him a Peruvian passport, which they sent to the Soviet prison authorities in the hope that it would secure his release. Now all his countrymen were leaving the camp and he was left behind – one never knows. . . .

My turn came, and again an N.K.V.D. official tried to persuade me to stay and work as a free citizen. Meeting with my refusal, he handed me the allocated two hundred roubles for the journey. The money did not last long. I thought I had it tucked well into my felt boots, but it was stolen the same day in the steam bath-house. It was a quick bath; I found little water, which was already cold, but by God it was an expensive wash!

After many hours I reached the railway terminal on foot with a group of others and boarded the familiar cattle train. The winter was in full swing. With me was Leib, "forever grateful" for saving his life.

It was evening and for some time we sat in the darkness of the wagons talking about our experiences and our future. In the end we got hold of some wood and our group sat around the iron stove with its warm pleasant glow. Tired from the march and happenings of the day,

I fell asleep in a huddled position; a shrill whistle and a jolt woke me up. We were moving towards Kotlas. I smelt a roasted lamb and saw smiling faces chatting animatedly around the red-hot stove; they were voraciously swallowing big portions of lamb. I listened to their conversation from the corner of the unlit goods wagon and realized that whilst waiting for the departure of the train, these people, led by one of their travel companions who once was a butcher, stole and surreptitiously killed a lamb.

Kotlas was full of newcomers in transit, some already having waited several weeks for transport as the war had strained Russian resources. People were talking of the influx of refugees to the South causing hunger and various diseases among old and young. I saw a number of them who had changed their minds and were returning to the Far North.

At last, I was able to board a train in the direction of Kuibyshev, eager to join the Polish Army which was being organized in the nearby Buzuluk. It was a goods train, full to overflowing with Polish people and their families still in their fufaikas, some in rags and rotting clothes.

During this journey I witnessed a horrifying epidemic of measles which brought unbelievable mortality, especially among the very small children. At every few stops the small bodies had to be removed from the train and left behind. A nightmare. Grieved, hysterical mothers often refused to part with their dead children. Other travellers tried to calm them telling them it was the only way. Where persuasion failed, the body was taken by force. Tempers frayed; sometimes the unfortunate mother was cursed. Being able to write in Russian, I filled in the necessary forms. This was the only help I could give. Some railway authorities refused point blank to take the bodies – "We have several already and can't take any more, try at the next stop".

We passed Perm, then the Ural Mountains leaving Europe and entering Asia. In Chelyabinsk, where we stayed for several hours, I was able to get in touch with the Medical Authorities who provided me with essential drugs for the rest of the journey.

I returned to doctoring, aiding another doctor – a Major K., still in civilian clothing. In the meantime we were told that owing to lack of facilities recruitment into the Polish Army had slowed down, dealing only with professional soldiers. Instead of travelling to Buzuluk we went further south to Asiatic Russia, through Kazakhstan along the Aral Sea – the fourth largest lake in the world – the River Syr Darya, the edge of the dry and barren Kyzyl-Kum* Desert and arrived in Tashkent, capital of the Uzbek Soviet Republic and the largest city in the Soviet Central Asia. Many towns with strange names flashed in front of me – Orenburg, Aktyubinsk, Aralsk, Kzyl, Orda, Arys . . .

When I left the north in early November it was already severe winter with heavy snowfalls; now, more than two weeks later, it was sweltering heat. A few days earlier, when in the train, I took off my shirt to keep cool somehow. It was because of this heat that the children's bodies had had to be disposed of without delay.

Looking out of the train I realised how vast and varied Russia is. Taiga and forests cut off by the Arctic Ocean in the north, deserts in the south, steppe in between. I was now some three thousand kilometres from the Arctic and already used to the Mongolian faces, high cheek bones and slanting eyes of the Uzbeks in their embroidered skull-caps and padded khalats. Women wore black dresses and carried bundles on their heads in oriental fashion. I admired wonderful melons and grapes which people were buying, but which I could not afford. I had "kipietok" – hot drinking water available and free at all stations instead. Everywhere were masses of refugees from the West, fleeing from the Germans; railway lines were blocked by trains with evacuated equipment, a great deal of it was dismantled machinery.** At one of the railway stations I spotted transported carriages from the Moscow Metro. I also came across a stationary train full of wounded Russian soldiers, casualties from the front. I felt compassion for them; some were so very young, pale looking, heads covered with bandages soaked in blood, others on crutches.

It struck me that I had no hatred against the Russian people; they suffered more than I did. They were given law, order and injustice. They never knew freedom – their individual liberties had been taken from them a long time ago. They walked on the edge of a precipice and lived in fear, ruled by an autocratic aggressive oligarchy and secret police blessed by their archpriest Stalin, a despot who used Draconic means of threats, harassment, arrests, show-trials, executions and the like! Now they were cannon fodder. Their rulers were killers, slave drivers, brainwashers, unbelievable unbelievers. Three million atheistic Communists imposed their will on two hundred million citizens and gave them dull, insecure, degraded lives – liberation of the Russian serfs granted in 1861 was now forgotten. Blunted by the lack of

* Kyzyl Kum. Red sands.

** Whole factories were moved across the Urals.

liberty, deprived of self-respect, they became resigned to their lot. Who still believes that Russian peasants and workers are the masters? They have rid themselves of the old exploiters only to gain more unscrupulous ones. The old hated élite made place for the new one, even less lovable. The "moujiks" still play the same role but under a different name. We were all under the same rule of brigands.

My journey to the South took longer than would be expected from travelling de luxe. My train stood for hours at many stations, priority given to army transports and supplies.

In Tashkent, again, masses of people – refugees, local Uzbeks and their neighbours – Kazakhs, Kirghis, Tartars, Tajiks, Armenians, even Afghans. Oriental looks, oriental colours, dirty narrow streets, mud built houses, bazaars, mosques and minarets and, away from the native quarter, the modern town.

I travelled some 260 kilometres south-west to Samarkand which in the fourteenth century was the capital of the Mongol Prince Tamerlane, the descendant of Ghenghiz Khan ("Mighty Ruler"), now with a population of one hundred and thirty-four thousand. Tamerlane lies buried here beneath the azure dome of Gur-i-Emir.

I found myself in the oldest city in Central Asia, dating from the fourth millenium B.C.

Samarkand has a magic sound – it is said that in its vicinity the Sultana Scheherazade spent a thousand and one nights with her husband, arousing his curiosity in her tales and so achieving a reprieve from execution.

Leib, my old patient from the camp's infirmary, was still with me, making himself useful. I wished to take a glance at Samarkand so he offered to be in charge of my wooden case with some precious goods still left inside.

I went to the town and found an open bazaar where I sold a jumper and a pair of slippers given to me by Major K. for this purpose, also my own fur cap. Self satisfied with the transaction, I bought a bowl of katik* at the same bazaar and then found a bookshop where I purchased a text book for beginners in English. Sitting on a bench, in the shade of an acacia tree, I opened the book and learned my first few words in English – Comrade, Communist, Capitalist, Imperialist, Proletariat, Working class, Red Square, Collectivization.

I was soon strolling through the winding streets of the native quarter looking for the tomb of Tamerlane, my new friend – the book – in

* Katik. A kind of buttermilk.

72

my hand. When I returned to the station it was already dark. Tired, but pleased with myself, I laid down on the floor next to Leib who said, "You must snatch some sleep, doctor, I will look after your case." Thanking him I soon fell asleep. When I awoke a few hours later, they were both gone, Leib and my case, for ever!

In the morning, near the status of Adam out of Paradise, I boarded a train to Kagan, Major K. still with me. He was accompanied by his wife and two daughters who were freed from deportation in Kazakhstan. The family felt sorry to hear about my loss and the Major gave me one of his shirts and some roubles – the proceeds of my transaction for him in Samarkand.

By now we knew that thefts and robberies were a mode of life. They were happening all the time – in the trains, on the streets, in the railway stations and in the czai-khanas,* committed by adults and by children. The Major placed his case, full of the family's belongings, on the luggage-rack in front of our seats so that we could keep a constant eye on it. We arranged to watch the case in turn and not for one moment was it left unobserved. The journey proved to be a bumpy one and the suitcase was jolted about, as we were. A lot of laughter and noise was coming from the next compartment. When on arrival in Kagan the Major lifted the case down, he found it half empty – the youngsters from the next compartment had cut a hole at the back of the case and taken as many things as they could. In spite of this loss we all smiled helplessly at the ingenuity, skill and audacity of these young people.

In Kagan I parted from the Major and his family. My first steps were to the steam bath-house where, among a crowd of refugees, I waited hours for my turn. When it came, it was agony to pour the hot water on my dry itchy skin, which had not seen a wash for several weeks, but when I left the place I felt revived and my deloused garments more comfortable. In the streets I saw mostly refugees; the local population was swallowed up by them and only discernible when on a camel. I was on the old camel route leading to China, but now replaced by the railway. By this, so called Silk Route, silk and tea were brought in from China in the old days. The Afghanistan and Pamir Mountains were not far away, and it was some hundred and fifty kilometres to the North-West Frontier of India. Reindeer and horses were replaced by camels, often a dromedary – it provided transport, milk, meat and even hair for weaving.

* Czai-khana. Teahouse.

73

Camel meat is tough and rather sweet but, after long privation, I thought it delicious and it was hard to come by. I watched strings of camels striding unhurriedly and swinging from side to side to the sound of their bells, regimented and devoid of initiative and zest, like their owners.

I watched a local funeral at which women were crying hysterically and pulling at their hair. I learned later that they were not the relatives, but professional mourners. This was not as odd as having professional sneezers in old Japan – to hear a sneeze was supposed to bring good luck. After some prayers the women departed and the men left on camels with the coffin.

For us, newly-released prisoners, without passports, it was impossible to obtain work, Russian refugees having priority. Consequently it was difficult to find bread. For several days I ate "makucha", the food for camels, living on hope.

The first night I slept in the open. After a very hot day I woke up in the early hours to find myself shivering, the ground covered with frost. I walked to and fro flailing my arms, blowing my hands and rubbing them to bring back the circulation. Impatiently I waited for the teahouse to open and rescue me. I slept the next few nights on the floor of the teahouse, with several others; before I could lie down, I had to hand money to an old Uzbek, the proprietor of the establishment. My money was running out. People around me lived by deceit, embezzlement and theft, but I could not bring myself to do it. Besides, I still remembered the North, the others were desperados. All decency had disappeared. I remember a man borrowing a blanket from his friend only to sell it forthwith at the nearest bazaar.

I took a train in search for work elsewhere. I chose a night train to provide me with the coveted night accommodation. There were only two people in the compartment when I boarded the train and I was able to stretch out on the hard bench, my few belongings in a bundle under my head. I awoke with a start in the unlit compartment. Someone tried to snatch my humble possessions from under me. There was no one else in the carriage besides the intruder and myself. I had only a spare shirt, a pair of socks, two handkerchiefs, a tooth-brush, a piece of soap and the English text book, but it was all I possessed and I fought for it tooth and nail! He gripped my throat, almost strangling me, and twisted my wrist but not being able to shout for help I kicked his shin and hung on. He fled empty handed. In tears from the pain and shock of this experience, I left the train at the next station resolved to make my way to a

74

place I had heard a lot about, Bukhara. It was a comforting thought that a Polish Delegation was installed there.

This town, once an independent state normally harbouring sixty thousand people, was now swollen with refugees. I saw yet another old dusty town, drenched in sunshine, with its maze of narrow streets, mud walls, sun-baked bricks, and open canals full of stagnant water which served the district for drinking and sewage. However, this place was more picturesque, with the snow-peaked mountains on the horizon, with its many mosques, minarets from which the wailing call to prayers was heard, the twelfth century tower – Minari Kalyan – from where condemned men were hurled to the ground not so very long ago, shady orchards, cherry gardens, vineyards, cultivated tobacco plants and melons, and in the distance the new Bukhara – in the Russian European style.

The Russians brought changes into the town. Most of the walls with its towers were pulled down and only a few mosques and colleges remained. Some changed their functions being converted into a palace of culture, a hotel, an office or a billiard saloon. I never saw an Uzbek with a prayer mat kneeling down, face towards Mecca, as in other Moslem countries. Bukhara Jews were never seen with prayer books on their way to the synagogue even on a Saturday. Yet the Jewish community there was the oldest in the world. Places of worship were erased all over the country. Marx called religion "the opium of the people" which must be discouraged.

The influx of refugees, lack of proper sanitation and accommodation, extremes of climate and famine brought the inevitable typhus epidemic with its frightening mortality. Russians had a love-hate relationship with this disease. It helped them to defeat Napoleon's army, and it reappeared in the turbulant years of the Bolshevik revolution, killing three million people. In fact, most of the great wars were accompanied by this disease which got the nickname "war fever".

I reported to the Polish Delegate and Dr. N. who dealt with medical matters. I was asked to call on sick Polish people, which I did. I saw young men with dry skin, flushed cheeks, rapid pulse, temperatures exceeding 40°C. complaining of intense headache, malaise, dizziness; they were soon in a stupor. I did not need to wait for the rash to appear to make a diagnosis, the question was how to help them. In those days there were no antibiotics* which could reduce mortality, no vaccine

---

* Chloramphenicol and Tetracyclines.

and no DDT* insecticide to protect against the disease. Many of these patients were soon dead, whether they reached hospital or not. It was a lousy country. Pediculus *humanus* corporis – or simply a louse – and man have a special relationship. The cycle involves man – louse – man, never an animal; the louse dies of its infection and fails to transmit it to its offspring. To keep lice alive Professor Rudolf Weigel of the University of Lvov, the pioneer of typhus vaccine, had to ask his assistants to breed the parasite on themselves in little cages. In 1928 a Frenchman, Charles Nicolle, received a Nobel prize for the discovery that typhus is transmitted by lice.

Typhus did not save the Polish Delegate and his Secretary, both of whom died. Dr. N. was gravely ill, but survived. One saw mass funerals daily, ten to fifteen coffins in procession. There was also a high mortality from diphtheria and emaciation among children; the Delegature could help very little.

I once visited a children's hospital where a large ward was crowded with small patients, some gravely ill; their parents, mostly refugees, were carrying out nursing duties at the bedside. In the centre of the ward, I saw a woman-member of Komsomol** delivering a political propaganda speech. I looked round and noticed the distressed faces of the parents bent over their children, oblivious of the speaker's presence.

I found refuge from this gruesome reality in the local library – spacious, full of light and well stocked with books. Here I browsed over the places to which fate had thrown me and of which I knew so little due to my lack of enthusiasm at school! I realised, a little late, that I was not a martyr to geography and history after all. I read that Marco Polo referred to Bukhara as "this most noble and grand city", that it was on the old Silk Trade Route between Europe and China, also trafficking in spices, jewels and slaves, and the most celebrated place of learning in all Asia. It once possessed over a hundred religious colleges and 400 mosques. It was destroyed by the Mongol Conqueror Ghenghiz Khan in 1220 A.D. and later rebuilt, only to be invaded by the Russians in 1866, and Samarkand two years later. Ghenghiz Khan's empire stretched from Persia to Peking and from Siberia to the Indus. He is said to have admitted that it would take two years to travel across his domain. His descendant Tamerlane spent all his life in military cam-

* DDT was first produced by a Swiss, Paul Mueller, but was not available commercially until 1942. It was used with great success early 1944 in Naples, nipping in the bud an outbreak of a typhus epidemic.

** Communist Youth League.

76

paigns and overran Northern China and Russia, subdued Persia, Georgia, Tartars, took Syria with Damascus, defeated the Turks, fostered justice, learning and the arts, and brought the Jews in from Mesopotamia. His grandson, Batu, advanced through Poland and Hungary and reached the Adriatic coast, events resulting in great migrations from Asia into Europe. Another grandson, Ulug Beg, was a great astronomer.

I also learned of Bukhara's cruel past and its wicked rulers. There were Emirs who used to have some three hundred wives. A story is on record of execution of the English Colonel Stoddart and the Irish Captain Conolly a hundred years ago. Stoddart offended the Emir by riding in his presence and refusing to kow-tow to him. They declined to save themselves by becoming Moslems. Before their deaths they were put in a pit and tormented by reptiles and scorpions specially bred for such a task. An Italian – Orlandi – was slain being unable to prevent the Emir's watch from stopping . . .

When I was too tired to absorb more knowledge, I read the newspapers lying on a large table, mostly "Pravda". A statesman, I believe it was Machiavelli, once said that words were invented to hide the truth; this certainly applied to "Pravda" – the Russian word for "Truth". I read in the papers that the "poor" British people had to queue for sugar and were living as in Dickensian times. There were no such queues in Russia – there was no sugar! I saw an ingenious way of drinking tea by a family sitting around a table just looking at a cube of sugar hanging on a string, that way preserving it for the next occasion! "Pravda" never mentioned censorship using the word "state control" instead.

Thirty years later, Mr. Heath, then the Prime Minister, was asked by a Russian reporter about oppression of Catholics in Northern Ireland, and was said to have replied, "And how do you manage your problem with the Jews?". The Soviet press was and remains completely subservient to authority, integrity not being its strong point.

The library also had medical books, and one day I picked up a text book on tuberculosis. I read it with great interest, Forlanini's break through in the treatment of this scourge fascinated me. I followed the technique of artificial pneumothorax in minute detail. It occurred to me that I might be able to get a job in a sanatorium and, after finding such a place in Bukhara, I enquired if a doctor was needed. "No", said the Administrator of the Sanatorium after finding out who I was, but

77

seeing my disappointment he added, "I might need an orderly". "I don't mind", I hastened to say. The job was immediately available and so that same afternoon I started to distribute medicines, take temperatures, change beds, accompany a doctor on his rounds. I hoped to be able to fill my empty stomach but it was not to be. I was given a small salary and food was not provided. I worked from 8 a.m. to 1 p.m. hurrying to a café afterwards, a large queue in front of me – early comers who earned their money by theft or swindle had no difficulty in getting there on time. Usually, when my turn came, there was no meat left on the menu, only a thin soup and kasha. I spent the nights in a disused mosque with two other refugees. We huddled together as the nights were very cold and tossed to decide who would sleep in the middle.

Soon my companions were in hospital, both with typhus. Each time I developed a headache I took my temperature but it was normal. A false alarm – the result of my hunger, I suppose. I escaped typhus. I imagine the lice preferred their flesh to mine but I did not wish to take any more chances. I decided to find a job on a kolchoz,* away from Bukhara.

I found one some fifteen kilometres from the town, where I was told to dig potatoes. I could not have been much good at this because on the following day, when I asked to see the President of the farm, to whom I explained I was a medical man, he was pleased to switch me to the First Aid post to look after his people. I was invited to a celebration after the killing of some sheep and found myself in a large hut in which the President and the governing body, all men, were on the floor, sitting cross-legged in a circle. I joined them, a plate and a finger bowl on the side of each of us. Soon a huge plate of delicious smelling mutton was placed in front of us. My nostrils widened and I breathed in the exquisite aroma. I saw my hosts helping themselves with their "washed" fingers from the centre plate. The hands dipping into a communal dish, the bearded faces and the not too clean garments stopped me reaching for the mutton. I explained to the hospitable President that I had a temporary indisposition, that what I smelled and saw was too intoxicating to bear . . .

After three weeks of my "new appointment", I started to run a fever, was unable to eat and lost several pounds in weight, which I could ill afford. I became so weak I had to stay in bed and in the end was taken to hospital by horse and cart. I found myself in a long

* Kolchoz – Collective Farm.

78

narrow ward with twenty other people.

My immediate neighbour was a professional soldier from the newly formed Polish Army which had been under canvas all winter. He was brought to the ward with pneumonia and was obviously dying. There were a few more Polish soldiers in the ward as the Army Medical Services were not yet in existence. A Russian doctor appeared, looked at my tongue, touched my tummy and "diagnosed" typhoid – a fashionable illness in this area at that time; only several years later a chance X-ray revealed that in fact I had a tuberculous chest infection at the time. However, the rest did me good and after about two weeks in the ward my appetite returned with a vengeance; my meagre ration of bread, soup and kasha was not sufficient to satisfy it. No one could expect another helping, but we were able to share the extra bread left untouched by dying patients; the staff distributed the daily ration of bread at each bedside table without looking at the patient, who could be unconscious or dying.

Then one day – a surprise! Major K., in Polish uniform, came to visit the sick soldiers and was astonished to find me in this crowd. He told me of recruitment in the nearby Kermine and promised to expedite my admission. He kept his word.

I soon left hospital, and after being vetted by the Colonel of the Polish Medical Corps, I reported to the recruiting centre. These preliminaries took three days, and being without means, I had to sleep rough. Although the days were very hot, it was freezing at night. I envied refugees who had roubles and could sleep in the chai-khana. The second night, well after midnight and half frozen, I went near the chai-khana, waited outside for a "paying guest" to come out on urgent business, and on his return I followed him in under cover of darkness and ducked into the warmth of the teahouse. I lay down on the floor, in an atmosphere of stench from perspiring bodies, but oh so glad to be in the warmth. This "bliss" lasted only a few hours as I was soon awakened by the angry voice of the Uzbek who had collected money from his "patrons" the previous evening and recognized me as an intruder. I was kicked out forthwith. The same thing happened on the following night and I was glad when my turn came at the recruiting centre. I did not need to repeat this performance. I now slept in a tent with a few others awaiting my assignment. At last I had "accommodation", and my days of starvation were over. Only a few days earlier, when I got hold of a morsel of camel's food, I was given advice by a Russian, "Beware of colitis". What I really needed was not advice but bread!

For the next two days I carried those who had died from typhus to the grave – just a huge hole in the ground – and late in the evening, after common prayers and bugle call, I laid down in a tent on a blanket, close to my neighbour for warmth, immediately falling asleep from exhaustion. In the morning I noticed that my neighbour could not stop scratching. Being a doctor I asked him to let me look at him. There was no doubt whatsoever that he had scabies* – "the itch".

Then the big moment came and I left to join my unit. A man who had the same assignment as myself, and had become acquainted with me only a few hours earlier, invited me for a "drink", which in fact was tea, to the chai-khana already well-known to me as a farewell gesture to our civilian lives. I went with him to this place without any trepidation, an invited guest, and drank with gusto the hot tea poured from a large decorative teapot by my new friend. The ceremony completed, not a drop of tea left, my benefactor with a roguish smile hid the pot under his shirt and left the chai-khana to sell it at the nearest bazaar. In this way he took the final parting from his civilian life. I did not reproach him, in fact I was glad someone had robbed the greedy inconsiderate Uzbek bastard.

Various people tried to join the Polish Army. Not all of them were honest, some gave false names, religion and occupation just to gain access to it. The Military Authorities had a difficult task on their hands weeding them out.

After half-an-hour's walk I reached my destination – the Polish Field-Ambulance – situated in pleasant grounds with many trees providing welcome shade; the brook with its strong current and refreshingly cool water was a godsend. The date was March 25, 1942. Immediately upon my arrival I was presented to the Commanding Officer, a Captain K. I stood to attention and saluted in the best manner I could. It was my first military performance, and my legs were very weak. Questioned by him I reported that I had received my medical Diploma in Vilna in 1938. I was directed to a bathroom where I discarded my dirty battered clothes to my great relief, as they were a constant reminder of my unhappy experiences. Provided with a piece of soap, an item denied me for some considerable time, I plunged into a bath full of lovely hot water.

Reborn and happy I found myself whistling for the first time in the last two years. I put on new clean linen and a soldier's uniform, all received from Great Britain.

* Scabies – A contagious skin disease due to itch mite.

I began my military career as a private, never having been in the army before. I confess it was an ordeal. Every time I passed a "higher rank" – even a lance corporal – I had to salute. It was an exacting exercise, and when I eventually rebelled by pretending not to see an approaching corporal, I was stopped, shouted at and ordered to salute him ten times. I had only myself to blame, and I in turn could not take it out on anyone else for I was the lowest rank . . .

From then onwards I was trained to be a soldier and my medical upbringing had to be forgotten for some considerable time. Life in the military camp was taken up by assemblies at various times of the day, when one had to appear, in a flash, with all one's belongings before a Sergeant Major or some Corporal who examined us from the front and the rear in minute detail. Keeping the tent in perfect order, "spit and polish", long marches*, sometimes during the night, taking part in manoeuvres, doing sentry duties and the like, filled our day. Morning started with bugle call, the hoisting of the Polish flag and common prayer; then a wash in the brook and queueing with a mess tin at the field kitchen for breakfast. Meal times were our principal attraction as we had not yet recovered from our hunger. Frequently civilians – the families of soldiers – joined in.

There were more than a dozen doctors in the camp who had never been in the army before. We had to learn blind discipline and to obey orders without question. Higher education was now a handicap.

We underwent rigorous training, a task given to a young Lieutenant, a dapper figure, a professional soldier with a mixture of firmness, punctiliousness and bluff, and without tact. We were not left in any doubt that we were on *active* service. He had forgotten that we had just arrived from labour camps, that we were living in a hot climate and that some were in their fifties. We were ordered to run, to throw ourselves down on our faces and to jump up at his command only to repeat this performance again and again, hardly able to get our breath. We soon heard his shrill voice: "March! Left right, left right, left right . . ." in increasing tempo. We were watched to see who would crack first. Our Lieutenant was a total soldier, we were infinitesimal by comparison.

He shouted at us: "You are no soldiers!", "You are soft!", "You have no guts!", "I will never shake hands with any of you!". By now I learned it was a relief to obey orders without having to think, that com-

* We had to march and sing, although we did not feel like it; our new masters knew that one can not sing and think simultaneously.

81

pulsion and bullying were giving better results than encouragement and persuasion. At all times we were told in the most minute detail, what to do and when to do it! It would be wrong to say "We *never* had a dull moment!" I had had a basinful of being told, and of regimentation, an extension of my Russian experience. No one understood my deep-seated yearning for the freedom that was denied to me for so long. Yet it would be unreasonable in the circumstances to reason with any unreasonable demand. We began to feel inadequate and insignificant. I have often woken up in the middle of the night tortured by nightmares of a missing button, unpolished boots, or unpressed trousers. No doubt we underwent a mental surgery of a kind. We must have had superb mind-benders! I began to understand why a German "Captain from Koepenick" decided on masquerading, Jaroslav Hasek on writing "The Good Soldier Schweik" and Franz von Suppe on composing the "Light Cavalry", all poking fun at the glorification of soldiering. Later on I developed an admiration for Barnes Wallis, not only for his inventive mind, but also for his refusal to wear a uniform . . . How nice it would be, I thought, to be born in the state of Andorra, $28\frac{1}{2}$ kilometres in length, with a population of 5,200 (600 of whom live in its capital), natural frontiers, unarmed police and *no* army. I could look after flocks of sheep, goats and cattle or work in one of Andorra's half-dozen tobacco "factories" . . .

The drill went on until one of us had a heart attack. Our Lieutenant was disgusted. He himself was a man of steel and it was common knowledge that he was soon to be drafted to London to be parachuted into Poland. Colonel Okulicki, the Chief of Staff of the Polish Forces, had also volunteered to be dropped into Poland and was temporarily with our unit when we left Russia.

I soon discovered that I had developed "the itch" – a gift from the recruiting centre. In spite of everything, I was reluctant to report it, as it would mean my leaving new friends and my new "home" for a while. I had had enough of wandering, so I got hold of sulphur ointment which I rubbed into my skin at night outside the tent, in secret. Naturally, I avoided close contact with my fellow men. The treatment was successful and after a few days I stopped itching. Unfortunately, our Quartermaster noticed how greasy my underwear had become and reported this to the Commanding Officer, who must have thought I never washed!

One cold morning I stayed too near an iron stove which was erected in the grounds, my behind next to it for warmth, and burnt a hole in

82

my trousers, which I had to patch. This clinched my military career. I never rose above a second Lieutenant; we were mutually disappointed – my bosses and myself.

My Company was once ordered to be present at the execution of a soldier sentenced to death for armed robbery. When he was brought into the field the sun was just rising. He was tied to a stake and before he was blind-folded, he exclaimed "Oh, what a beautiful morning", then there was a salvo, and soon his body was taken away. The picture of this first and last execution witnessed by me lingered in my memory for a long time.

One day we had a visit from General Szarecki, a medical man, and General Bohusz-Szyszko. The latter arrived in Russia from London as head of the Polish Military Mission. He knew Russia well as he had lived there before and witnessed the Bolshevik Revolution. Until now he was a legendary figure to us, and we often marched singing a song about his bravery.

The Germans invaded Norway on April 9, 1940. In May General Bohusz-Szyszko led a Polish Brigade which captured Narvik, a Norwegian port near the Arctic Ocean, the vital link by railway with Sweden from where the iron ore was shipped to Germany. It was a combined operation involving the British, Norwegian and French troops; General De Wiart, in command of the British Expeditionary Force, and the Poles were again comrades in arms. The German onslaught upon the Western Front necessitated the evacuation of these troops numbering twenty-four thousand. It was not a futile exercise – the German Navy was put out of action during the vital summer months when Hitler, after the conquest of France, threatened to invade Britain.

Now General Bohusz-Szyszko was with us – still a young man, tall, well built, of military bearing and jovial. He was interested in talking to doctors, enquiring about our experiences. By his own ingenuity he had acquired a tin of Will's Woodbines with a cooling mint aroma. He passed these round and we all enjoyed the "fag" after a long denial.

The Easter of 1942, the first we could celebrate since 1939, will always remain in my memory. Easter is the most observed holiday in Poland and we felt the festive atmosphere in which old memories revived.

The Chaplain arrived and the Poles were overcome by religious feelings. Soldiers, bareheaded, heads bowed, and kneeling in prayer in the open, reminded me of pilgrims seen in my childhood, waiting for a miracle.

We sat on the ground, helping ourselves to delicious sausages, hard boiled eggs painted in various colours, cheese and white bread. The white sugarlamb with a flag beside it (an old tradition) was missing – the only reminder of the war on this festive day. Significantly we celebrated the spiritual and physical Resurrection of Christ which happened some nineteen hundred years ago.

In mid-July we heard that our army would be evacuated to the Middle East. The wonderful news spread like wildfire, but in the early days it was difficult to believe it was true. Soon the Uzbek people were greeting us with smiles, saying: "You lucky chaps, you will soon be over the Border".

High ranking Russian officers visited our camp to bid us good-bye. It was a big occasion and we played host well. A concert was given in honour of our Russian guests, the main attraction being a Polish violinist. He played superbly and our guests were visibly impressed. A few days later, when the violinist was strolling in the streets of Kermine, a limousine stopped by his side and he was forcibly taken away. He would probably never have seen freedom again, but for another soldier, who saw the incident and reported the matter to the Polish Headquarters. Initially, the Russian authorities denied any knowledge of the event but, confronted with the eye witness, admitted that the man was taken away owing to "mistaken identity". He was released with apologies. He told us that when the Russians let him go, he ran down the steps looking back for fear of being shot at.

The long awaited day came at last on August 15, 1942. We boarded a train to Krasnovodsk, a port on the Caspian Sea. This was not yet the end of our ordeal. N.K.V.D. men boarded the train and took a few soldiers away. There was no time and no means of redress, yet at last we reached Krasnovodosk. Here a Russian ship "Molotov" was awaiting us. She was filled to overflowing with troops and we were sitting on each others laps, uncomfortable, but radiantly happy and full of expectation.

The ship started to move. A military band played the Polish and Russian National Anthems. Russian military men stood to attention at the quayside, saluting; we smiled and waved as if leaving our best friends. We were too happy to be angry.

In world affairs British and Soviet troops entered Persia on August 25, 1941; on September 16, the pro-German Shah abdicated to be succeeded by his son. On December 8, the United States of America

84

entered the war, and its national war effort rose from a mere 2% in 1939 to 40% by 1943. The Russians were in full retreat; on August 23, 1942, German troops had reached the Volga just north of Stalingrad and were only fifty miles from the main oil fields of Caucasus. In the same month Churchill landed on a Moscow airfield for talks with Stalin. He arrived from Cairo where his visit had had a twist to it. Churchill's charming hostess, wife of the British Ambassador in Cairo, Sir Miles Lampson, was the daughter of an Italian, Dr. Aldo Castellani, who was at that time helping Mussolini in medical matters arising from the war. He was made Surgeon General in Ethiopian campaign and later raised to the rank of Marchese. Winston Churchill became Prime Minister on May 10, 1940 – at the time of Hitler's invasion of Holland and Belgium – only to leave the office when the war ended. The Battle of Britain, which began on July 10, 1940, was won by the British and Allied pilots, Polish squadrons among them, after less than seven weeks. In their Spitfires and Hurricanes they shot down some 2,400 Luftwaffe planes. Polish pilots accounted for 203 enemy aircraft.

9

Through Kurdistan to Iraq

The world is as ugly as sin – and almost as delightful.
Frederick Locker-Lampson
Wem Gott will rechte Gunst erweisen, den schickt Er in die
weite Welt. *Joseph Eichendorff*
(On whom God wishes to bestow a favour, He sends into the
wide world.)

The ship loaded with Polish people headed for Persia, also known as
Iran. The Caspian Sea looked dead, desolate and the shores like
no-man's land. On crossing the sea we found ourselves in the Persian
Port, Pahlevi, and came under British Command. Much has changed
since Vyacheslav Molotov, Commissar for Foreign Affairs, pronounced
that "The bastard of the Versailles Treaty has forever ceased to exist",
since Benito Mussolini's announcement, from the balcony of the
Palazzo Venezia in Rome, that Poland was liquidated, and since the
secret protocol (September 28, 1939) of Hitler and Stalin agreeing to
institute terror designed to suppress Polish freedom and to quench any
flame of protest. They were all wrong; where there's a will, there's a
way. Some one-and-a-half million Polish people were deported* to
Russia, and many died. Only a hundred and fifteen thousand were allowed to leave the country and they were now starting life afresh carrying the Polish banner with self-awareness, determination, courage,
devotion and unshakeable faith, resuming the struggle against Hitler's
Germany which had *only begun* in September 1939. They remembered what their "Strong Marshal", Pilsudski, had once told them –
"One who does not know how to endure defeat, is not worthy of victory."

All sections of Polish life forged themselves into well-disciplined
units contemptuous of death. It was an immense diversity of people –
various occupations, classes, religions and political affiliations. Among
them were farmhands, factory workers, carpenters, cooks, butchers,
clerks, landowners, industrialists, artists, clergy, military, and mem-

* The Soviet authorities became expert in deportations; in 1944 more than 400,000
Crimean Tartars were uprooted and sent to Central Asia.

bers of other professions. They were Catholics, Protestants or Jews, nationalists and socialists, men and women. They all blended together to keep alive their own ideals and to pursue relentlessly their pagan adversary with its master race ideology, a totalitarian state and the hated swastika. They were the backbone of the Polish Nation, resolved to repay the brutal enemy in kind and to regain their country; the patriots without patria (Latin for fatherland). To quote Mickiewicz, a Polish poet and an exile like Chopin: "The Fatherland is like one's health, one only learns to appreciate it truly once one has lost it". They survived a precarious existence when there was no ray of hope and remained very much alive because the human is the most resilient animal of all. They showed incredible endurance, now strengthened by singleness of purpose and self-surrender to their cause; they bounced back to life like balls thanks to their resourcefulness. They will win somehow!

Persia is an Islamic country, a kingdom covering an area seven times that of Great Britain, with only one third of its population. We were outside Russia, but still in the Russian zone of occupation, and the chai-khanas here did not differ much from those I had already seen.

I heard that Persia had a strong militant communist party – Tudeh – and yet we were in an entirely different world. In the busy outdoor bazaars with stalls full of goods, a free enterprising people, full of vitality, were shouting at the top of their voices, a kind of advertising I suppose, and bargaining with the customers.

I looked in amazement at the various foods including oriental pastries, a gamut of delicious fruits – pomegranates, apples, pears, grapes, figs, nuts, raisins, etc. and strange vegetables such as red peppers.

The evacuation was well organized. Although we were there only in transit, we were provided with comfortable accommodation and fed well. A week later, wearing a new uniform, I found myself in a convoy of open lorries with reckless but superb Persian drivers, who took us through an impressive mountain range. They were negotiating at breakneck speed hairpin bends, often at a great height, along the edge of precipices and dangerous passes with the greatest of ease. I was holding on to an iron bar attached to the lorry, my hair swept by the wind, absorbing the breath-taking scenery. We passed Kazvin and reached Hamadan touching on mountainous Kurdistan, north-west from us. The town had narrow, somewhat tortuous streets, numerous bazaars, and harboured the tomb of the celebrated philosopher and physician,

Avicenna, who died there in 1037. His medical encyclopaedia "Quanun" remained Europe's standard medical text for 400 years.

Hamadan also has the tomb of Esther, a Jewess who thwarted Haman's plans to exterminate her people. We were told not to make long stops for fear of bandits. Kurds were turbulent people, intolerant of authority, and their history had been one of warfare and rebellions. Given hope of Nationhood after World War I, they saw Kurdistan divided among Turkey, Syria, Iraq and Iran. They remembered Saladin, their great Armenian warrior of the twelfth century, who unlike another oriental ruler, Stalin, knew the spirit of conciliation and generosity towards captives.

Our next stop was Kermanshah, a town pleasantly situated in a valley, then followed the Zagros Mountains with impressive gorges and a village with flat roofed mud houses bordering on Iraq, before we arrived in Khanaquin, a frontier town at the foot of the mountains.

We passed on our journey strong chinned, dusky skinned natives on foot, on donkeys and on camels. It was a tremendous drive. We had the feeling of having stepped from a nightmare into a dreamland of the Orient.

We pitched our tents in the desert slowly getting accustomed to the sweltering heat. We were now wearing light khaki shirts, shorts and tropical helmets. The day started with reveille at 6 a.m., disposition, wash, prayers, breakfast, roll call and lectures, followed by the all important siesta lasting from nine till five, thus preventing heat stroke. We also learned to drink large quantities of water with salt added.

After a short spell of idleness, I was drafted to a convalescent home under canvas for several hundred of our soldiers, with an Indian unit in attendance. British authorities gave full consideration to their religious beliefs. I observed a large tent allocated to a single Indian private, a Sikh of a particular sect, who could not share his roof, this in spite of the hardships of war.

Like my medical colleagues from Kermine, I was still a private, which led to complications. The British Commanding Officer of the convalescent home suggested that I be given an officer's rank according to the post held by me, for a limited period, but this was refused as being unprecedented in the Polish Army, and so I, a private, ate in the Officers' Mess at the same table as the Major, the Captain and the Lieutenant.

The Indian cook was superb, and I was impressed by the quiet and efficient manner of the servants in their native costumes. The food was the principal medicine in the whole camp. Soups were as thick as glue and each day I heard the Sergeant giving a most unusual command, "Everyone gather to collect liver".

On entering the wards I was met by a soldier of the highest rank among the patients, usually a Warrant Officer, who, standing to attention and saluting, reported the number of soldiers present. I was embarrassed for I knew how a Warrant Officer must have felt when he had to stand to attention before a private.

Christmas Eve arrived, and we invited our British hosts for supper. Polish borsch with mushrooms and dumplings was served, followed by other traditional dishes. Afterwards we sang carols. Our guests were impressed. The very pleasant evening came to a halt when two soldiers who had had "one too many" appeared bleary-eyed, reeling and singing at the top of their voices songs that were neither religious nor conventional. Each fondled tenderly the neck of his bottle. It was a lover's touch! No doubt the climate had affected our soldiers. I saw a few in a dangerous stupor, possibly the quality of drink obtained from private sources had something to do with it as well.

Soon I was in a cadet school, where we underwent an intense and exacting military training. Fortunately it was early spring without too much heat. We learned to present arms, to clean rifles, to drill, to polish our boots highly. We also attended lectures held by military experts and medical specialists — like Colonel Sokolowski — Chief of the Military Accident Unit in Warsaw before the war. In my humble opinion, that is if a soldier can have an opinion, our Sergeant Major with a voice and manner of a bull rather overdid things — legs spread, hands on his hips and shouting at us, but then it was his job to teach us to obey orders without further ado and to instil discipline. The course helped the authorities to screen people. One "doctor" was exposed. He happened to be an apothecary assistant before the war and this gave him the idea of masquarading as a doctor for a while. In spite of the rigorous life I found the place agreeable and made many friends.

In June 1943, now a cadet officer, I was drafted to a field ambulance. I carried out sick parades and held lectures for soldiers, teaching them preventive measures against our newest enemy — malaria. Special patrols were formed to find infected areas and everyone was issued with a fine mesh mosquito net. We were able to fight that enemy thanks to the discovery by Ronald Ross in 1897 that a particular kind

89

of mosquito named Anopheles* carried malaria to humans. In a tribute to him, it was said that he made a third of the world inhabitable. Before him, it was thought that the bad air – "malaer" – rising from the swamps was responsible for the disease. Malaria had been a big killer; among its victims was Alexander the Great – the King of Macedon and the magnificent warrior who died in his thirty-second year, 323 B.C., also the greatest Italian poet Dante who succumbed to "marsh fever" in Ravenna in 1321.

In the nineteen-thirties the uninhabited Pontine Marshes, south of Rome, were drained and the land reclaimed after freeing the area from malaria. It was turned into a prosperous farming community and the new city Latina created. Even so this endemic disease continues to exist; some 200 cases are brought to the British Isles each year from abroad and the number is rising. A significant proportion remains undetected.**

Our unit was situated in the desert, near the town of Kirkuk. The air was oppressive, very dry, with a smell of oil – we were next to oil refineries, an oil pipe line and natural gas fires; breathing the hot air was most uncomfortable. My nose felt as if all the nasal sprays available and so often abused these days were forced on me. For the first time we cursed the sun seeking shelter in our tents and taking cold showers improvised by large tin containers, originally used for packing dates, in which we pierced numerous holes. When the sun left us for the night, the howling jackals and "laughing" hyenas came close to our camp. These beasts were a lesser menace than the Arab boys, always ready to steal.

Besides riches there was a lot of poverty here and we were besieged by persistent beggars thrusting their dirty, ever-ready hands in our faces saying the word "Bakhshish" again and again.

We had yet another adversary – the sandstorms from the East known as "Khamsin"*** – a hot wind blowing thick clouds of sand, usually in the spring, within a period of some fifty days. On one occasion a large tent in which four of us slept was blown to the height of three men, with two of us hanging on to the pole; minutes earlier we

* Anopheles means "hurtful" in Greek. The mosquito's bite transmits malaria, and a suggestion was made that it was the culprit of the Greek decline. Only the female seeks blood necessary for its eggs and flies as far as 8 kilometres (5 miles), if needed, to find it; like the human louse the mosquito looks for human blood. Animals do not suffer from malaria.

** In 1973 a death from malaria was reported in this country, the patient was erroneously treated for influenza, and similar cases are on record.
*** Khamsin means fifty.

could see the noisy whirlwind approaching. On such occasions, even when sheltering in the tent, we were covered with sand, which penetrated into our eyes, ears, nose and mouth.

Baghdad with its river Tigris, heavily infested with flukes,* was not the town of fable that I had always pictured. Gone was the image of "The Thousand and One Nights" which reflected its splendour and prosperity in the "golden" ninth Century under the Caliph Harun al-Rashid.** In the dirty dusty streets I noticed a number of blind men and women – the result of trachoma – a disease of filth rampant in this part of the world. I spotted large scars on bare-footed people and destructive facial lesions due to yaws, also oriental sores – "*Bouton* de Baghdad" – yet another outcome of poor hygiene. I wonder if the French would call it Baghdad *Button*! I also saw pale emaciated children with a yellowish tinge, having large tummies, sad looking, obviously ill – the victims of chronic malaria and kala-azar.*** Many people were hollow-eyed and in rags. Smells came from the gutters. Poverty was not a rarity.

I was impressed by the Baghdad bazaars, full of glittering trinkets, but also displaying real gold – sometimes in small bars – and I saw women being sold as wives. Places of ill-repute were set up in the town in three grades – for officers, for sergeants, and for other ranks; extension of discipline outside barracks, I suppose. They became a refuge in which one could be absolutely sure that there would be no superior to salute, but they seldom offered sexual fulfilment.

It struck me that most of the foreign products for sale were of German manufacture. I remember from the pre-war years how German merchants were able to flood our markets with their goods, even scientific books were offered on easy terms.

A man from my unit introduced me to a well-to-do Iraqi family; over a cup of tea the head of the house, who managed to speak a little English, as we did, mentioned with reverence the name of a Polish corporal who had recently left for Palestine. This departure was much regretted by our host, who said, "The corporal was a maestro, a virtuoso . . . in bridge, all Iraqi friends lost to him". Smoking a long pipe he switched the conversation to politics. Not aware of our experience, he praised the Soviet system. "What do you know about it?" asked my friend, and our host brought out a Soviet propaganda leaflet with glossy illustrations depicting the happy and carefree lives of farmers,

* Parasitic worm.
** In 1258 Baghdad was captured by Mongols.
*** Visceral leishmaniasis, also called black fever, or Dumdum fever.

91

factory workers and scientists in the Soviet Union, with eulogizing accounts and impressive figures. "You can have the whole of Russia!", I said magnanimously . . .

South of Baghdad, between the Tigris and Euphrates, stretches Babylonia – where once stood the most famous city of antiquity – in the vicinity of the modern town of Hilla. On the alluvial plain called Edin the Bedouins pastured the flock of their Babylon masters. Elaborate irrigation by a network of canals carrying off the water of the Euphrates to the Tigris made it very fertile and thus densely populated; it was the most advanced land in the world, enjoying the golden age under the great 18th Century B.C. King Hammurabi. Somewhere here "the Lord God planted a garden eastward in Eden" well watered and beautiful, where "every tree grew that was pleasant in the sight" . . . but this was a very, very long time ago. According to the Hebrew calendar precisely 3,744 years, although the excavation of the oldest village Jarmo in the Babylonia region points that it would have been in existence some 6,000 years, and fossils reveal three billion years of life on earth! Now this whole area is desert-like, with only a few biblical reminders.

The tower of Babel, a structure some twelve metres high and carved in sandstone, is an appropriate edifice for expressing confusion among people jabbering hopelessly in various tongues, whose impious attempt to mount to the heavens and challenge God himself was thwarted this way, or so the myth says. Some believe that this structure is a fake, that a hole in the ground to be seen in the modern Essahan is the only remains of the tower. Old wall ruins, part of the ancient defences of Babylon erected by Nebuchadnezzar, the "Gate of Ishtar" and relics of the great temple of Marduk, said to be in the centre of the city, are the only indications of the mighty rule of that King, who once brought destruction to the Temple of Jerusalem and took many Jews into captivity.

10

Palestine

A people cannot be saved except by itself.

Theodor Herzl

We did not find our stay in Iraq too hard to bear. From time to time we were visited by Polish entertainment groups giving concerts, variety shows and plays, a lively farce "Ladies and Hussars" by Fredro* being the most popular one. Among the artists were outstanding names of the Polish entertainment world from the pre-war era – the conductor Wars, the poet and composer Hemar, the singer Ordonowna, the comedian Krukowski and others. After the performance we joined in singing the Polish National Anthem "Poland is not lost while we are alive". But we had to be on the move again. This time for Palestine, across the desert of Iraq, a part of Syria and the River Jordan, to Ghedara and Rehovot, overtaking caravans of Bedouins with goats, donkeys and camels.

For some time now malaria caused us much trouble. A great number of our soldiers became infected and a yellow appearance was a common feature due to the disease itself or the tablets** which we had to take as a preventative measure. A number of our men brought this disease from Uzbekistan. Still good humoured, we called ourselves the "Chinese Army". I was busy looking for malaria parasites under the microscope in the numerous stained blood samples.

One hot day I was called to an officer who had an attack of malaria; he felt very ill and between frequent bouts of vomiting complained of an intense headache. On entering the tent I saw his batman standing over the bed, which was protected by a rubber sheet, pouring cold water over him with a watercan. The patient's teeth were chattering. I took his temperature, it was over 40°C. Afraid he might become delirious, I ordered him to hospital. A beautiful Dalmatian dog was whining at his bedside. The officer implored me to look after the dog in his

* Alexander Fredro – Polish Comic Dramatist in the 19th century.

** Synthetic atebrin and plasmoquine. Quinine, previously used, was extracted from the cinchona tree. It was in short supply – Java and Sumatra, rich in cinchona plantations, were overrun by the Japanese.

93

absence. I was delighted to do so.

The Dalmatian took to me as I took to him. People turned their heads seeing this animal strolling alongside me. I got used to the attention we were getting from passers-by and so I did not think anything of it when one day a military policeman gave us his full attention. He was carrying a briefcase from which he took some notes, glanced at them, then at the dog, saluted, and stopped me to ask a few questions. "Is this your dog?" "What is his name?" "Where did you get him from?" "How long have you had him?" He was dubious when I told him that the dog's name was Felek and it belonged to an officer who at present was in hospital. The military policeman informed me that the dog was on the wanted list, that its name was "Ralph" and that it belonged to a British Colonel stationed in Syria. He asked me to give my particulars and to leave the dog. The next day a surprise – "Ralph", alias "Felek", ran away from the police quarters straight into my tent. A happy reunion took place but, sad as I felt about it, I took the dog back. The officer in charge of my case was at a loss and asked me to take it back with me until I heard from them. The following day a military policeman ran into my tent panting from the exercise and asked me to come immediately to the police quarters as the British Colonel was on the telephone from Syria enquiring about his pet and wishing to talk to it. When I picked up the receiver, an anxious voice asked to let the dog bark into the telephone. Hearing it bark the Colonel exclaimed, "It is my Ralph!" The proceedings were speeded up. It turned out that the dog was taken by our troops who were passing through Syria when "Ralph" was running unescorted along the road. As it did not happen in Soviet Russia I was acquitted, a free man! The British Colonel was happy to have his pet back and did not wish to pursue the issue any further to find the culprit. Everyone was aware that our soldiers had left their families and friends behind and turned their feelings towards animals. In our midst there were, besides a number of dogs, two bears, some monkeys, parrots, pigeons, rabbits, guinea pigs, etc. We all had one thing in common – we were homeless.

We missed Poland's green pastures and its woods full of singing birds, and were glad to find olive and eucalyptus trees, citrus plantations, vegetable fields and even sunflowers cultivated with the help of artificial irrigation; the restful, green, shady trees were welcomed after the sun-scorched deserts. We were back in civilization.

My first trip was to the Dead Sea, which lies 394 metres below sea level. It is rich in minerals, mainly potash. As I was about to jump from a spring-board, I heard a warning "Shut your eyes!". The salt water certainly would have hurt them. Once in the sea I was unable to submerge. It was a strange feeling to be buoyed up as though I were a cork. When I came out I was covered with salt and had to take a thorough shower. It was interesting to see the biblical Sodom inhabited by workers engaged in extracting minerals from the Dead Sea. I remembered the story of Lot's wife who turned into a pillar of salt, and of the destruction of Sodom and its twin town Gomorrah by God for debauchery. In 1957, extensive natural gas reserves were found near Sodom and the biblical event could well be explained by explosions of such gas. As to Lot's wife, it was possibly a salt deposit formed into a rough rock, which by chance had the shape of a woman. It sounds less dramatic but more convincing. I nearly missed this interesting trip. Our company had not sufficient transport facilities to take many of us and so the Warrant Officer had the task of discouraging us; he did it very well. He announced in a matter of fact manner that a tedious venture was forced upon us which would cause a lot of hardship to the party. He concluded, "Should there be some brainless volunteers, they must gather in front of the lorries". After that, not many of us stepped forward.

I was very much taken by the beauty of Haifa, the city built on Mount Carmel, from which one views the crescent-shaped harbour and the blue waters of the Mediterranean. The rather flat city of Tel-Aviv, founded in 1909 by sixty Jews of Jaffa, appealed to me less, but it was an interesting thought that the conglomeration of white modern houses, the imposing Boulevard Rothschild and the many green trees and bushes in Allenby Road, Ben Jehuda Road and Dizengoff Square stood on sand dunes. This new town adjoined Jaffa, an old port founded by the Phoenicians, Arab in character, with mosques and picturesque markets; its biblical name was Joppa.

The big moment came when I was able to visit the Holy City of Jerusalem, then the capital of the British Mandated Territory of Palestine.

Its population of over one hundred thousand comprised Moslems, Jews, Christians, Druses, Samaritans, etc; the day of rest for Moslems was Friday, for Jews Saturday and for Christians Sunday. I was fond of the mountainside with its olive groves and vineyards. I pondered while walking through the narrow streets and crooked alleyways of the old city, or looking at the Mount of Olives, Mount Zion, the shrines of various religions, the tomb of Christ, the Mosque of Omar, churches and synagogues and the venerated Wailing Wall, the remainder of

Solomon's Temple.* The tomb of Christ was different to what I had imagined – it glittered with gold and in it congregated Christians of many denominations. I saw Catholic, Protestant, Greek and Eastern Orthodox priests and those of the Coptic rite ("Coptic" means "Egyptian").

I visited Hadassah Medical Centre – a teaching hospital attached to the Hebrew University on Mount Scopus. In the streets I saw Arabs in their burnous, oriental Jews from Yemen and Tunisia, Orthodox Jews, some with long curls, wearing black caftans, boots and wide brimmed hats or peaked caps, women in sombre dresses with long sleeves and black stockings as I saw them in the ghetto districts of the old market in Czestochowa and Warsaw Nalevki. On occasions one could spot large flat fur hats worn by the Hassidim sect (mystics) of Poland, much out of place in this hot climate. Through the same streets walked girls in khaki shorts, or corduroy trousers – the native born "Sabras" – and the Jewish Colonists in blue shirts and shorts. They were born here and wished to die on their own soil; asked if they had lived in Palestine all their lives, they would answer with a sheepish smile "No, not yet". I met Palestinian Jews in British uniforms from units serving with the British Army. All Jews greeted each other with, "Shalom", which means "Peace"; Arabs did the same in their own language, saying "Salaam alaykum". The Synagogues were frequented by elderly pious people; the young ones had no time for it and remembered a rabbi only when they wished to get married, as civil marriage did not exist in that part of the world. If anyone speaks of a generation gap, or better still of a rebellion, this is it.

During my strolls I saw many races – Europeans, Africans, Asians – among them some highly sophisticated and some primitive people, and I heard many languages – Yiddish, Polish, Russian, German, English, Hungarian, Greek, Oriental tongues and, of course, Hebrew. The Polish language was often heard – Poland had a large Jewish community; over the years a number of them emigrated to Palestine – Chaim Weizmann, Israel's first President, David Ben Gurion, its first Prime Minister, Bronislaw Humberman, the world famous violinist who founded the Israel Philharmonic Orchestra in 1936, Jascha Heifetz, another great violinist, were among them. Artur Rubinstein, the celebrated pianist, was Polish born and once lived there. No doubt the tough environment shaped their characters. The tongue most used by

* It was destroyed in 70 A.D., after Rome crushed the revolt of the Jews led by Bar Kochba, bringing about their dispersal.

96

young Jews was Hebrew, a language transformed from the ancient scripture of the bible into the modern daily speech and the national language. I saw a small boy, the son of a Polish major, playing happily with Jewish children and conversing with them in Hebrew to the astonishment of his father.

In Jerusalem I visited a Mission Hospital for leprous patients run by Sisters of a German Order; three-quarters of the patients were Jews, the rest Arabs. The Sisters of Mercy did their best to save these doomed people. I talked to a woman patient, advanced in years, who once lived in Poland. She was mutilated and grossly disabled − her deformed hands, which had lost feeling, were useless, the face disfigured. She was half-blind, her nasal bones had vanished and it was difficult to outline her mouth; she had to be fed by the staff. The woman was mentally alert and interested in news of Poland. She praised the Sisters for their concern, kindness and devotion. Amazingly she had no complaints apart from her headaches, which she had recently developed; her other disabilities she had accepted a long time ago. She contracted this disease in the old days when there was no effective treatment; since then substantial progress has been achieved.

Sulphone drugs have been used since 1943, the best one of this group by the name of Dapsone being known for over twenty years. Several other remedies are in use and the newest antibiotic, Rifampicin, is the safest and most effective, restricted only by its high cost. In recent years the crippling disabilities caused by leprosy can be effectively reduced through advances in surgery. The stigma of incurability, the false notions which caused exclusion from society, have waned over the years. It needed a saint like St. Francis to mix with the lepers and to cause his rich and noble friend, Bernard of Quintavalle, to follow his example. The legend says that Bath was founded by Prince Bladud, father of King Lear, expelled from court being a leper.

It is reckoned that there are still some 15 million such sufferers in the world, now showing less despair and having a glimpse of hope. I talked to one of the Sisters, a kind, middle aged woman. There was something holy about her. Answering my questions in German, she told me that none of the staff was afraid of contracting the disease − "We do the Lord's work, and so we cannot be punished". "No, no-one has gone down with leprosy, but we have to leave the place after two years, the work is too exhausting". It crossed my mind that the disease begins insidiously and may smoulder for years before it manifests itself. I admired these German Sisters and remembered what Roul

Folereau, the founder of the World Day for leprosy sufferers, once said – "Civilization, if it means anything, is loving one another". How strange that at the same time other Germans, incited by the evil of Hitlerism, were committing torture and mass murders on able and healthy people, useful to the community, many of whom were in their prime of life. They were subjected to criminal experiments, shot, hanged, burnt alive, starved to death, gassed or massacred. The Nazis killed some six million Poles, half of them Jews. At Babi Yar, near Kiev, they murdered tens of thousands of Russian Jews, old and young alike.

In Jerusalem I admired the devout German Sisters of the Mission Hospital. In Poland the Germans committed the most heinous crimes for more than three years. Through the Warsaw streets a Polish doctor marched in front of two hundred Jewish children from the orphanage he had founded and patronized, to the transfer point from where they were transported to the extermination camp of Treblinka.* They were wearing white brassards with the blue star of David. It was early August 1942. The doctor knew their fate. Offered release, he refused to save his own life by abandoning the children as he felt that his presence would help these wretched innocent creatures,** he loved so much, in their last tragic hours. He was sixty-three years of age, a paediatrician of repute, a Polish patriot engaged in welfare work most of his life, the author of several children's books under the name of Janusz Korczak. His real name was Henryk Goldszmit. In one of his short fable stories, "Three Journeys of Little Hersz", he wrote how the Lord, angry with the Jews, took pen and paper to sentence them to death, but the letters of the alphabet thwarted this by escaping and going into hiding. The author must have been psychic.

The real events, however, were more formidable than his tale. After the war I heard the gruesome story of my university colleague, Lucy G., the only child of a well-to-do family. Her father, a bacteriologist, was taken hostage by the Germans and shot and she found herself with her ailing mother on a train heading for the gas chambers. Being a doctor and entrusted with the medical care of the occupants (German thoroughness and Nazi perfidy!) she had some freedom of movement and soon discovered the real purpose of this journey. Lucy decided to escape, but her mother, suffering from deep depression, was unable to grasp her daughter's plight. There was only one thing left for Lucy to

---

* Treblinka – the notorious Nazi camp set up in July 1942 where 800,000 were exterminated in one year.

** Hundreds of thousands of children perished during the extermination of 1942.

98

do — she administered a lethal dose of morphia to her mother and jumped off the "death train". In London, Szmul Zygielbojm, who escaped from Poland after his wife and children had been killed, wrote as a member of the Polish government in exile to the President and Prime Minister of his government "in protest against the passivity with which the world is looking on and permitting the extermination of the Jewish people." He then committed suicide on May 12, 1943.

There was nothing original in Hitler's accusations and cruelty to the Jews — Amalekite Haman tried to do the same thing at the time of the Hebrew Exodus from Egypt, and at the very end of the 19th century, Plehve, the Russian Minister of the Interior, nicknamed "killer of Kishinev", engineered a ruthless wave of pogroms resulting in many deaths. In between, the Jews experienced the Spanish Inquisition, accusations of ritual murders, the Dreyfus affair and pogroms in many lands.

Being in the army, I did not know of recent happenings in Poland. In Palestine, there was turmoil and underwater currents among the Jews, and illegal immigration took momentum. A handful of Polish soldiers of the Jewish faith, officers among them, were persuaded to desert and hide in the Kibbutzim — the communal farms. Haganah, a defence organization, was becoming stronger, and the Stern and Irgun extremists were secretly preparing to show their teeth.

On the wider arena, the Russians fought fiercely, left without choice. Hitler announced that German soldiers guilty of breaking International Law would be excused. On his directive the war was conducted with unprecedented harshness — the Soviet Commisars taken prisoner were shot or hanged, mass murders were committed, the civilian population was starved; no wonder the opponents of the oppressive Soviet régime also rallied against the common enemy — Germany. Even so, some eight hundred thousand Russians willing to bear arms side by side with the Germans against the Stalin régime formed a liberation movement under General Vlasov.* The Russian leaders attempted to negotiate a separate peace with Germany in 1942 and early 1943. By October 1942, the Soviet resistance stiffened, bitter street fighting went on in Stalingrad itself, and the great battle raged until February 2, 1943, when General Paulus and his army surrendered and were taken prisoners by the victorious Russians. The Russian advances continued — in October they crossed the Dnieper, by

* Vlasov was hanged by Stalin in 1946. He was 45. A great many Russians — men, women and children — were forcibly repatriated to the Soviet Union after the war, to face execution or forced labour camps.

November much of the Ukraine had been liberated, and on January 6, 1944, they had crossed the Polish frontier. At the Teheran Conference, Stalin, when presented with the sword of Stalingrad, said, "In Russia it is dangerous to be a coward".

We Poles left Russia just in time. Stalin would never have agreed to our departure after their successes at Stalingrad.

11

Reaching Italy

This beast is very wicked; when it is attacked, it defends itself.
Jean de la Fontaine

North Africa, Crete and Sicily were under air attacks from the Allies, the next targets were Taranto and Naples.

On June 20, 1942, the Afrika Korps and Italian Divisions, under the command of General Rommel, captured Tobruk and two days later entered Egypt. At El Alamein they hoped to break through the Nile, but they lost the battle – launched by General Montgomery on October 23 – to the British leaving dead, a great many prisoners and their haunting song "Lilli Marlene".* The Afrika Korps was on the run, Tobruk was recaptured. On November 8 the Allies landed in North West Africa and on July 9, 1943, in Sicily. Sixteen days later Mussolini was arrested after a stormy meeting of the Fascist Grand Council, and on September 8, the Fascist Party was dissolved. Italy surrendered and Germany occupied Northern Italy – it was the finale of the Italian Empire proclaimed by Mussolini on May 9, 1936, after a successful Ethiopian Campaign.** In the Atlantic the U-boats had to retreat because of great losses. On the enemy home ground, Barnes Wallis's "dam buster" bombs destroyed Germany's great Moehne and Eder dams on May 17, 1943. The attack was carried out by a single squadron of the R.A.F. sending floods down the valley of the Western Ruhr for eighty kilometres, putting out of action coal mines, factories and a large military airport; roads, railways, bridges and power stations magically disappeared. But at a price – nearly thirteen thousand were drowned, most of them non-German slaves and prisoners of war (a Russian P.O.W. camp was in the valley below the Eder) – the futility of war!

At the Teheran Conference, at the end of November 1943, Stalin

* It was first used as the signature tune of the German Army radio station in occupied Belgrade, sung by Lale Anderson, the German singer who died on August 29, 1972.

** Orde Wingate, the brilliant British warrior, did well behind the enemy lines in Ethiopia and later on passed his experience to the Jews harassed by Arab attacks.

struck a mighty bargain with President Roosevelt, and Prime Minister Churchill had to agree despite foreboding. Churchill's plan for an Anglo-American invasion of the Balkans was rejected and the decision taken to support Tito and his Communist Partisans, 250,000 strong. The sphere of interests among the Allies was initiated, with all the consequences that followed; it was understandable that the Poles in exile became anxious. A few months earlier, on July 4, they lost their military leader and Prime Minister – General Sikorski – in an air crash off Gibraltar. Only a month previously he had inspected the 2nd Polish Army Corps in the Middle East. At the conference in Cairo in December it was decided that the Allied invasion of France would be the supreme operation for 1944, and that "nothing would be undertaken in any other part of the world to hazard the success of these operations".

At this turning point of the German fortunes of war, only in Poland did they continue to be successful, aided by Lithuanians serving in the auxiliary police force and known as shaulis (Lithuanian for soldier). The Paviak prison in Warsaw was notorious for crimes committed there by the Nazis; Jews were herded into ghettos* from where mass deportations took place to the death camps in 1942. Luckily more than 100,000 died earlier from disease and starvation, only 250–300 calories per person being allowed. A military underground organization, the "Home Army", responsible to the Polish Government in London, was formed the same year; they used the Warsaw sewers as a life-line for arms into the ghetto. On April 19, 1943, the uprising in the Warsaw Ghetto broke out, led by the Jewish Fighting Organization under the command of Mordechai Anielewicz. They had only 300 fighters armed with a few dozen rifles and pistols, home-made grenades, fire bombs and . . . knives, but they were a match for the Germans and were able to stop their tanks. Anielewicz followed the example of his forefathers – Joshua, Gideon, David, Bar Kochba, Berek Joselewicz. After twenty-seven days of heroic resistance in the unequal struggle the uprising was crushed on May 16. Germans shelled the Ghetto with artillery, used poison gas, set fire to it and took the survivors to the death camp at Treblinka. People who jumped from burning houses were killed outright on the pavement, and the injured arrested on the spot. About 7,000 Jews lost their lives. 56,000 were captured and only seventy escaped through the sewers, sometimes neck-high in water which was near boiling point from the heat of the

* The Warsaw Ghetto was set up in October 1940.

fire above. A few found shelter in Polish homes, in spite of German threats. Naturally the tragedy of the Jewish children hounded by Nazis aroused the greatest commiseration. It is reckoned that about 3,000 Poles were killed for helping the Jews.

Like everywhere else in the world, there were some people devoid of conscience who acted as informers or blackmailers, extorting a pay-off for their silence. There was nothing left of the ghetto except an eight-foot high wall, and, fittingly, the Gensia Street jail, which stood solidly among the ruins within the walls. At Treblinka the prisoners staged yet another fight before they perished; their personal effects were sent to the Reich – artificial limbs, women's hair, gold melted from gold teeth . . . The "Krankenkasse,* which for years has been providing the Germans cheaply with golden teeth, must have run out of them! There were many more death camps in Poland. Three-and-a-half million Jews lived in pre-war Poland, but they now form its smallest minority – under 30,000. Even to-day it comes as a shock to know that it actually happened.

The rigorous military training of our units was nearing its end – the army was now mechanized – some twenty thousand people from all walks of life were trained to be drivers; the rest learned how to fight the enemy.

We moved into Egypt, preparing for transfer to the Italian Front. In our last days in Palestine we witnessed a fight between a scorpion and a large colony of ants near the camp. The venomous creature, ten to twelve centimetres in length, its segmented abdomen ending in a flexible tail carrying the sting and poison gland, was striking forward, its tail arched over its back. The little ants were fighting back, creeping over their own kind which were already lying motionless on the battle-field, in an heroic attempt to reach the dreadful scorpion. We saw them seized by the powerful enemy, paralyzed by its sting, and torn to pieces. This went on for hours and millions of ants perished, but in the end the defeated scorpion lay dead among the huge number of corpses; a handful of the little creatures which survived mounted the dead body. We applauded, seeing ourselves in a similar situation.

Before leaving for Egypt, many soldiers had to part with their pets. The dogs had to find new owners. Some were accepted at police training centres and a bear was presented to the Tel-Aviv zoo.

We were soon in the desert again, this time at Qassasin, in the

---

* Health insurance.

vicinity of Tel-El-Kabir. En route, we crossed the Suez Canal near El Qantara and saw a ship passing through, and had a quick glance at Ismailiya. Later on I was able to follow the trail of the mighty Pharaohs – the Sphinx portraying the Egyptian King Chephren, the pyramids, of which the largest one was built by King Cheops for his own tomb some four thousand seven hundred years ago, Memphis and Saqqara – south of Giza – the burial grounds of the Pharaohs and their noblemen where well preserved wall-reliefs depicted scenes of life in ancient Egypt, a reminder of its past glory.

I strolled through Cairo, and was interested in the old quarter with mosques and minarets, winding alley-ways, mediaeval courtyards, open markets, bazaars full of people, some with crates loaded with fruit, others with trays full of bread balanced on their heads. On foot or on wheels, tradesmen shouted their wares; artisans were hammering copper, and in this crowd – grunting camels, braying laden donkeys and bleating goats. The old quarter was full of life, teeming with people and flies in sweltering temperature. Egypt has a dry climate and in my early days rich people, suffering from kidney diseases, were sent there; there was little else doctors could offer. The residential quarter had wide streets like the Kasr-El-Nil, hotels, of which the Shepheard Hotel was usually frequented by the British, many cafés and restaurants. I liked Groppi's, where I enjoyed excellent coffee and pastries, the mint tea not being a favourite of mine.

Walking along Soliman Pasha thoroughfare, I heard a frantic hooting and three cars passed at breakneck speed – it was King Farouk, then twenty-three, and his entourage, no doubt not a very popular monarch. Nine years later he was overthrown and forced to quit Egypt, leaving behind him the sumptuous Abdin Palace in the centre of Cairo with some three-hundred-and-sixty rooms and crystal sparkling everywhere. When King Farouk died in exile in 1965, weighing twenty stone, he was buried at night, in secrecy, in Cairo, next to one of his forefathers in the Mohammed Ali line, as was his last wish. The grand Mohammed Ali Mosque still reminds people of their rule.

Sometimes I was approached by a beggar or a vendor unfolding "dirty pictures", that means dirty to mind and hands, in a most furtive manner. On being refused, he was not deterred, and often produced the death mask of King Tutankhamun whose tomb was discovered by the British archaeologists, Howard Carter and Lord Carnarvon, in 1922.

Before leaving Cairo, I visited a cabaret in the suburb of Heliopolis. There I saw performing belly-dancers – an oriental art which I had not previously encountered.

In January 1944, our unit was transported to the Port of Alexandria (founded by Alexander the Great), for embarkation to Taranto in Southern Italy. I found various troops on the ship – Poles, Scots, Americans – well-disciplined, ready to fight the Germans. We remembered what Churchill said on September 5, 1942. "All of us are defending a cause of freedom and justice; of the weak against the strong; law against violence; mercy and tolerance against brutality and ironbound tyranny". We were crossing the Mediterranean in convoy, at one point being near Crete, then in German hands.* An aircraft circled in the vicinity guarding us, mine sweepers were ahead of the ships, and a destroyer hovered in attendance. However, not only soldiers were aboard the ship. Their pets were with them and I noticed a dog, a turtle, a rabbit . . . In a later transport a bear was shipped to Italy. Its name was Voytek, a mascot of the Polish 22nd Transport Company, whose badge depicted a bear carrying a shell against the background of a steering wheel. Voytek shared with them the whole campaign, ending its eventful life in the Edinburgh Zoo. Its exploits inspired the animal story "Soldier Bear", published after the war.

While on the ship, I was attached to a British Colonel in charge of Medical Services, being mainly a translator for my compatriots. Sitting behind the desk next to the Colonel at the morning sick parade we heard a gentle knock, then a pause. The door opened slowly and a peaked cap appeared round the door. Eventually a corpulent figure slouched in, hands in his pockets, chewing gum. "What's wrong with you, man?", bellowed the Colonel, his eyes twinkling, his moustache twitching in amusement. The "soldier" had ear trouble, but could not answer – his mouth was glued with gum – and so he leaned over the Colonel, slowly extracting a hand from his pocket, and holding his painful ear, shoved it under the Colonel's nose. He was the first American I encountered; I believe he was a war correspondent.

On the fourth day we landed safely at Taranto, greeted in yet another tongue few of us understood. The date was January 27, 1944. We were again in Europe. After some marching we reached our camp, not far from the town. I was with a Field Ambulance of the fifty thousand strong 2nd Polish Corps, incorporated into the British Eighth Army under General Leese. Besides the British and Poles, there were

*·Crete was taken by the parachuting German troops by May 27, 1941.

Americans, Canadians, New Zealanders, South Africans, French and Moroccans, Greeks, Indians (Ghurkhas in their midst), also Italians. General Sir Harold Alexander was Commander-in-Chief of these Allied Armies in Italy. The Command had the objective of opening the road to Rome. Our Allies fought since mid-January near Cassino, the stumbling block, and on the 22nd landed some troops between Anzio and Nettuno, but the Germans put up a stubborn resistance.

During the next few weeks, while our soldiers were still arriving in Italy, I was able to get acclimatized. I was curious about the country to which Goethe referred with affection as "the land where the lemons flourish". With a colleague of mine I visited a café in the town, listening with fascination to the sound of the melodious Italian language and watching people raising their hands and voices to such an extent that I motioned my friend to leave the place, thinking a brawl was imminent; he laughed – "These people are only having a friendly chat, it is their Latin temperament". Having studied medicine in Genoa before the war, he was able to understand them. I started to pick up some Italian words, – "Buono" (good), "cattivo" (bad), "tedesci" (Germans). I already knew the expression "E vietato sputare nella carrozza" (Do not spit in the train), which I learned in my early days when travelling on inter-continental carriages.

An excursion to Naples, occupied by the American Fifth Army on September 30, 1943, was arranged. On arrival, I had the feeling that I had been there before; the view of the Bay of Naples from the hill of Posillipo, with its villas and gardens, somehow reminded me of Haifa. In the background loomed dormant Vesuvius whose last eruption took place only the previous year. One had no idea that a mere fourteen days later it would erupt again and continue for several weeks. Harold Macmillan describes* "great flames shooting out, and hot lava running in two red-hot streams down the mountain side . . . All the sea was glowing red in the reflection of the lava and flames from the cone . . . The next day the volcano was belching out rocks, stones and ash . . ."

In the town I noticed with interest the enormous glass-roofed passage of Galleria Umberto Primo lined with shops and cafés seething with soldiers. However, Naples of 1944 was not the gay place known to the world through the Neapolitan songs popularized by Enrico Caruso and Benjamino Gigli, and the famous words, "Vidi Napoli e poi Mori" (See Naples and then die) were due to a wrong translation – the real

* "The Blast Of War", Harold Macmillan, London, Macmillan, 1967.

meaning being "See Naples and Mori" (a small village near the town). I walked through the narrow, dark, dirty streets and back alleys full of stench, deprived of sun and warmth, with drying linen hanging from the windows of squalid dwellings and across the street. I saw places full of rubble and destruction, all the time watchful of children ready to pick my pockets. The streets of Naples were taken over by "scugnizzi" – homeless urchins trafficking in American cigarettes on the black market, pilfering, and often pimping for the teenage girls on the look-out for soldiers; they lived in the streets and slept on the pavements. I was glad when we were taken back to our camp.

12

Chasing Germans and Italian women

Heroes exterminate each other for the benefit of people who
are not heroes.   *Havelock Ellis*

In mid-February heavy fighting broke out in the Cassino area. The ancient monastery, turned by the Germans into a bastion, and the town below with a population of about 25,000 were both bombed, shelled and reduced to rubble. Enemy positions on Monastery Hill and surrounding mountains blocked the Liri valley and the highway to Rome. The powerfully equipped crack units of the German 1st Parachute Division stubbornly resisted all the attacks; they fought with weapons and propaganda leaflets in which they listed the names of fallen fighters, prompting the enemy to desert – "The prisoners will go home, the dead will never return". But it was of no avail. I wondered why they did not quote Achilles, Homer's character, that "it is better to be a living serf than King of the dead". It all started when General Tuker, the Commander of the Fourth Indian Division, combed the bookshops in Naples for information about the Monte Cassino monastery. In a book dated 1879 he found that in the nineteenth century the monastery was converted into a fortress, and reported to his Corps Commander that Monte Cassino was a modern stronghold and had to be dealt with by modern means. It was situated on the very summit of Monte Cassino, at a height of 1,700 feet.

With two N.C.O's I was sent to the British Military Hospital in Vasto, reached by rail, to tend the Polish patients passing through on the way to a Polish Hospital. The first one had acute gonorrhoea, the second – syphilis, and the third an obscure feverish illness which brought mental confusion – not all our forces were yet in business.* Penicillin, now the accepted treatment for the first two illnesses, was not yet at hand. Hence the man with gonorrhoea was treated with sulphathiazole, a drug synthesized in 1938. Looking back, I remember that the only case of acute gonorrhoea seen by me in the Soviet labour

* Some Polish Forces were engaged along the Sangro River at the beginning of February, 1944.

camps was treated with permanganate irrigations – the only treatment available apart from silver protein solutions – ending in inevitable epididymitis, a then common and very painful complication. The patient was a commercial artist who commuted between several labour camps; others had no opportunity or strength to pursue such activities. It is easy to understand the origin of the Polish lay term "tripper" (phonetically adjusted to the language) for this disease.

During my studies I was told of many sequelae of gonorrhoea – prostatitis in the male, inflammation in the pelvis and adnexae in the female with subsequent sterility or extra-uterine pregnancy, gonococcal ophthalmia of the new born, arthritis, endocarditis . . . It was a routine measure to put silver nitrate drops into the eyes of a new born baby to prevent possible impairment of vision due to corneal scarring, should they be infected by gonococcus.

In resistant cases fever therapy had to be applied – a ten hour session at 40.5 to 41°C.* by means of T.A.B. vaccine given intravenously. Sometimes bougies had to be used – slender cylinders introduced into the urethra for dilation. In my student days I was told a story illustrating the presence of mind of an ageing professor, who introduced a bougie intending to leave it for ten minutes but, turning to other patients, had completely forgotten his first case. Thirty minutes later an orderly rushed to the professor reporting the man to be in great pain and perspiring profusely. The composed professor, covering his embarrassment, took his pocket watch out very slowly and calmly said, "I will be right down, Peter, the time is not up yet, the bougie should remain two minutes longer" . . .

The patient with syphilis was already showing evidence of generalized infection – he was pale, had slight fever, complained of persistent headache and sore throat. I noticed a faint rash on his body. Clearly the case could only be dealt with by a specialist. As for the third man, I had not a clue what was wrong with him and I couldn't even say he was talking nonsense – I was told by the psychiatrist of my University that the patient never does this, his pronouncements are an important medical sign! I turned over the pages of Manson-Bahr's text book for tropical diseases, but it did not help me. I then enlisted the help of a British Colonel, the medical specialist. He examined the patient very carefully, shaking his head from time to time, and in the end he requested his papers to jot down the diagnosis – "G.A.K." I learnt many abbreviations in the army – R.T.U. (Return to Unit), M.T.

* 105.9 to 106.9°F.

109

(Malaria Tertiana, or mess tin for that matter) and the like, but this was a new one to me. I felt too embarrassed to ask the Colonel. I went to Captain P. telling him of my predicament, but he only laughed and said, "The old man always writes this when he is in difficulty", "G.A.K." means "God alone knows". We both had a laugh.

Captain P. was a good sport. When I first met him, I apologized for my bad English. He put me at ease saying "I understand, old chap, I'm not English myself". "But your English is excellent," I interposed; "Well", he said, "I am a Welshman". I brought back from my British assignment many pleasant memories. I spent a few happy hours watching an E.N.S.A. performance in the Vasto theatre. I found the audience, comprised of British troops, delightful; gone was the restraint I was told so much about, the artists had an easy task to communicate with the responsive, appreciative group. The soldiers enjoyed it to the full joining in the singing of "Bonnie Banks of Loch Lomond", "Oh! what a lovely bunch of coconuts", "Daisy, Daisy" and the popular "Lilli Marlene". Many more songs followed. I heard them for the first time and was fascinated to learn that they were as romantic as those of the Poles. I soon found myself humming "Sally", "Goodnight Sweetheart", "If you were the only girl in the world", "She's a lassie from Lancashire" . . .

On May 3, 1944, Polish National Day, the Poles were more determined than ever to fight the Boches. On the night of May 11 – their troops positioned on the left flank of the British Eighth Army – they attacked the fortified mountain of Monte Cassino, some six kilometres in width and eight in length, after earlier successes at Monte Croce and at Monte San Angelo. Hand to hand fighting took place in a rocky terrain, made more hazardous by thorn, gorse and gulleys. The attack lasted until the following afternoon. Six days later they again went into action in close co-operation with the British 13th Army Corps disregarding losses from mines, traps and crossfire and took the fortress on the morning of May 18. There was no need for the Polish troops to storm the monastery as the last of the German garrison had withdrawn during the night, leaving only a German officer and thirty other ranks behind, most of whom were wounded. The green valley presented a terrible sight; it was littered with corpses lying in a blaze of sunshine among pillowboxes, anti-tank obstacles, dug-out mines, stones, craters, rubble, splintered trees, white corn and masses of poppies. Here and there fallen enemies lay across each other beside pieces of bodies, fragments of uniforms, helmets, tommy-guns and spandaus. It was

110

"The Valley of Death", strangely silent and unreal. The scene was immortalized in a beautiful, but very sad Polish song.

The Cassino town was captured the same day by the 4th British Division. The Poles now moved down the southern slopes of Monte Cassino. Further attacks followed. They surged through the broken Gustav Line, constructed by the Germans right across Italy, towards the next defences – the Adolf Hitler Line whose name the enemy soon changed to the Dora Line, not to discredit their Fuehrer ... In Kipling's words – the victors were men in a world of men – bitterness heightened their inborn courage. They already looked upon Hitler as a Samson shorn by the Allies. But it would be wrong to say that Hitler's wings were clipped as he was anything but an angel. On May 25, after another five days of fighting, the Poles took Piedimonte, a town turned into a fortress by the Germans, and the infantry conquered the 1,669 metres high Monte-Cairo. Owing to the successful action of the combined Allied troops the road to Rome was open. The Polish victory was achieved at the cost of 3,784 casualties, of whom one third were killed. An achievement? Saying, "We won", was a peculiar calculation of wartime, perhaps even diabolical, its meaning was distorted. At the cemetery of Acquafondata the survivors bade farewell to fallen comrades in silence. Symbolically no bells rang, the monastery was in ruins; with the Polish flag lowered the soldiers saluted their dead. It was a necessary sacrifice. They defended the cause of freedom and justice by fighting the Nazi evil with the old slogan on their lips: "For our liberty and yours". They lost everything and acted with fury; some of them could not bear the sight of blood before. And yet it was so futile. Many young precious lives were lost which prompted the royal consent of King Victor Emmanuel for a Polish military cemetery to be established on Monte Cassino. The Monastery was destroyed,* only to be rebuilt by the people who caused its ruin. Founded 529 A.D. by St. Benedict, it had been sacked, destroyed** and rebuilt twice before.

Photographs were taken for posterity. Horrors, dead and heroes were on both sides. They went out purposely to inflict injuries, to kill and maim, and the ground was splashed with Polish and German blood alike. Not all the "Jerries" were barbarians, neither side could claim a monopoly – the British had Montgomery and Peniakoff of the

* Only a fragment of the north wall remains as a memento, next to the rebuilt monastery.

** By Longobards in the 6th Century and Saracens in the 9th Century.

111

"Popski" Private Army, the Germans – Rommel and Skorzeny; there were numerous examples. The young soldiers did not give their lives of their own choice, their lives were taken away from them. A number of them received *posthumous* awards. Many others, on crutches, were unable to stand to attention and those with shattered arms to salute when honoured. Some were deprived of seeing their awards through loss of sight.

There were rare moments when hatred was set aside, like a spontaneous firing truce on Easter morning observed by Allies and Germans, which brought a short-lived, almost idyllic peace. It was sad to realize that the Polish Army had lost as great numbers from hunger and illness when it was stationed in Soviet Russia as in the fighting; between February and June 1942 3,600 Polish soldiers had died there, and possibly in May 1940 some 10,000 Polish prisoners of war, most of them officers, were massacred in the Katyn Forest near Smolensk in Byelorussia.* They were brutally murdered, with their hands bound and a bullet in the base of each skull. Afterwards the bodies were closely packed in a deep pit, head to feet like sardines in a tin; the clods were smoothed and little conifers planted to conceal the crime. Elsewhere in Russia another 5,000 Polish bodies were buried in similar circumstances. Eventually the Russians erected a monument in the Katyn forest, near the mass graves of the Poles, with the inscription: Here are buried Polish imprisoned officers murdered by German Fascists in the Autumn of 1941. Can we really believe the Soviets?

At the time when the Americans were swiftly advancing on the road to Rome, now open to the Allied armies, and entered the city on June 4,** our medical men were busy tending the wounded. The medical staff were vulnerable too, a casualty clearing station received a direct hit, in spite of a large Red Cross sign being displayed on the tents. Two surgeons and a chaplain were killed and three other doctors, a nurse and twelve patients wounded. The last two weeks of May I spent in an advanced post of the C.C.S., through which ambulances carrying war casualties were passing in an incessant stream, bumper to bumper. At the Main Dressing Station the seventy-year-old chief Polish surgeon, General Szarecki, carried on operating day and night. I entered each ambulance, checking the condition of the wounded, seeing that they were sufficiently sedated, that the bleeding was controlled or if they

* German armies penetrated into Russia on Sunday morning, June 22, 1941.

** Rome was spared from damage. The German Field Marshal Kesselring forbade the blowing up of bridges over the Tiber because of their historical value and because they carried pipes and cables vital to the city's life.

were in need of immediate transfusion, making sure that the wounded men were fit for further travel to the transit military hospital in Campobasso. I checked papers pinned to each one, making short notes.

We worked from dawn till late at night – an exhausting and sad task. A great number of casualties had legs blown off from mines, often from small "schuhmines" which would tear off the foot of anyone who trod on them. Others had multiple injuries from shrapnel or various gunshot wounds. I recognized a young cadet officer I had met much earlier, who was seriously wounded by a bullet which missed his thigh and penetrated a vital organ. I made a point of seeing this unfortunate man some time later, a courageous person with high principles. He was engaged to a Polish A.T.S. girl, but decided on his own initiative and against the opposition of the distraught girl, to break off their relationship.

A young soldier complained of intense pain in the thigh where he was wounded. The bandages were soaked with exudate of a mousy odour, his limb was swollen, tense on palpation. I felt crepitus; the pulse was rapid, he shivered. I bid goodbye to him with a sunken heart; it was obvious to me he suffered from gas gangrene, and possibly septicaemia. I did not know of any treatment which could save his life. Alexander Fleming, who identified penicillin and experimented with its broth, said in a letter published in the British Medical Journal in 1941 that the production of it for treatment of septic wounds was not practicable owing to the lack of stability and the difficulties of preparing it. The Oxford team of Florey, Chain, Heatley and others managed to overcome these problems, but because of the war situation and the bombing, part of the team had to be transferred to the United States where they continued their work. I had no idea of the miraculous results achieved in 1944 with penicillin when used for war wounds. Before that time the wounds rarely healed by "primary intention", with some luck they could heal by "secondary intention" but often they had no intention of healing at all! Only much later I learned that two days before the battle of Monte Cassino Poles received twelve million units of penicillin, enough to save a few. Perhaps the young soldier was lucky after all.

The first phase of fighting by the Second Polish Army Corps was completed and they were temporarily withdrawn to the rear. They had "the honour of striking the blow", "with God's help and blessing", "covered with glory", "their proud days", "the victorious battles", "military feat", "their triumph", "gallant soldiers", "the bravest of the brave", "a job well done", but in fact it was bedlam, absolute hell, and we were not in the least jubilant. The Commander of the 2nd Polish Corps, General Anders, went through the same experiences as ourselves of being imprisoned in Soviet Russia; he left Moscow's Lubianka prison utterly exhausted, able to walk only on crutches. This soldier of repute, eight times wounded, now received the Companionship of the Order of the Bath, the American Legion of Merit and the Cross of Virtuti Militari, equivalent to the Victoria Cross (for the second time). I was awarded the Bronze Cross of Merit with Swords and the Cross of (luckily not at) Monte Cassino. Was it glory of death or death of glory, so hardly won, so costly in human life and suffering, that was indelibly inscribed in our minds? I had the feeling the medals I received were *commemorative* ones and so I have hidden them since . . . to forget.

I was drafted as an auxiliary staff to a Polish Hospital crowded with wounded. I was told by an inspecting Colonel of the Medical Corps on one occasion to wrap up a gangrenous foot with cotton wool, to improve its circulation. Next day another doctor with the rank of Captain directed me to expose this foot, as only a diminished consumption of oxygen might be able to save it. Not being a born soldier, I carried out the Captain's order – after all one cools the organs and tissues for preservation. It only shows that in the medical profession, as in any other profession, differences of opinion do exist.

Among the injured was the German Captain captured at Monte Cassino. When taken prisoner, he was ordered to lead the Poles through the mine fields, as he had full knowledge of their location. He stood on a mine on purpose, wishing to kill himself as he was not able to fulfil the duty entrusted to him by his Fuehrer. He lost a leg and I attended to him as he was among other wounded soldiers.

I soon heard wonderful news – on the night of June 5–6 the British and Americans made successful landings on the beaches of Normandy – D-Day had arrived! It was a prelude to their drive through France and the Low countries to the heart of Germany. In the excitement I told the news to my German patient. To my surprise his face brightened. "This is wonderful news," he said, "This is what we Germans were waiting for". I was puzzled, but not for long. The Captain explained that his Fuehrer was saying for months that Germany's destiny would be decided in the West – "at the Atlantic Wall the enemy will be annihilated and our secret weapons will bring Britain to its knees". As it happened, Hitler's much propagandized Atlantic defences had been breached within a few hours. Todt* workers and the forced labour of Russians and Poles were used there, and it was madness to hope that they would help Germany. "Do you believe what you are saying?" I interrupted. "Doctor", he said quietly, "You believe in *your* propaganda and I believe in *mine*". This was the end of the argument. By June 12 nearly 327,000 men were ashore, and on June 26 the formidable fortress of Cherbourg capitulated. Hitler put his hopes into the secret weapons – on the night of June 13–14 the first pilotless aircraft, known as the flying bomb, "buzz-bomb", "doodle bug" or "V-1" landed in the South of England. The attacks continued for the next few months, causing damage and many casualties in spite of the capture of some launching sites and bombing of others by the R.A.F.

On September 8 the first "V-2" landed at Chiswick, London, and the flying bombs continued to fall throughout the rest of the year. They were temperamental weapons. On June 17, when Hitler had a conference in an elaborate bomb-proof bunker built in the summer of 1940 as his headquarters for the invasion of Britain, (incidentally never used), an errant V-1 on its way to London landed on top of this bunker. The Fuehrer left it immediately, not stopping until he got to the safer one in his mountain retreat at Berchtesgaden. There he dreamt of launching the fabulous guns of V-3 which were to have been fired on London. Barnes Wallis' bombs took care of that – the concrete monsters, six metres thick, harbouring secret weapons, were wiped out.** He went to France to see for himself what his "tallboys" had done. Wearing a dirty old raincoat and grey slacks, he was almost arrested by an American Major who took him for a spy.

Symbolically, on June 15 the legendary German General Rommel, the "Desert Fox", was seriously wounded when his car, on the way from the Normandy front to his headquarters, crashed into a tree after being attacked by a low flying allied fighter plane; his combatant days were over. It was now the Nazi war-lord's turn; five days later, after eleven-and-a-half years reign of terror, the bid was made to bring Hitler and National Socialism down and a bomb went off in his headquarters in East Prussia. Hitler's right ear was deafened, his legs were burned, his right arm temporarily paralyzed, but he survived to exert a bloody mediaeval vengeance. He promised it to his opponents, and he kept his word for the second time.

* Dr. Fritz Todt – the engineer in charge of building the Atlantic Wall, and the man who built the pre-war autobahns and the Siegfried Line.

** Missiles establishment was moved to the forest near Blizna, in Poland, making it safe from air attacks.

The plotters were hung on meat hooks like cattle, a noose of piano wire was placed around their necks and they died in agony in front of movie cameras. The film was rushed to Hitler the same evening, he enjoyed it not once but several times. The "poor" man was badly in need of carnage to satisfy his instincts; one would not expect it from a vegetarian.

People's Courts with their macabre trials, modelled on those of the Russians, operated for a long time after. Everyone, even remotely implicated, was liquidated and all his relatives persecuted. About 5,000 people were killed. Some, like Field Marshals Rommel and von Kluge and General Beck were forced to commit suicide, General Stuelpnagel attempted to kill himself and, blinded, was led to the gallows. Among the executed were Field-Marshal von Witzleben, Colonel-General Hoepner, Colonel-General Fromm, Colonel Stauffenberg . . . The tyrant ordered that the condemned be refused the last rites of the Christian church. Exhausted by his own blood-thirstiness, he mourned: "The German people are unworthy of my greatness". No wonder he hated the race whose Ten Commandments included "thou shalt not kill", "thou shalt not bear false witness against thy neighbour". One hears a cruel man called a beast. It is not fair to the beast for I cannot imagine anything as cruel as Hitler. Arrogantly, any man imagines himself as a "Homo sapiens" (wise man). I prefer to reserve this adjective to animals, and I would replace the word "beastly" with "*menly*".

During the last two weeks in June, Polish troops were switched to the right flank of the Eighth Army in the Pescara area, and after a short rest began to pursue the enemy, reinforced by the British armoured units and the Italian Liberation Corps. On June 17, the Chienti, Potenza and Musone rivers were crossed, the battle of Loreto fought, and on July 18 the Carpathian Lancers entered the important port of Ancona, advancing 120 kilometres up the Adriatic coast; the enemy, taken by surprise, left the port undamaged. The German morale began to falter and our troops captured some 350 deserters, most of them in civilian clothing. The Poles collected fresh laurels, took 3,000 prisoners, suffered 2,150 casualties, of whom 388 were dead. The Jerries, who by now were very good at retreating, had fallen back 240 kilometres to the Gothic Line in the Etruscan Apennines, running from Pisa to Rimini and constructed by the Todt Organization with forced Italian labour in the Autumn of 1943. Anti-tank obstacles and mine fields stretched for six kilometres.

116

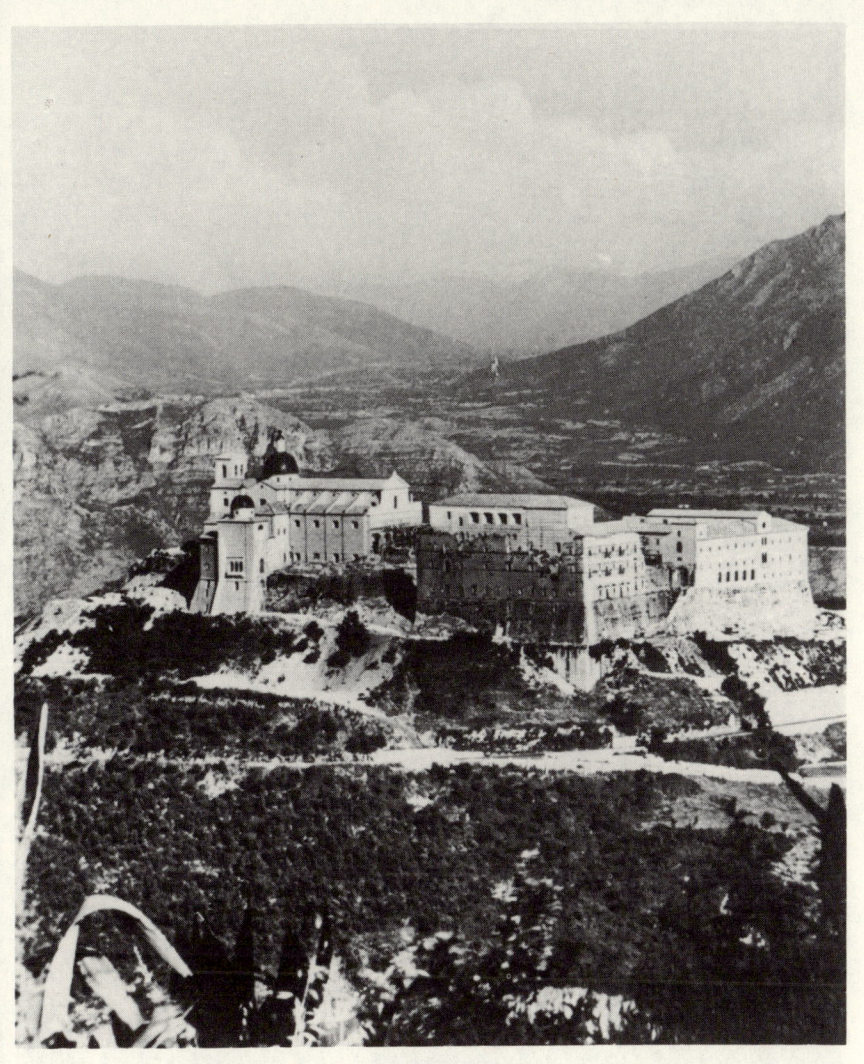

Monte Cassino

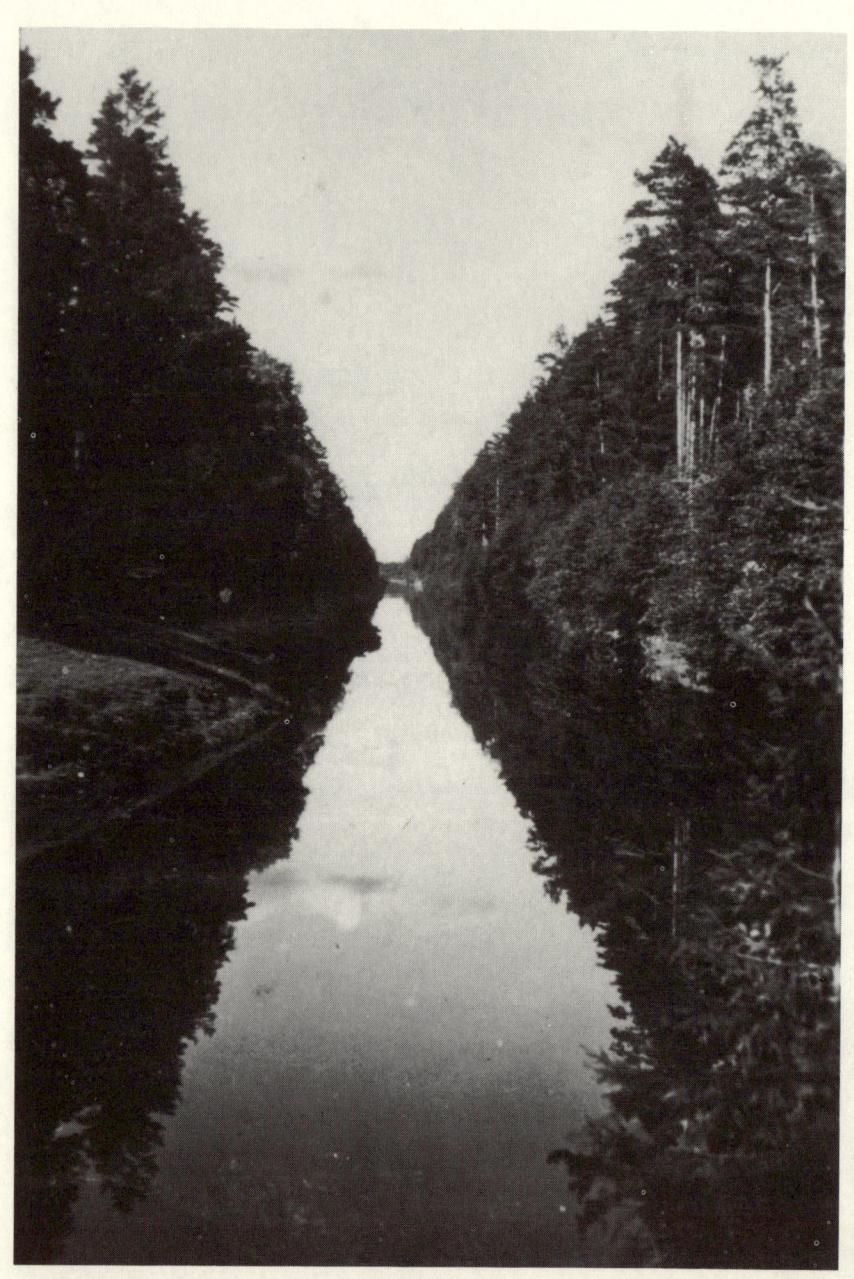

Augustov Canal

I was put in charge of a team and instructed to open an infirmary and a preventive post in Ancona for our troops who had been withdrawn from the front to this area for rest. My first task was to find suitable accommodation and I tried to achieve it in a *civil* manner, but it did not work – people were not at all helpful. We eventually found a house with its doors shut and, not getting any response to our knocking, asked the neighbours of the whereabouts of the owners or caretakers. They pretended not to know. I shouted in desperation, "La chiave, dove la chiave", then ordered the soldiers to break and enter. As soon as the hammering started, a frightened fat Italian, no doubt fed on spaghetti, wind-blown, with sweat running from his brow, appeared with the keys. The conquest was achieved without firing a shot!

In the cellar we found the owner's membership card of the Italian Fascist Party and several photographs, including an autographed one of Benito Mussolini with a little boy on his shoulders. No doubt the house belonged to an important member of the Party who left in a hurry. Scattered on the floor were coloured propaganda postcards depicting "victorious" Italian troops at the gates of the Kremlin and the like. The captions read, "La Russia dei Sovieti non puo giocare, senza pericolo mortale" (Soviet Russia can't jest without being in mortal danger) and "La marcia su Mosca che sara infallibilmente vittoriosa" (March on Moscow, which will be infallibly victorious).

We were now able to dedicate ourselves to work. Our team had not much illness on its hands and preventive measures took most of our time. It was soon clear to us that not a great many soldiers aspired to the order of chastity and self-denial . . . Bishop Ignacy Krasicki, the illustrious Polish writer in the 18th century, was a good psychologist with a great knowledge of his people when he ridiculed the monastic life in "The Battle of the Monks"!

Fraternization with the local population was an easy task and we intermingled socially. At the end of the eighteenth century the Polish military leader, General Dombrowski, led his countrymen in the Lombardy campaign for the liberty of Italy and Poland, and our National Anthem relates their march from Italian to Polish soil. The Polish people have remained Italophiles ever since. The Italians, in turn, have shown friendliness towards us; in Loreto Basilica one of the altars had a painting, the theme of which was the Polish victory over the Bolsheviks in 1920.

A great number of Italians were glad to see the back of the Germans anyway and greeted the victors with enthusiasm – clapping their hands, throwing flowers, offering wine to the soldiers and shouting: "Bravo, ragazzi". Italians are a peculiar race – I met devout Catholics who frequented the church and were active Communists, others, with holy medallions dangling from their necks, engaged with gusto in guerilla warfare.

Women, although vivacious and easy to talk to, were virtuous – they observed chastity or had remained faithful to their husbands for life (divorce was not allowed in Italy). They were a creative force. Beatrice inspired Alighieri Dante; Lauras, a married woman, influenced Francesco Petrarch; Maria d'Aquino was Giovanni Boccaccio's heroine; the actress Eleonora Duse shaped the destiny of Gabriele D'Annunzio, and another actress – Marta Abba – that of Luigi Pirandello. They usually had pretty faces, beautiful eyes and not too good figures, unless they were well under thirty, when they could have a brilliant appearance. The Polish women were able to preserve their figures a little longer and were also renowned for their elegance. A great many Italian women were well bred, well educated and possessed undoubted charm and individuality; they seldom talked shop. They belonged to the upper-middle class, Italy lacked a middle class as it is known in Great Britain. Of course, there were prostitutes as well, the war swelled their ranks, but then one could find them all over the world.

Poles and Italians have much in common – they are Continental, unlike the British. The Italians even carry the Polish white and red flag to which they added their own green, possibly to symbolize the beauty of the Italian countryside. Most of them are devout Catholics, generous, hospitable, kind-hearted, warm and sensitive. They are also virile, chivalrous, good-humoured, artistic and fond of music. Extroverts who love food, drink and company, and able talkers but poor listeners, with a flair for arguments. They are too temperamental, impatient and stubborn to await their turn. They interrupt any conversation, everyone speaks at once, and voice as many views as there are people present. The strongest voice drowns out everybody else's and wins the day! Where monologues reigned supreme and people were not aware that there might be other points of view, discussion was out of place and futile. They reminded me of hungry birds with their beaks open. I seldom experienced a quiet gathering.

Interested in foreign culture and languages, Poles and Italians respect foreigners and, unlike the British, are eager to meet them (xenophobia is not among their fears). Both are more critical of others than themselves (one hears: "I wish people would show as much goodness as I do"), both are more often than not impetuous, reckless drivers, in which the Italians excel. Both are resourceful but inconsistent, both shake hands with everyone, unlike the British, but the Poles grip harder. Both feel happiest when in the company of women and have the reputation of being good lovers. They show their approval of shapely girls by a whistle, but the Italians, although they meet such girls in smaller numbers, are more in tune – they give them a gentle loving smack on the bottom when the Poles whistle rather wistfully, like a blackbird sitting on eggs . . . The Poles kiss the lady's hand and let her pass first, the Italians kiss their hands and cheeks and leave them behind. Poles and Italians have the same maxim: woman loves to be discovered by man! They are so sure of it that they would not dream of depriving a woman of their company. It has never occurred to them that this might be unwelcome and could be opposed by the opposite sex. The truth, however, is that man is the one who longs for success with women. Both nations are individualistic – they by-pass the rules and queues, do as they please and do not care for punctuality – time is not liras to them.

Poles and Italians alike are keen to dwell in the past, but when the Italians refer to their relentless lovers as Casanovas – the amorous Venetian adventurer of the 18th century – the Poles go further and call on Greek mythology, naming them Adonis – Aphrodite's lover. They are both fond of exaggeration and lack the British reserve and manners, but what is wrong with that! Aristocracy had great influence on both nations, as in Great Britain.

They have their differences too. Poles like travelling to Italy, and in it, but the Italians prefer to stay put (save Columbus). The Italians drink vino, the Poles vodka, and get drunk more readily. Poles do not beat about the bush to a point of rudeness and intolerance, and when provoked they fight, Italians prefer to gesticulate so vigorously that it tires the watcher who feels compelled to retreat; the Poles fight because they are proud people, the Italians are too proud to fight. They are more graceful than the Poles – even when they are doing nothing, they do it gracefully and happily. When in distress the Poles call God, the Italians their own mother – "mamma mia". If a generalization is ever possible in our quickly changing world, I would describe the Italian counterpart in the shortest possible way – *he is a Pole*, a clear-cut distinct race. I should know – I was born a Pole myself.

13
Carry on Soldier

When you think about the defence of England you no longer
think of the chalk cliffs of Dover. You think of the Rhine.
That is where our frontier lies to-day.
Stanley Baldwin (30 *July* 1934)
A gentleman is one who never strikes without provocation.
Tom Masson

Ancona was a good starting point for the assault on the Gothic Line.
The troops soon reached the Matauro river and on August 25 the
British Eighth Army surged over it. I was put in charge of medical personnel with two ambulances and ordered to accompany a group of cavalry regiments. Two days previously, I escaped capture by a hair's
breadth. I was given a jeep and a driver, and told to find a suitable location for a first aid post some eleven kilometres ahead. We had driven a
good ten kilometres through deserted countryside when we noticed a
hamlet. I went to the nearest hut, not far off the road, and was confronted by two Italians looking at me with great surprise. My uniform
was obviously unfamiliar to them. They realized my predicament and,
having their sympathies with the Allies, pointed to the other huts,
warning me that the "Jerries" were still there. The information given
to me by my superiors was too optimistic. I do not need to describe the
hurry in which the driver reversed the jeep and sped off!

Two days later, together with two ambulances I followed the cavalry regiments to the forward positions. We were heading towards the
river Foglia and Pesaro; a combined operation of the 2nd Polish,
British and Canadian Army Corps was taking place. The column
pushed forward some eleven kilometres and came across several
wrecked farmhouses without meeting any resistance. We were told the
area was clear of Germans for another few kilometres. Suddenly the
troops were fired on from the surrounding hills which caused heavy
casualties. Unexpectedly mauled, they had to retreat some seven kilometres. Apart from eight killed – whom we covered with blankets and
handed over to the padre (rightly in the rank of a Captain) – there

120

were several gravely wounded, and it was decided that I and the ambulances should stay with them. We moved the casualties, mostly from the Household Cavalry Regiment, into a nearby derelict building. The injured men behaved superbly, there was no panic. One of the soldiers with a large chest wound only gritted his teeth when I packed it and I had the impression he did not wish to show any softness in front of a Polish soldier.

Soon we had two more deaths. The rest of the injured were now lying quietly, being sedated by morphia or cognac, and awaited transport under cover of darkness. We were at least seven kilometres in front of the front line. The building was heavily shelled, the very walls shook around us, and we thought we had had it! Soon the "Jerries" would get us dead or alive; our nerves were on edge. When the shelling stopped, the sudden stillness made us feel uncomfortable. Soon we were alerted by an alien sound — it turned out to be a door banging in the wind . . . As it happened, the "Jerries" had no intention of taking prisoners — theirs was a delaying action. When night descended, we evacuated the wounded, leaving the dead covered with blankets. On the return journey we came across the body of a soldier from the Italian Corps of Liberation which must have been sent in front of our advance. It was the nearest I got to the enemy and the fighting.

We now found a new location, not far from the regiments still in the rear. I discovered an inhabited, undamaged farmhouse, but the people there were not very friendly — I got the impression that they were pleased to see us in retreat. They tried to find out if the Germans were following us — no doubt they had Fascist sympathies.

I decided to give a fillip to our soldiers after the past days' experiences and tried to buy some wine from the owner of the farm. He shook his head, shrugged his shoulders, spread his arms in a gesture of desperation, and making repeated clacking sounds peculiar to the Italian language,* he said, "Non c'e piu niente, hanno tutto rubato i tedeschi, siamo poveri" ("no more, the Germans have stolen the lot, we are poor"). "Bad luck boys", I said, "let's have some ersatz coffee". We were "enjoying" the coffee and biscuits when one of the medical orderlies entered and asked me to step outside. He pointed to a horse in the farmyard who was pawing at the ground covered with straw. On close inspection we found a ditch full of flasks of wine. The news spread like wildfire, and the soldiers were allowed to take as many bottles as they wished. We had a merry evening, with lots and lots of singing. When

* The nearest translation in English would be tut, tut.

the farmer came running to me, red in the face, his arms flying in all directions, I refused to have anything to do with him. I summoned one of the soldiers who had a smattering of Italian and instructed him to tell the farmer that we would pay for his "vino". When he winced, I shrugged my shoulders, and with repeated clacking sounds, now familiar to me, I said in Italian of a kind, "Non c'e piu niente vino . . . i polacci . . .", then I looked with affection at the horse, wondering what treatment he would get from his "padrone". At last, the battle was won!

Two weeks later I received an official letter from the A.D.M.S. office. I opened it full of expectations – a commendation for my exploits? Alas, I was hopelessly wrong! The Quartermaster's Office requested a full explanation of why several blankets were missing, a great number of thermometers had been broken, and two bottles of cognac emptied. I soon recovered from the shock, sent the necessary information, and awaited the next assignment, which arrived a few days after my return to the Field Ambulance.

My Unit continued to be on the move – Pescara, Roseto, Fermo. From here I was posted to the Polish hospital wing, where I was kept busy tending the wounded, most of whom had "Bristol bottles" hanging at their bedside. I was still "other ranks" and envied the army chaplains, all of them with the rank of Captains upwards, and A.T.S. who were graded in accordance with the status they held. A little earlier General Szarecki, a surgeon, sought medical help because of an acute ear infection. A specialist called on him, leaving his white coat behind and disclosing to the surprised General his rank of sergeant. This was soon remedied for all the doctors in the army. And so one day I had a visit from my immediate superior, Major T., who informed me of my commission to a Second Lieutenant on September 1.

It was my last promotion in the army, and it was good to know that Hans Reiter, a German, who described a disease named after him, did not rise above the rank of a lieutenant, like me. The patients noticing a little metal star on my epaulettes, smiled and congratulated me. A few weeks later I had an urgent request to return to my unit, then stationed in Porto Recanati. My plea that I was still needed in the wing was rejected. I found out in no time that I was coming to a "dolce far niente". I imagine they were desperate for another hand in bridge, or another possible reason may have been the wish to exercise authority. It could not last, I was not the best of players . . .

Much was happening in other parts of Europe. On August 25 Paris was liberated after General Leclerc's Armoured Division came to the assistance of the fighters within the City who had risen in revolt six days earlier. The Polish capital was not so lucky. The Russians led a successful offensive in Byelorussia and took its main town Minsk on July 3. They soon crossed into Poland, entered Vilna – my University town – on July 13, and Lublin ten days later; shortly after the Western Ukraine, including Lvov, was over-run. Masses of Germans found themselves prisoners of war on Soviet soil.

Despite all the crimes and atrocities the Germans had committed, some Russian people were reported to show commiseration, and one heard utterings "Just like our poor boys . . . also driven into the war". But all was not well. In Lublin the Soviets installed a Polish National Committee for Liberation, of a communist brand, which yielded to the Russian demands for a revised Polish–Russian frontier over the protests of the Polish Government in London. The Soviets made them the Government of Liberated Polish Territories.

An uneasy compromise was reached at the Moscow Conference attended by Churchill, Stalin and the Polish Premier, Mikolajczyk. Advanced guards of the Soviet Army, led by General Rokossovsky, had already reached the right bank of the Vistula and the outskirts of Warsaw. On July 29 Moscow radio called upon Poles to take up arms and to fight in the streets of Warsaw. The Polish Underground Army, also called the "Home Army", started the rising on August 1 at 5 p.m. It was led by General Komorowski, called "Bor". He succeeded General Rowecki who had been arrested on June 30, 1943 by the Gestapo and liquidated. The operation aimed at securing a strong bridgehead for the Russians on the left bank of the Vistula. The Germans were caught by surprise and Polish colours were soon flying on many liberated buildings. Ill-armed though they were, they took almost the whole city on the left bank of the river. The Germans kept Praga and other districts of the town on the right bank, but were cut off. At this juncture the Soviet Air Force disappeared from the sky, only reappearing early in September. The Soviet artillery became silent; the Russians had a series of setbacks at Radzymin, north of Warsaw. The request for arms and intervention of the Soviet Army soon reached the Polish Premier, who at that time was negotiating with Stalin in Moscow. In September, Soviet aircraft made several drops of arms and food, but no important attack was launched by them, and they refused British and American planes permission to land behind their lines. On August 14 Moscow disassociated itself from the rising throwing the responsibility on to the Polish Government in London and the insurgents; the Soviet Union had no interest in seeing patriotic elements, striving to achieve freedom and sovereignty, strèngthened by a successful uprising.

The Germans fought back. The Luftwaffe began systematic bombing of Warsaw. A brigade, formed from paroled German convicts and Russian turncoats, appeared on the scene. They burned prisoners alive with petrol, hung women upside down from balconies, impaled babies on bayonets. Even for the German Command it was too much to bear: the Brigade was ordered to the rear and its Commander shot. The insurgents, lacking arms and ammunition, and fighting against heavy artillery and tanks equipped with explosive charges, incendiaries and flame throwers, lost the suburb of Mokotov, where I once lived. On September 27 they had to abandon other positions but prolonged the struggle in the sewers of their city; on October 3, after sixty-three days of fighting, they were compelled to surrender. 22,000 combatants and almost 200,000 civilians lost their lives and General Komorowski and the surviving defenders were taken into captivity. On October 9 Hitler ordered that the city, which numbered 1,350,000 inhabitants before the war, be razed to the ground. On January 17, 1945, when the Russians entered Warsaw, they found it demolished – just a heap of ruins, a deserted and dead place, without a single human being. For three months preceding Hitler's order, Warsaw had been systematically destroyed by the Nazis. Special Hitlerite units called "Vernichtungs-kommandos" destroyed schools, museums, libraries and theatres. They set fire to streets and blew up memorials, palaces, churches, power stations, gas works and bridges. General Komorowski's post as the Commander of the "Home Army" was taken over by General Okulicki, whom I met in Russia after our release; in March 1945 he was again arrested with fifteen others and tried in Moscow; his travels took a full circle.

The Allied offensive in the west, in the Autumn of 1944, brought the liberation of Belgium, Luxemburg and nearly all France, German towns were systematically bombed and devastated. On the Italian front the Americans forced the passes of the Apennines and the British were engaged in heavy fighting in the region of Rimini, reaching the Rubicon at the end of September. I remember from my school days that Caesar crossed the same river with his legions in the winter of 48 B.C., in the march on Rome. Doing so he said "Alea jacta est" (the die is cast). It was the right move which enabled him to defeat the enemies who plotted against him in the capital, so averting mortal danger. Ever since, "Alea jacta est" and "One crossed the Rubicon" have been universally known sayings. The Rubicon as such does not merit remembrance; like the biblical river Tiger, both have no force, no beauty, no sparkle.

We now had a new ally – the Autonomous Republic of San Marino with a territory of thirty-eight square miles, which declared war on Germany in September; it had an army of two hundred, now strengthened by eighty men, and a police "force" of fourteen. The little town, twenty-two kilometres south-west of Rimini, perched on the 750 metres height of Monte Titano, with a population of 14,500, was used by the Germans for artillery observation posts. San Marino, which had enjoyed independence for several hundreds of years, was now sheltering masses of refugees. On September 20 the Camerons of the 5th Brigade entered the city after the loss of thirty-six men killed and wounded.

The second Polish Corps was once again put on the left flank of the Eighth Army directed toward Forli; the new sector was mountainous, with winding tracks. Rations and ammunition had to be transported by mules; the Engineers were putting "Bailey" bridges over the swollen rivers and operating mine detectors. The Poles occupied Santa Sofia and took Monte Grosso on October 22. In December they took part in two battles at Faenza, where Mussolini went to school; it was entered by the New Zealand Division on December 16. On the push they reached the Rabbi River near San Zeno which passes Predappio, some three kilometres from the village of Dovia where Mussolini was born on July 29, 1883. In later years his impressive profile was carved in the mountain peak near by and could be seen from a long range. Seeing his chin thrust forward, his lips pouting, I could imagine the man whom the masses idolized in the 1930's, telling them in a theatrical pose "I will care for you, I too have known hunger". They trusted him. Glasses from which he had drunk and pickaxes which he had used during his tours were prized as holy relics. Their attitudes were understandable – bridges, canals, roads, schools, hospitals and orphanages were built, swamps drained, forests planted, archaeological works financed, not only on the mainland, but in Sicily and Sardinia as well. In 1929 Mussolini signed the Lateran Treaty with the Holy See, to the relief of the Italians. But great poverty continued to exist, only now beggars were kept off the streets by the police . . . Fascist censorship banned books of many notable writers including Robert Graves and

125

Axel Munthe. Among people who raised protest against Mussolini's régime was the famous conductor Arturo Toscanini, who preferred to leave his country, also the renowned Benedetto Croce.

By the end of December the Senio river was reached, but by now the troops had to fight in snowstorms, and the roads were blocked by the severity of the winter. Before the Allies could break into the Po Valley, the operations had to be halted. This happened at a time when the German troops were deprived of their able commander, Kesselring, who sustained severe head injuries in a road accident on October 25.

At the end of October I was sent to a British Military Hospital where I assisted other doctors in attending the wounded, Poles and Germans alike. The two wards allocated to them were crowded and the injured lay side by side; naturally, my first duty was to our soldiers. When I attended a German sergeant with a shot gun wound which broke his arm a day after his admission, he was most grateful that I had found time for him. He was a nice man, a school teacher by profession, who had no interest in the Nazis. Entering the wards for the first time, I was met with an unusual scene. The Boches, already attended to at the Casualty Clearing Station, their broken legs in plaster of Paris, were unaware of being a mobile propaganda of anti-Hitlerism. Someone had written in indelible pencil on their plasters: "Hitler Kaput", "Fritz is a Nazi swine", "What a Kamerad" . . . "Jerries" lying with their shattered legs in plaster, were not able to see these comments. During one of my rounds a medical orderly drew my attention to a Polish soldier of the Jewish faith who had serious injuries after being blown up by a mine. His face was covered in bandages, only the tip of his nose sticking out uncovered; both arms and legs were in plaster. Next to him lay a big, swarthy, fierce looking German with a haemothorax* caused by a bullet, but who was in good shape. The Polish soldier motioned to me with one finger which happened to be uninjured, moving his lips painfully, his voice almost inaudible, and when I bent over him I heard him whisper haltingly, "Doctor, mo-ve th-is bloo-dy Ge-r-man aw-ay, or I wi-ll ki-ll him"! It was pathetic. I noticed that just talking completely exhausted the poor man.

To my horror I observed that, in spite of all the attention given to our soldiers, the wounds of the Germans were healing much quicker. It was soon brought home to me that by frequent changing of dressings and keeping wounds clean, we interfered with nature. Luckily for the Germans we did not have much time for them! Pus is a liquid product

* Haemothorax. A collection of blood in the chest cavity.

126

of inflammation made up of white cells (leukocytes) which ingest micro-organisms and other substances, so aiding the healing process. This was recognized by Elie Metchnikoff* towards the end of the last century. We had to mend our ways!

On one of the rounds with the British Major, a neurosurgeon, we stopped in front of a young German soldier with a bullet in his back which caused paralysis of the legs. The Major asked me to tell the German that he would operate on him the next morning. The soldier shook his head and bluntly refused. The Specialist, his face stern, requested an explanation of this stupid behaviour. I passed the Major's request on to the soldier, only a boy, who told me they had been warned by their officers that the enemy would do everything possible to kill his adversary, "Don't trust anyone, even a doctor". He had tears in his eyes. When I gave this explanation to the Major, he softened and talked through me to the soldier like a father to his son. We were able to convince the poor wretch and he was operated on the following day. The neurosurgeon told me he was confident that the operation would be successful. Once more we were confronted with Nazi propaganda, and found that the monumental lies of Goebbels were sometimes difficult to dispel. His assertion that the enemy does not take prisoners but shoots them occasioned incidents when wounded German soldiers fired on stretcher bearers who rushed to their aid.

In the operating theatre I saw a soldier with blocked kidneys. He had been previously treated with a sulphone drug used for many maladies; he may possibly have disregarded his doctor's advice to drink large amounts of fluids, or he could have been exposed to a hot climate – in any event the drug which was administered to help him, killed him. There was no way to unblock the kidneys and he soon died from uraemia. Since then much safer sulphone drugs have been introduced and such mishaps do not occur any more. Adverse reactions to various drugs, however, can happen. The medical profession calls diseases unintentionally caused by a drug given to help a patient, iatrogenic diseases. They might be caused by lack of knowledge, too much doctoring or too many doctors involved. The term "physician" stems from the Greek word physis (nature); it shows that the abuse of drugs is against the very nature of a doctor and can lead to an unnatural outcome of iatrogenic diseases! One hopes that an ever-widening knowledge will be a safeguard. The Committee on Safety of Medicines and

* For discovering the curative nature of the inflammatory process, Metchnikoff won the 1908 Nobel prize for physiology and medicine.

127

the yearly publication "Drug-induced Diseases", some 400 to 500 pages, alert physicians to iatrogenic dangers. Risk is sometimes unavoidable but it should be prudently balanced against the benefits one hopes to achieve.

I had many happy times during my stay with the British. First – the Officers' Mess into which I walked with reverence – like going into a church. Several tables, covered with impeccable white cloths, had a lavish display of cutlery. The solemn mess waiter, in a long swallow-tail coat and black tie from his previous days, was an Italian, but everything else was British. I was bewildered by the variety of plates, spoons, knives and forks and at a loss when and how to use them according to the conventions of British etiquette. I was afraid I would pick up a roll belonging to my neighbour as I was accustomed to it being on my right . . . I observed the half-astonished, half-amused looks of my fellow officers watching me cutting a roll instead of breaking it, or putting a napkin under my chin. I watched them with amazement too – eating with a fork upside down, ordering fruit juices as a starter, drinking horrible tasting gin and commenting, "By Jove, it's *awfully* good". The polite, obliging waiter tried to teach the officers a little Italian. Raising a knife he would say, "Coltello"; "Knife", said a British officer; "Si, Si", said the waiter – "Coltello". "Knife", repeated the officer stubbornly. Unperturbed, the Italian continued, "Questo e la forchetta . . ., e quello . . . le cucchiaio". "Yes, Yes", said the officer, "A fork, a spoon". In the end the officer had won, the would-be teacher turned into a pupil – from then on it was only knife, fork and spoon, the waiter had learnt it! I seldom heard the British talk politics, unlike the Poles. I was in the Officer's Mess listening to the wireless on December 17 when I heard the news of a major offensive in the Ardennes led by Field Marshal von Runstedt, in which he was able to penetrate some eighty kilometres deep into the American lines, and in which Hitler had staked his last reserves, so delaying the Allied advances for six weeks.* This situation was overcome with the help of the 8th Indian Division, borrowed from the Eighth Army. There were several officers in the mess, but no one was interested in the happenings. I was the only listener. Soon, when the news was over and the football results were read out, everyone rushed to the set with pencil and paper. I remember another occasion when everyone listened to the radio and that was His Majesty King George VI's speech on Christmas Day. It

* On December 22 the Commander of the German Armed Corps sent a note to the American General McAuliffe demanding surrender of Bastogne and received a one-word answer which became famous: "Nuts".

was touching to watch the reverence and concern of the listeners because of his impediment – everyone sighed with relief when the broadcast ended without a hitch.

I spent the end of winter and the early spring of 1945 as the Medical Officer of a Polish Cavalry Regiment. I found the atmosphere convivial. Most of the officers were gay and socially-minded; many were professional soldiers before the war who once belonged to the gentry and talked wistfully of the days when horses dominated their lives. Watching them sitting astride wooden stools, glasses in their hands instead of reins, engrossed in a jovial conversation reminiscing about the good old days, brought back to me the familiar image of the colourful figure of a cavalry man – his chest full of medals like a jeweller's display case, breeches adorned by red stripes along the outer side, high, black and shiny boots on bandy legs, jangling spurs, and the indispensible sabre, a pom-pon hanging from its hilt. The cavalry was a military élite, a force apart. A captain would be most offended should one call him that; he was of course a "Rotmistrz". It was like calling a surgeon a Doctor, instead of a Mister. The other ranks were Uhlans, more colourful than their counterparts. The distinction stemmed from much older days when cavalry charges dominated battlefields to the sound of bugles. The tall, four-cornered headgear of the Uhlan carrying the emblem of an eagle and the theatrical-like attire from the past epoch were portrayed by Kossack and other painters, or displayed on chocolate boxes; often horses were included to adorn the picture. But the romanticism went out of business – horses were replaced by tanks, the gentlemen riders transformed into tank crews, the Uhlan regiments into armoured cavalry and the cavalry charges into tank warfare. Even then they looked upon other formations with a condescending air, but they held the medical profession in high esteem; as with most primadonnas, I discovered a neurotic trend in "gentlemen riders".

I was billeted with an Italian family who, I found, were very united. The old "nonna" (grandmother), a widow, was held in reverence. She was the first to sit at table, and her grandchildren never attempted to get up until she rose. She was undisputed boss and busied herself in the kitchen etc., no doubt enjoying her advanced years. I constantly felt the presence of this family – they talked loudly, laughed a lot, behaved in an excited fashion and displayed many charming gestures. During the first few days I noticed that they were uneasy having "Signor tenente" in their midst, but this reserve soon disappeared and their volatile behaviour made me feel at home. Slowly I was able to comprehend what they were saying. My hosts addressed me now as "Dottore", and the children began to bring their problems to me. One day little Giulio burst into my room complaining that his older brother had *tried* to smack him. "Really?", I asked, "How do you know?", "Because. . . . he smacked me"! said Giulio crying. The mother was an attractive brunette with sparkling black eyes, fresh complexion and coral lips often forming into a smile. Her shapely, long-limbed figure was accentuated by a short-skirted black dress. She was a gentle person, speaking in a much softer voice than the rest. Clarissa, as she was called, was well educated and spoke reasonably good English. She volunteered to give me lessons in Italian, naturally with her husband's consent! I was delighted.

The winter was no longer bleak now that I had an attractive pastime. My teacher was proud of her heritage and gave me a taste for the interesting places in Italy, stressing the differences in the way of life, people's characteristics and language between the industrial North and the rural South. Each day I learned new words, new phrases. During one of our lessons she discussed the word "povero" (poor). "We say povero, poverino, poveretto, poveraccio, poverello, poverone . . ." I was impressed and exclaimed "What wealth!", and immediately perceived the absurdity of such an expression. As the weeks passed I began to grasp not only the language, but also the Italian gestures such as patting the stomach to indicate hunger, lightly flicking the chin with the back of the fingers and saying "Non me importa niente" to express indifference, raising the thumb to the lips as an invitation to have a drink, or twisting the index finger against the cheek – an expression of great satisfaction. And so the rest of the winter passed in bliss among a happy family, even though a foreign one. I appreciated my luck after years of deprivation and it saddened me when I had to take leave of my Italian friends. From mid-February the weather changed and soon the glorious warm Italian sun returned to stay for many months.

I had only one unpleasant experience among many happy ones there. I developed toothache and was advised to visit an Italian dentist. "Mal di dente", I said, pointing to my trouble. "Si, Si," he muttered and started the awful drilling. I withstood this assault and was told to come again. It developed into a routine – I had drillings twice a week for three solid weeks, each time a little deeper, each time more painful. I noticed a smile on the dentist's face when he was looking at my contorted features. No word of pity or apology. I myself was uncomplaining, I wished to try anything to save the tooth – after all it would not grow again. On the sixth visit the dentist informed me he would have to take it out. "E peccato", he said with a shrug of the shoulders, but it was obvious to me he was not the least sorry. I was furious; my mouth was too sore to shout and throw abuses and it was lucky for him I was a doctor and unarmed. I felt he got the better of me and a little revenge for the defeat of his country . . . Many years after I appreciated the progress made towards painless treatment in dentistry.

The 2nd Polish Army Corps, all its units brought up to full strength, was by now ready for another assault. These were strange reinforcements. They consisted of men who had recently arrived from Poland after various Odysseys and who belonged to the "Home Army". This was disbanded on February 7, 1945 by decree of Mr. Raczkiewicz – the President of the Polish government in exile – to appease the Russians. Some of these men participated in the Warsaw rising. The largest contingent consisted of Poles called up to the German army, who were captured on various fronts, mostly in Normandy and Italy and found suitable, after screening, to fight with us. This trend started as far back as 1943, during the Tunis campaign. They certainly exposed themselves, besides the risk of war, to the death penalty should they fall again into enemy hands. These reinforcements were of importance; the Allied resources in the Italian campaign were strained. General Alexander lost seven divisions and seventy per cent of his air force to the operation in the south of France. Alas, the Italian campaign ceased to have strategic priority.

The offensive was launched on April 9, 1945 with a tremendous artillery bombardment and support from the fighter bombers. It started with the tragic mistake when the Americans bombed the Polish troops who were waiting to attack and caused heavy losses. Afterwards we used to say, more humorously than grudgingly, "When the Germans are bombing, we Allied troops hide from the planes, when the British are attacking, the Jerries hide, but when the Americans are sighted – both Germans and Allies keep out of sight". The 2nd Army Corps had reached the far bank of the River Senio to the north of Imola and by successive daily attacks broke through the defences on the rivers Senio, Santerno and Salustia, and the chain of canals, particularly the Gaiano, where the fighting was as fierce as that at Monte Cassino. The centre of Bologna was reached in the morning of April 21 where the Polish troops, coming from the east, met the Americans of the 5th Army arriving from the south. The ex-German soldiers of Polish origin took part in the fighting. Harold Macmillan described the scene on his arrival in Bologna on April 23 and said that "Two well-known Liberal leaders, shot by the Fascist Black Brigade just before the retreat, were lying in state in the Town Hall against which wall they were executed and a large crowd was filing past the two open coffins". Photographs of many victims were displayed there and I saw many more in various Italian towns later on. Time was running out for the enemy, who was driven back to the River Po and the Plain of Lombardy only to find that the bridges were destroyed by Allied bombing the previous autumn. Soon came the coup de grâce – the Allied armies crossed the River Po and on April 28 Germany signed an unconditional surrender of all German forces to the Allies, which included the Soviet High Command, with effect from May 8 – VE Day. At last the Hitler-land was battered into submission. The Germans made a great effort to surrender to the British and Americans rather than to the Russians! Unfortunately, the bold concept of Churchill to press eastwards after crossing the Rivers Po and Piave and seize Trieste and the Istrian Peninsula, with the aim of reaching Vienna, was rejected to please Stalin. It could have altered the political destinies of the Balkans and Eastern Europe. As it happened, the inevitable "iron curtain" began to fall.

The Allies had lost 312,000 killed and wounded of which 59,000 belonged to the Eighth Army – the price for containing fifty-five enemy divisions, but the German losses were much higher. The Poles had lost 2,220 killed and 8,800 wounded. At the foot of Monastery Hill at Monte Cassino they left an ever burning flame to remember their dead, but there were many more graves scattered over Italy – at Casa Massima, Loreto, near Bologna . . . These were the only tangible results . . . But the Poles sustained far greater losses in their native land.

In the early stages of the last offensive I was drafted to the Centre of the Polish military police at Urbino. I had a batman with me – a resourceful twerp who spoke with a distinct Russian accent. I had no doubt that he was in fact a Russian who fought with the Germans but was clever enough to pass for a Pole when he was captured by the Allies. It was only human to let such people be "Poles" – their return to the "fatherland" would mean certain death.

Urbino was entered by the 1st Royal Sussex battalion on August 26, 1944, cheered by its inhabitants. The town is picturesquely situated on a hill and has a mediaeval character with its narrow, crooked streets and old houses dominated by the Ducal palace. In the square stands a monument to Raphael. The modest house where he was born and spent his boyhood was turned into a museum. The officers, lacking the jovial, "happy-go-lucky" air of the cavalry men, were rather sombre to the point of being dull. Some were in the habit of using the precise, concise language of a trained lawyer. The war interrupted university for some of them. One such officer consulted me because of an acute earache. I prescribed the standard phenol drops in glycerine to ease the pain. The next day, however, a spontaneous perforation of the ear drum occurred and the patient connected it with the treatment he had received. I was accused of negligence and subjected to cross examination by his colleagues. They requested that I drop some of the liquid, which I had instilled into the patient's ear, on to my skin, to prove it was harmless. I did, and the case was dismissed. The incident reminded me of the behaviour of some medical students in their first years of study who like to play doctors.

By now Venice was in Allied hands and a group of officers went there on a short leave. Excited at the prospect of seeing this lovely city, they consulted me for . . . preventive measures. They were no doubt successful as I heard little of the beauty of Venice on their return. Venice was once a place full of secrets, renowned for its masked and fancy dress balls, with the reputation of a gay and wicked city swelled with courtesans and the most "celebrated" brothel in Europe on the Rialto. It was also the town where Casanova lived and loved.

In the capacity of Medical Officer I had the task of carrying out checks on newly taken German prisoners, with the purpose of finding those who had SS marks tattooed. I was sitting behind the desk shouting "Next" when a German prisoner in green uniform marched in and, springing to attention, clicked his heels with military precision and, raising his right arm, greeted me with "Heil Hitler". He stopped abruptly when he realized his blunder. He had done this too long and too often – it was in his blood. I lifted my eyes and roared "What the devil's this, where the hell do you think you are?", aware that the Boche could only grasp my tone and not my words. He became red in the face and mumbled something incomprehensible. I ignored him. "Next!" I shouted. The door opened slowly and a German sergeant quietly walked in, without any attempt to display military bearing. I looked down at my list and called his name. "Kuck!" "Sir", he said in a ponderous voice, with a mixture of condescension and impertinence which only a German aristocrat can show, "My name is von Kuck, a distinction of nobility . . ." I got very annoyed with him. He did not know I had lost faith in aristocracy anyway! I repeated firmly – "Kuck, there are no VONS here and never will be!" At that moment I recollected the insulting behaviour of the two German fliers whose capture I witnessed when they baled out over Warsaw.

The Military Police were undergoing rigorous training which included intricate exercises on motor cycles. For several weeks I had requested that an ambulance be allocated to the Centre, but without success. One day I was called to the scene of an accident where a motor cyclist lay on the ground near his heavy Norton, unable to move. I found that both his legs were paralysed, no doubt due to a broken spine. Thanks to the local surgeon I was able to mobilize a civilian ambulance and got the man to the Military Hospital. I noticed that the surgeon, an elderly man held in high esteem by the local population, was addressed as Professor. I found later that this is the usual title of a surgeon, equivalent to our "Mr.". After this episode I did not have to wait long for an ambulance and driver to be allocated to the Centre. It gave me an opportunity of learning to drive. After a few lessons I was at the wheel, with the driver at my side, busily negotiating the narrow crooked streets of Urbino, when an Italian took all his time to cross the road hoping, I imagine, to bring me to a halt. I was not prepared for such an eventuality, the man was in my way; I panicked and instead of slowing down I accelerated. The frightened adversary ran for his life, fortunately successfully. Thinking that I did it on purpose, he turned towards me shouting and raising his fist. He must have been a Fascist . . . Since then I have learnt to press hard on the brakes.

One hot, lazy day I decided to take my "crew" to the river by ambulance. The Foglia flows some nine kilometres beyond the town. On arrival we filed out of the ambulance, one by one, to the amazement of the few onlookers expecting to see a stretcher casualty. We rushed down to the river to refresh ourselves and, looking at the stream, pondered that less than eight months ago our troops crossed it in different circumstances – under fire.

Watching soldiers in training, I took a liking to motorcycling and obtained permission to join a course. The result was I had a minor accident severing the lateral ligaments in my left ankle, which necessitated an operation. I left my post for the Military Hospital in Bari, southern Italy, finding myself at the other end of the syringe – the needle's end. I was soon lying on an operating table and a colleague, with whom I was with in Russia, pushed the needle into my vein. I counted only to five

134

or six and out I went.

Much has changed in the field of anaesthetics since William Morton began to use ether in 1846. I had the benefit of an intravenous agent Penthotal used on me to induce general anaesthesia, followed by the Boyle anaesthetic machine to administer the required gases. I only remembered someone touching my face and saying repeatedly "Wake up, wake up". I felt it was an intrusion and did not wish to be disturbed as it would rob me of my sleep and dreamland. However, bereft of will, I followed the "intruder's" request and lazily faced the light with half open eyes. Complete relaxation and well-being took care that I did not resist – it would bring an effort I was unprepared for. At long last I was brought back to reality and found myself lying in a ward among other casualties, my leg in plaster up to the knee. I had no nausea, no vomiting, no headache, no hangover. After a few days I was allowed to get up on crutches and to visit patients more unfortunate than myself, a few waiting to be flown out to Britain for special treatment owing to the seriousness of their condition.

I was soon able to walk outside the hospital grounds with others, most of whom were on crutches and in plaster. We watched civilians passing by and heard an occasional remark – "Poor boys, injured in fighting. Eh! la guerra". I felt a fraud. After a month I was back with my unit, fit again and given the task of contacting an American Military Hospital near Genoa where two Polish soldiers were lying with serious injuries sustained in a road traffic accident. I was given an ambulance and a driver, also two stretcher bearers, should the injured men be fit for transfer.

A colleague of mine who obtained his medical diploma in Genoa before the war implored me to visit the girl he left behind with a broken heart, or so he thought. He also gave me a gold sovereign to change into liras. The American hospital impressed me for it was well equipped and very well run. I found the Yankees courteous and helpful. Unfortunately the condition of my two patients deteriorated and we all agreed that they were not fit for transportation. I was soon in Genoa, which surrendered to the Partisans on April 26. I was curious to see this chief port of Italy with its old university founded in 1471, the birthplace of Christopher Columbus and the Italian Virtuoso Nicolo Paganini. I was told earlier that his coveted violin was still in Genoa.

We parked the ambulance on the Piazza Giuseppe Verdi, as the narrow streets were inaccessible to our vehicle. The square was surrounded by a number of figures in a Fascist salute, standing on the stony "fascinae" of the lictors, the symbols of Roman authority, giving the impression of greeting us. The Genoese watched us with curiosity — I think we were the first Polish soldiers in this town. I proceeded to the address given to me earlier by my colleague. On the way I admired picturesque narrow streets, lanes and alleys, mediaeval churches with striped facades of black and white marble, palaces and villas — once the homes of partricians. I eventually found the house, walked up two flights of narrow, winding stairs and rang the bell. A pleasant woman opened the door and looked at me with surprise when she heard me saying I had a message for her. We spoke in English. She asked me in, we sat down in a well-kept lounge and the woman looked at me inquiringly, waiting for the message. When I mentioned my colleague, she grew red in the face and said furtively, with embarrassment, "Please, tell your friend I am a married woman, I have two lovely children and a good husband". She got up and said "Arrividerci". I had no chance to mention the gold sovereign which I dutifully returned to my disappointed colleague. I heard him say "Eh, la vita".

14
Like a Holiday

> If a man could have half his wishes he would double his
> troubles.   *Benjamin Franklin*

During the next few months I visited several interesting places in Northern Italy. First I went to Bologna, admiring its arcaded streets, interesting churches and its landmark of two towers, both out of perpendicular. Bologna has a famous University founded in the 11th century and a number of Poles from the Forces were accepted there when the war ended. They had illustrious predecessors like Dante and Petrarch. Among the famous professors at the Bologna University was Marcello Malpighi, the 17th century anatomist, Luigi Galvani, the 18th century physiologist, and the poets Giosue Carducci who lived in the 19th century and his pupil Giovanni Pascoli. In Ravenna I admired the famous mosaics which survived undamaged and I saw, of course, the sarcophagus of Dante. In Milan I found a great deal of destruction caused by bombing in the vicinity of the splendid Piazza del Duomo, from which a number of streets radiate in all directions. The beautiful cathedral was intact. Several years after the war a Canadian who took part in the air raids on Milan told the following story. On revisiting the city he was stopped by a car park attendant who handed him a ticket. The Canadian waved him away with "I am not paying for this ruddy car park, I helped to build it myself . . .". The Italian was puzzled.

The Scala Opera House in the city centre, which once held an audience of 3,600 and where Toscanini reigned supreme, was wrecked. Giuseppe Verdi is buried in Milan; he died there in 1901. Piazza Loreto has gained notoriety since the mob hung the bodies of Mussolini and his loyal mistress Claretta Petacci along with other Fascists there on Sunday, April 29, 1945. Mussolini was shot on the previous day without trial by Partisans. The atmosphere in the Piazza was highly charged. The dead swung from the girders of a half-built garage, one woman fired five shots into Mussolini's body to avenge her five dead sons, some spat at him. In his last letter to his wife Rachele,

137

Mussolini wrote, inter alia, "Surrender to the Allies who may be more generous than the Italians . . ." He knew very well that his own people stopped idolizing him a long time previously. The Italians did not care for his Salo Republic under the German auspices. The executions of his son-in-law, Galeazzo Ciano, and those of the 78-year-old Marshal De Buono* – Mussolini's oldest friend – and four other prominent members of the Fascist Party were the last straw. Edda Ciano, Mussolini's only daughter, fled from her father to Switzerland disguised as a peasant woman. And yet the happenings on the Piazza Loreto angered me. There is a saying: "The mob has many heads but no brains", and I hasten to add – no heart either.

Next I visited Lake Garda, in its beautiful setting, and the majestic Dolomites. Amidst the dignified stillness and impressive views I was able to put aside my memory of the horrors of war for a while and to find some peace and tranquility. I spent my next leave in Venice and was allocated accommodation at the Excelsior Palace on the Lido. A special lift was laid on from the hotel to the beach which enabled one to cross under the street ready for bathing. The food was excellent, the waiters of the highest order – each speaking at least three languages. A visiting painter portrayed me for posterity. It happened after an exquisite dinner and the artist caught my air of contentment.

The marvellous surroundings did not prevent me from having an occasional meal at the Hotel Danieli, another resting place for officers. In contrast to the modern Excelsior it was a 14th century palace of the Doge. It lies a stone's throw from the Piazza S. Marco with its beautiful Basilica and Palazzo Ducale, and the Ponte dei Sospiri (the Bridge of Sighs). In front of the hotel colourful gondoliers congregated inviting passers-by to their gondolas tied up to the striped mooring poles and gently swaying with the lapping of the water. From under their boater-shaped hats with wide red ribbon emerged the sun tanned faces, and snow white shirts reflected the brilliant sunshine, a contrast with the scorched hairy arms. The gondoliers are the guides of Venice – "the Queen of the Adriatic". Proud and knowledgeable of their heritage, they reminded me of the fiakers of Vienna and Vilna. Sitting on the roof terrace of the Hotel Danieli I admired the enchanting view of the Grand Canal and the Lagoon, watching the gondoliers thrusting the pali (mooring stakes) into the water and their gondolas bobbing up

* Marshal Emilio de Bono led the March on Rome in October 1922, which put Mussolini in power.

and down from the swell of passing vaporettos and motor boats. In the evening, on the same roof, a string quartet turned my meal time into an unforgettable experience. I went by a vaporetto down the Grand Canal, preferring to watch the bobbing gondolas rather than share the experience of their occupants. I was fascinated by the old palaces emerging from the water, among them the Ca'd'Oro – the Gothic 15th century "palace of gold", and narrow dark canals. Venice sits on tiny islands linked by numerous bridges, its main "street" – the Grand Canal. No wonder that some years later I heard a quip relating to a shapely olympic swimmer – "she must have been a street walker in Venice". I alighted at the Rialto Bridge, one of the landmarks of Venice, and explored the nearby market. The celebrated bordello situated on the Rialto ceased to exist a long time ago. I was given to understand that some Contessas specialized in running such houses adding dignity to the establishment. The decadent Venice of the past was a playground for the flippant.

I was warned about the smells from the canals, but this was not my experience. Perhaps Venice loses some of its attraction in the winter, perhaps the life for its inhabitants is not always an easy one – its present population is practically the same as it was in the 16th century. However it is rich in beauty, paintings by masters like Bellini, Carpaccio, Titian, Tintorreto, and has many interesting shops. For years I admired this city from Carpaccio's paintings and I was not disappointed at seeing it in reality. Before leaving Venice I had my last glimpse of the graceful Piazza S. Marco and thousands of pigeons. I said to myself "Arrividerci Venezia!"

Soon I was able to see Florence – the city of Dante, made famous by the Medici dynasty – the patrons of art. Its splendid palaces, the Duomo, the towers, the galleries and museums are known world-wide. Florence is the guardian of the works of Michaelangelo, Raphael, Botticelli, Titian, Cellini, Giotto, Uccello, it is also the burial place of Michaelangelo, Machiavelli, Galileo, Rossini and the poet Alfieri. When Miss Nightingale was born in this beautiful city she was christened Florence. I noticed many signs of the recent war. Ponte Vecchio which crosses the river Arno was the only bridge to survive; Florence had a number of them. The corridor on its side connects Galeria Uffici with the Pallazzo Pitti but I was unable to visit them. I only saw the exterior of the Palazzo Vecchio and admired Michaelangelo's snow-white statue of David – which happened to be an exact replica – and the elegant Loggia dei Lanzi. I was walking through busy streets with

Gustav – my best friend who also was in the Polish Medical Corps – when a petite wizened old lady passed by with a pekinese dog under her arm. She looked as if she were born old. Being in a happy mood I made a facetious remark to my friend – "I wonder whom I should admire most – the lady or the dog". "Thank you very much for your compliment, officer" said the lady in a gentle voice, in Polish. I learned she had come from Cracow many years earlier to live in Florence. For a moment I felt rooted to the ground. With regret I decided it was time for me to leave this beautiful city. Nowadays I certainly would think twice before expressing loudly adverse opinion in my native language. When touring many European countries, even Turkey, I unexpectedly came across Polish people on numerous occasions when asking for directions. It reminds one of the exodus of the Jewish people and their dispersal.

Despite the German surrender, the army did not wish to dispense with my military services and I now rejoined my unit from which I was **sent during the winter of 1945 on a delightful skiing course near Courmayeur** in the valley d'Aosta. It was arranged by a colonel who was one of the principals of the Institute for Physical Culture in Bielany near Warsaw before the war. The valley is beautifully situated in the corner of three countries – Italy, France and Switzerland. Not far away are "The English Ladies" – the sharp peaks 3,604 metres high, and, in the distance, the majestic Mont Blanc 4,807 metres in height. **We had a wonderful two weeks, spending the days skiing and walking** in the mountains, and in the evening meeting interesting people in the local albergo. A great deal of smuggling and, possibly, political activities were going on in this corner of Italy. I observed suntanned faces still covered with frost, with skis and bulging knap-sacks, arriving straight from the border which they crossed illegally. They were expected and immediately taken to a far corner of the hotel where a furtive conversation took place.

I was soon back with my Field Ambulance which was stationed in Porto San Giorgio, working in an infirmary and living a few streets away. It was the usual G.P. stuff – colds, sore throats, stomach upsets, spots, minor accidents . . . One morning I attended to a rough type who had a painful bruise after being kicked on the shin. I gave him a pain-killer and explained it would take a few days before he could walk properly. The patient insisted on being taken to a hospital by ambulance for an X-ray saying "I am sure this scoundrel has broken my leg". I was weary of battles so I consented. The man was right, on the

140

way to the hospital the ambulance was involved in an accident and he broke the *other* leg in the process. It shows that the patient, who is the doctor's customer, is always right!

On another occasion a "patient" was brought to my lodgings late one night by two military police. He had offended the Major of his unit, and, before he could be put under military detention, had to be examined to ascertain whether he was under the influence of alcohol. A few hours earlier Lieut. S . . . came to me with a bottle of whisky, which was hard to come by. It was his birthday and he wished to celebrate it with me. Lieut. S . . ., a gynaecologist who had recently arrived from Poland, was a jolly companion. No wonder he persuaded me to have "just one," arguing: "There you are, you are always on duty". Of course, it did not stop at a single drink, and soon I acceded to his philosophy: "Drink and be merry for to-morrow we die". Suddenly we heard the ominous noise of an approaching jeep stopping under my window and seconds later the deserted street was ablaze with light. By this time I was in a mild state of intoxication; something had to be done. I retreated to the bedroom imploring my colleague, who was in a sorry state, to lie down on the bed. I instructed my batman to tell the military police that, in view of the late hour, I would examine the man in my bedroom and they would have to wait in the lounge for the result. It worked well. I only saw the prisoner, whom I subjected to routine questions to check his memory, but soon forgot which questions I had asked him. I put to him a tongue twister, which he pronounced more distinctly than I did, and finally requested him to walk across the room. All this time I remained sitting, afraid to rise in case of losing my balance. My companion, lying on the bed, was enjoying this farce, giggling discreetly. The arrested man soon grasped the situation and announced in a firm voice that he had not been drinking and further examination was unnecessary. All he had done was to tell the Major what he thought of him. Relieved at this, I ordered the man to leave and through my batman informed the military police that the prisoner was fit to be detained. I would send my report to his unit in the morning, I added, as it was such a late hour. However, I was unable to do so – among the many questions I put to the prisoner I had forgotten to ask his name and unit . . . Dr. S. came to me on two more occasions with "a bottle" and on each one I refused his invitation – once was enough!

Occasionally I took respite from routine by going to the nearby sandy beach for bathing or watching the fishermen who were sorting the fish, mending the nets and painting boats.

141

It was nice to see the signoras washing their windows and singing in beautiful soprano voices. Once I looked with curiosity out of my window into the courtyard on hearing a pleasant voice singing "Vorrei baciare i tuoi capelli neri" (I would like to kiss your black hair) to the accompaniment of a violin. I was astonished to see a girl of about fifteen playing it, and a boy, not more than twelve, singing beside her. They were poorly clothed, but had happy faces – in all probability an orphaned brother and sister. Even the war-time Italy had its charm. My thoughts went to the famous tenor Beniamino Gigli who lived near-by in a small town, Recanati, not long ago. I went to see his grand villa, but I was disappointed to find that it had lost its character. The tenor, who once delighted British audiences at Covent Garden, was not there, he had become a refugee.

One evening was indelibly imprinted on my mind. With three Polish officers, one of whom was a priest, I went to a dance given by the British. An Italian orchestra played some British songs, already familiar to me, but it was the first time I had seen the Gay Gordons performed. The British officers, among them many Scots in kilts, were partnered by Italian ladies, after a short tuition. The atmosphere was very gay and friendly, the heavy wine was replaced by heady whisky and gin. The table next to ours was occupied by an Italian couple. We watched them get up and dance. The man put his arm around the woman's waist and she smiled, disclosing her pearl-like teeth which contrasted with her raven hair; they were obviously in love. The signora had an exquisite figure and was smartly dressed. Her low-necked gown often slipped from her shoulders and accentuated her womanhood. The music stopped and we could not help but notice her beautiful legs carrying her gracefully to her table. One of our officers was following this delectable lady with his eyes, oblivious of anyone else, in abandonment. He looked like a man who had just given up all his possessions to be near her . . . He heard the woman's laugh like the tinkling of a silver bell and watched her flowing fringe, which from time to time fell over her eyes. She was bubbling with delight, her zest for life was infectious. The gaiety she displayed, her swan-like neck, her well developed breasts sufficiently exposed to give one a taste of her sturdy body, kept my fellow officer spellbound. She bent down and for a moment he thought that her breasts would fall out and drop like two toy balls on the floor. He saw in her a "female" woman, a woman and a half. Absent-mindedly he exclaimed: "She is great! What exuberance, what a figure, what breasts! One could play with them for hours . . ."

142

He did not mean to be disrespectful to the priest and apologized for disclosing his thoughts. The Captain-Priest was an earthy man and a good chum. He smiled and said he understood. "How did you like the gin?" I asked the impressionable officer, to take his mind off the woman. "It had quite a kick you know", he answered. Afterwards I wondered if it was the Italian lady or the British gin which stirred our imagination. Even a few days later, when I was examining a patient in the infirmary who was a heavy smoker and complained of breathlessness, I found myself jotting down: "A *breast*less man . . .". Yet, the woman may have been a bitch, a bitch usually looks attractive.

We had a number of newcomers from Poland in our midst. I remember a Polish woman who joined us in the early part of 1946 and who claimed to have been in the Polish "Home Army". I met this lady through a friend who knew her before the war. She gave the appearance of being a happy person, fond of company. Some weeks later I saw her again – a changed woman. She had a haunted look and told me she did not feel at all well and was awaiting admission to a military hospital. A few days after she was found murdered – the motive was never discovered. Much happened in subjugated Poland and some people carried their secrets with them wherever they went.

Once again I visited the city of Bologna. A friend who was studying at its University took me to "his" restaurant for a meal. The owner was a woman of considerable proportions. She had sparkling eyes, as black as her dress, rosy complexion and a pleasant face. Her size did not prevent her from bestirring herself about her clients – students from Polish Universities whose studies had been interrupted by the War. She chatted with each one, brought plates full of minestrone, pesci and pasta, urging them to eat and enquiring if they wished for more. She assumed the role of mother and in fact the students referred to her as "mamma".

On my return to the unit I found that the army barber was on leave and I had to visit a local "barbiere". I waited for my turn, listening to the incessant jibberish of the hairdresser. When I eventually took my seat he asked, in a voice loud enough to awaken the dead, how I would like to have my hair cut, gesticulating vigorously at the same time. He might have thought I did not understand a word of Italian, or he might have taken me for a half-deaf half-wit. He rubbed me up the wrong way, but I knew enough Italian to defend myself. With an air of superiority I commanded: "Sensa parlare!" (without talking) "Ha capito?". He understood.

In Porto San Giorgio I witnessed a delightful tradition – a newly-wed couple left the church and walked with relatives and guests through the streets introducing themselves to the inhabitants who cheered them from their doorways and windows. This custom was carried out in most small Italian towns.

It was time for me to have a holiday, and at last I was able to visit Rome, taking Gustav with me.

We looked with reverence at the many carefully preserved relics of ancient Rome – the triumphal arches, like those of Emperors Constantine and Titus, the latter commemorating the destruction of Jerusalem and quashing the Jewish rebellion, with reliefs representing the victorious procession and the spoils of the temple; the Trajan's column which is the Emperor's monument and tomb, with scenes from his campaigns; the column of Marcus Aurelius embellished with reliefs relating to Germanic wars and his equestrian bronze statue. We gazed at the ninth century burial places in the Forum, the Pons Fabricius from 62 B.C. over the Tiber and many palaces.

We went to watch a musical performance in the Baths of Caracalla, impressive ruins from 223 A.D. They had been luxuriously built and could accommodate 1,600 people. The Baths were once a place of meetings and entertainment. One hundred years later Diocletian erected magnificent baths on the Quirinal which could hold 3,600 bathers. Among the ruins of the Baths of Caracalla a scene of the great fire was superbly recreated. One got the feeling of being at the actual happenings – in ancient Rome, 64 A.D., with Nero displaying himself as an ambitious musician. I returned in memory to my school-days when I was taught of this emperor's cruel reign and death by his own hand with words of great vanity, "What an artist perishes with me!" His pretensions to divinity were quashed, as happened also to his assassinated predecessor Emperor Caligula.

In "Quo Vadis" I read of mass tortures to Christians. Now I was able to visit the imposing amphitheatre Colosseum, completed in 80 A.D., with some 80,000 seats, where combats took place and beasts were let loose on Christians. "The Dying Gladiator" is the permanent reminder of those fearful times. We visited the Catacombs – places of refuge and burial for the early Christians. In 312 A.D. Emperor Constantine accorded Christianity equal rights with other religions.

Much has happened since and when Gustav and I went to S. Peter's

144

we witnessed a tumultous welcome for His Holiness Pope Pius XII by pilgrims and visitors alike who filled the largest church in the world to overflowing. The great majority were soldiers from many lands and of various denominations. We heard the Pope speaking in several languages – I was told he was fluent in seven. After the Pope's address and blessing he was carried shoulder-high on a sedan-chair through the crowds, and many clicking cameras were heard above our heads. I saw the face of an ascetic-looking aristocrat in resplendent attire, flanked by red-robed cardinals and nobles of the church; it was more spectacular than moving. Years later I saw Pope John XXIII, a more earthy looking figure with a benevolent round face, plump and worldly. His address in Italian was translated into several languages. It all looked less spectacular, but somehow warmer. I had already heard of his rescue efforts during the war*, his understanding attitude towards other Christian denominations aiming towards unity, of inviting humble folk like circus people to his apartments – a gesture none of his apostolic predecessors had shown. Pope John believed in more than Christianity, he believed in man without reservation; anyone who can do this is a saint. He was revered and loved by all.

I revisited the Basilica the next day when free from crowds. The ancient basilica was built by Emperor Constantine in the early 4th century A.D. and rebuilt in the 16th and 17th centuries. Its splendour, opulence and vastness impressed me, but it produced an effect of showmanship and ostentatiousness which appeals more to the artistic than the spiritual needs. The mark was left not by the humble faithful artisans, but by the well-rewarded artists of world-fame such as Michelangelo and his pupils – Della Porta, Bernini and Bramante. I wondered how it was possible to communicate with God in these overwhelming surroundings. Gustav and I also visited the Vatican palace, which, like S. Peter's church, is the largest in the world. We admired the frescoes by Raphael among whose patrons were Pope Leo X and the papal banker Chigi. The artist's body lies in the Pantheon among the Kings of Italy.

The description of the exquisiteness of the Sistine Chapel needs a better man than myself to do justice to its beauty. Michelangelo, Botticelli, Perugino, Pintoricchio were among many masters who created this chapel on the orders of Pope Sixtus IV. The Pope also had the Ponte Sisto built, founded the Capitoline museum and restored the

* As the Apostolic Delegate to Turkey, he saved the lives of many thousands of Bulgarian and Hungarian Jews.

145

Trevi Fountain, but had to fill his treasury by the sale of spiritual dignities and favours. He enjoyed pleasures of power, luxury and nepotism. When Lorenzo de Medici refused to lend him money, he closed his account with them and transferred it to the rival Pazzi bank; Pazzi was later implicated in the killing of Lorenzo's brother Giuliano during High Mass. Not all Holy Fathers were holy. Pope Alexander VI lived in fabulous luxury for eleven years under the eyes of his son Cesare who murdered relations and courtiers who were inconvenient to him; it was said that all Rome trembled for fear of being destroyed by him. When Cesare could not assail with open violence, he resorted to poison. Father and son died eventually by accident after a fatal dinner with Cardinal Adriano of Corneto; the poison in the sweetmeat was meant for their guest. Apartments Borgia, painted by Pinturicchio, remind us of the luxury they lived in. How strange that Columbus bequeathed the prayer-book given to him by Pope Alexander VI to "his beloved home – the Republic of Genoa" commenting that to him it was the greatest of comforts in every kind of adversity. Surely it could not have been the villainous Pope, but his high office, which stirred the emotions of Columbus. On leaving S. Peter's we continued to admire the entrancing beauty of its square adorned by colonnades and two fountains of Bernini, with the obelisk from Nero's circus in its midst.

The Papal Swiss Guards in their colourful attire, reputedly designed by Leonardo da Vinci, were an expression of past power and riches. It is easy to visualize the ecclesiastical ceremonies, the pageantry, the lavish entertainment provided by cardinals, bishops, monsignori and wealthy feudal nobility in those days. During the carnivals, processions by torchlight were held and games in the Piazza Navona became remarkable for their war-like splendour. Chariots full of revellers in grotesque masks and buffoons were accompanied by men on horseback, and scandalous verses were heard.

The papal rule was supreme and it had done a great deal for the prosperity of Rome. To this and other ends the Popes engaged in battles, diplomacy, palace intrigues, bigotry, treachery, cruelty or benevolent despotism. There were virtuous and the not-so-virtuous princes of the church, some bestowing wealth on the church, some on people, others on their own families. Popes like Sixtus IV, Alexander VI, Leo X combined the enjoyment of artistic creations and antiquity with all other pleasures, and especially under Leo X the Vatican resounded with song and music.

There was a great deal of beauty outside the Vatican. Thanks to Bernini, Borramini and others Rome was embellished with elaborate baroque and a number of exquisite fountains in various squares. The famous Trevi Fountain always has many coins at the bottom from passers-by who hope that their wish will be fulfilled – an endearing custom but pagan in character, in fact an offering to the river god. The song "Three coins in a fountain" reminds the world of this romantic spot. Some thirty kilometres from Rome stands a villa built in 1550 for Cardinal Ippolito d'Este, its garden adorned by hundreds of delightful fountains at various levels.

The Roman decline was possibly caused not so much by extravagance, degeneracy and various invasions by Germanic tribes and Teutonic Vandals, as by plague and malaria. In spite of all this, Romans displayed great achievements and sturdy courage. The ruins of the aqueduct and the Appian Way show it; Appius Claudius created this road leading to Capua, an Etruscan town south west of Caserta, in 312 B.C. In Britain, they left ample evidence of their civilization and diligence after the invasion which lasted from 55 B.C. till 407 A.D. – the 75 mile long Hadrian's Wall across N. England proves it. The word Britain was derived from the Latin "Britannia" and the son of the Emperor Claudius (poisoned by Nero) was called Britannicus. When the Goths besieged Rome, the tomb of Emperor Hadrian was converted into a fortress. The great fire of Rome in 64 A.D., destructive invasions and the ransacking of the city by Germanic troops in 1527 only spurred its inhabitants to rebuild it and make it even more beautiful. Mussolini, like his predecessors, undertook extensive excavations and reconstruction. He planned a museum relating to Roman civilization, built Foro Italico with Olympic Stadium which is decorated with sixty marble statues of athletes engaged in various sports, donated by different cities. He himself lived in the XVth century Palazzo Venezia. All this meant to give the impression of grandeur. The "Duce" named the avenue leading from the Piazza Venezia to the Coloseum the Via dell'Impero. When visiting Rhodes in 1967 I was shown the Grand Master's Palace which the Italians restored from ruins to its previous splendour during their occupation of the island. They also created the magnificent gardens of Rhodini – all this in preparation for Mussolini who, as it happened, never arrived.

The Quirinal Palace, the papal summer residence in olden days, which I visited a few years after the war, is now occupied by the President of Italy.

The days of our "stay" in Rome passed quicker than we would have wished. On the last day we returned to Piazza Navona with its beautiful fountain, watching with interest the daytime bustle of the hurrying crowds – the shouting street vendors, the scruffy Italian soldiers, the undignified-looking priest in a dirty habit and sandals carrying a small can of petrol – so different from wealthy prelates – unruly children, busy looking men with wares – all noisy and sweating in the hot sun; just a humming human beehive. Layabouts were engaged in black market activities or seeking nefarious adventures, bare-legged women of the poorer class in black dresses and head scarves seemed to be in a hurry, but there were also small groups of people in slow motion – females of doubtful category, soldiers with nice or not-so-nice girls, elegant women strolling across the square, all overflowing with goodwill, glad that the war was over.

On arrival at Porto S. Giorgio a new assignment awaited me – I was sent to Innsbruck to carry out inoculations on the local Polish population, most of whom were students. I liked this town surrounded by mountains, its narrow streets and mediaeval houses and, I found that the smart bearing of the French occupying forces commanded obedience and respect.

I chose to go to the theatre the very evening I arrived. A big queue had formed in front of the box office and I heard a voice saying "All seats sold for three weeks". Undeterred I went to the front of the queue, requested a ticket for the same evening, and I got it. The people of Innsbruck looked at me with respect and servility, no one ventured a comment – they knew who had won the war!

Three days later I was on my way back to Italy. A few kilometres before reaching the frontier two civilians who were with us – and who were related to our soldiers stationed in Italy – left the lorry with the Officer in charge. Once over the border they soon rejoined us, all three smiling and saying how easy it was. Later the Polish Officer explained to me that the Italian frontier guard could have stopped the civilians and so he decided to take them surreptitiously across the frontier.

On my return I found that there was very little for me to do as our troops had already begun the evacuation. The Italian men had regained their composure and started to show that they were masters after all. Many innocent girls who had been seen with allied soldiers had their hair cut off, and most Italian women were now afraid to meet us.

I decided to visit Capri, where I arrived from Naples with a number of Italians. We stopped in Marina Grande, a small sea port under the rocky Mount Tiberio, in the blazing sunshine. A funicular was continuously taking a few people at a time to the top, the centre of Capri — a short journey through the vineyards and masses of oleanders. While waiting I was confronted with the Italian temperament. Everybody wanted to be the first to enter the funicular. They shouted, they pushed, and they fought. I saw a man hitting another over the head with a stick and I heard him curse. "Imbecille! Cretino!" shouted the assaulted man back. With one blow they destroyed my mood of romanticism and expectation as I looked at the marvellous sight of Capri from the sea below. But not for long.

As soon as I left the unruly crowd I found myself face to face with nature — the cloudless sky above me, the blue sea far below, in the midst of an uncanny stillness. I took to the place immediately and decided to stay there for four days. I enjoyed daily walks, the visit to the Villa Jovis and Monte Tiberio, the ascent of Monte Solaro with the superb view of the whole of the island, and the little town of Anacapri. I was shown Gracie Field's villa with the fitting name of "La Canzone del Mare" (The Song of the Sea), and another villa which belonged to a Polish major (he must have been an outstanding soldier to have won such an award!). I looked with curiosity at Monte Tiberio from where people were hurled over the precipice into the sea by order of the cruel and bloodthirsty Emperor Tiberius, who made his home in the nearby Villa Jovis. It was said that he, like Cesare Borgia, shrank from showing his repulsive features by daylight. I enjoyed the visit to the villa of San Michele in Anacapri, once the home of Dr. Axel Munthe whose book "The Story of San Michele" I had read when I was still in Poland. Before leaving this charming island of indescribable beauty for Sorrento, I visited the famous Blue Grotto. We glided over the calm sea into the grotto where the oblique rays of the sun turned the water a heavenly blue. The surrounding rocks provided a welcome shade and coolness from the scorching sun. I also saw the Grotto Bianca Meravigliosa.

I approached Sorrento full of expectation. The appearance of the town perched on the top of the high cliffs was most romantic when viewed from the sea. The song "Torna a Sorrento" (Return to Sorrento) which had spread the fame of the place all over the world and which I had heard many times, had increased my anticipation. I expected too much and I was disappointed.

My drive along the coast to Amalfi was a rewarding one. I passed vineyards, orchards, olive and lemon groves and went to see the beautiful "Emerald Grotto". It was full of stalactites and had a subterranean lake, the scenery surpassed only by the caves of Drach on the island of Majorca. The panoramic stretch was truly marvellous and I decided to return. Some years after the war, when I got married, I decided to bring my wife with me. We drove in a taxi from Sorrento to the charming little coastal town of Positano. The driver, learning that I was a doctor, asked me intricate questions about "thalassaemia" – the "Mediterranean anaemia". I must admit he knew more about it than I did. "You are very knowledgeable", I said. "Why", said the Italian, "I just read about it in a "Reader's Digest". It brought home to me how difficult it is these days for the doctor to be ahead of his patients.

When in Positano we met two elderly delightful Americans who had retired to this heavenly corner. One had been a pilot of distinction who was received at Buckingham Palace, his friend was an important member of the American Embassy in Copenhagen during Hitler's occupation whose hobby was to collect relics of Hans Christian Andersen. The latter told me of his experiences under the Germans which obviously were not pleasant. After the war he visited Germany out of sheer curiosity. It struck him that every jackboot-happy German with whom he came in contact disclaimed any knowledge of happenings under Hitler. After a long conversation with the affable hotel proprietor, the American began praising the fallen dictator sky-high to the astonishment of his host, whose surprise soon gave way to visible satisfaction. "Do you really mean this?" he asked, unable to mask the pride in his eyes. "Of course I do" replied the poker-faced American quietly. "Hitler overran Europe, almost defeated Russia and their Allies, put to death millions of people, and all this with his bare hands! He must have been a genius" . . .

The American remembered Hitler saying "I have not come into the world to make men better, but to make use of their weaknesses", and the acceptance of years of degradation by the German nation, bar a few instances, was fresh in his mind. The simple fact was that practically all the country turned into one of shame and disgrace, unwilling to know. The American's contempt was too deep for words – he knew that the great conductor Furtwaengler, the composer Richard Strauss, the famous writer Gerhard Hauptmann sided with the Nazis, taking the rest with them.

One hot afternoon we took a cab to Ravello. Some six kilometres before reaching Amalfi, we left the coast road and followed a steep track. My wife felt most uncomfortable in the horse-drawn cab, not on her own account but that of the horse. The poor wretch was puffing and blowing, sweat pouring from its flanks, its head drooping – possibly deep in thought. It looked as if the overladen animal would slip back, dropping us with the cab at the very spot where we had branched off! The clip clop of its hoofs was drawing out to c-l-i-i-i-p c-l-o-o-o-p, almost to a standstill. The burly driver assured us that nothing ever happened to his passengers. There is always a first time, I thought to myself, but as I pointed out to my wife, it would be unkind to abandon the cab – the strong Italian Communist Party teaches people: "That which does not work, does not eat . . ." "For the horse's sake", I said, "let's sit".

The cabman certainly could not boast of the magnificence of his horse and so, with great pride, drew our attention to his splendid brass lantern glistening in the sun on the side of the cab. "You an Englishman", he asserted. "I got it from London, you know, my son works at the Savoy". I realized in this remote corner of Italy how much the world had shrunk. In the end I decided to walk the last kilometre. It was a kind thing to do – the horse had already earned its meal, and anyway I like walking! And so we arrived in Ravello to the joy of us all – the passengers and the horse, which graciously accepted two lumps of sugar from my wife. The sun was still shining. It was a tiny peaceful town with small winding streets, and it was heavenly to be away from crowds. We were taken to a place from which we had a breath-taking view of the coast stretching for miles in front of us, the blue sea way down below. It was nearing sunset; gradually the sky and sea assumed a warm red glow. In the end it appeared as if everything around us was on fire – a view of views. A very memorable trip.

15

My start in Britain

One should forgive one's enemies, but not before they are hanged.
Heinrich Heine

If the Romans had been obliged to learn Latin, they would never have found time to conquer the world.

Heinrich Heine

But to return to the year 1945, I tired of spaghetti, pasta, food cooked in oil, cappucini and the Latin temperament, although not of vineyards, lemon groves, hill-top villages, sea and the sun. One may tire of people and their way of life, never of nature. I was ready for a change but will never forget the melodious Italian language and the cultural and scientific achievements of the Italian people. In the medical world alone there were luminaries like Eustachio, Fallopio, Malpighi, Valsalva, Santorini, Morgagni, Spallanzani, Scarpa, Forlanini, Banti, Bassini . . . The words opera, sonata and cantata came from Italy, as did delightful music.

During the last days of my stay in Italy I saw the film "The Great Dictator" which was shown to soldiers. It was produced by Charlie Chaplin and expressed disapproval of curtailing personal freedom. I saw the little man with the famous moustache turning and running back during a charge, saying politely "Excuse me" to the still advancing soldiers, his disarming smile his weapon against adversity. This innocent Jewish barber got clubbed when wiping his window on which the word "Jew" was painted. I watched an amusing scene in which the Dictator's train could not stop at the right place to enable him to step on to the red carpet. When an inventor of a new kind of parachute fell to his death after jumping, watched by dictator called the "Furor", the latter remarked, "I wish people wouldn't waste my time like this". Confronted with thousands of strikers, the "Furor" ordered them to be shot, explaining "I don't want anyone to be dissatisfied". In the end, we saw the Dictator lying face downwards on a sofa, bouncing a huge balloon on which the map of the world was painted, with his behind, only to hug it the next minute in an unsatiable desire to possess it all. When the balloon burst, the "Furor" broke down and sobbed.

A slapstick? Perhaps. Charlie Chaplin was as funny as ever, the story was not. It really happened. The rasping shrieking voice of the raging Fuehrer shouted for blood and his actions exceeded those of the actor a thousandfold. As with the stories of Korczak, the truth was much more formidable, much more brutal, much more incredible than fiction. Germany had no atom bomb but had the merciless Hitler, who was far more dangerous. Compounding impotence with madness, he attempted to drag the whole of Germany and the rest of the world with him. A thousand year Nazi rule, announced by this unparalleled felon, was cut short and his messianic mission to deliver German people to hell completed. He promised them world power or ruin and, as with Poles, the louse kept his word.

In 1940 the megalomaniac Hitler placed a colossal order for granite in Sweden, to be supplied after the war to rebuild German towns, but by then the client was dead, having shot himself on April 30, 1945. He never resorted to the old cry of the Kaiser — "Gott strafe England" (God punish England) — Hitler's terrible record prevented him from evoking God's name. The chief architect of destruction ordered his body to be burnt, knowing full well what reception the corpse would receive.

The Second World War had come to a close. Berlin fell to the Russians on May 2. The arch-liar* Goebbels, club-footed and spiteful, poisoned his family and then killed himself; notorious Himmler escaped justice by committing suicide; other inhuman Nazi lieutenants were sentenced to death along with traitors such as William Joyce, nick-named Lord Haw-Haw; only Krupp survived with his riches, not even being tried as a war criminal. Another dictator was still very much alive and announced that Soviet Russia had been transformed into a world power.

Everyone talked of the Russian heroism, none of Stalin's cruelty — until Kruschev arrived on the scene, Stalin was tabu. And yet he was the man who brought immeasurable suffering to his generation — the end justified the means, no matter how cruel. The Allied victory was only a part-triumph over evil. The Soviets were unreliable friends, determined not to reveal to the world what their ambitious intentions really were. Poles realized it more than any other nation, but no one was prepared to listen to them. I was once asked, in all innocence, if I

---

* During the war the German people joked that the lie has a short leg (Die Luege hat kurzes Bein).

had ever tasted caviar during my internment; after that I did not attempt to mention my experiences as obviously no one would understand.

At the Yalta Conference in February 1945 and at Potsdam in July, the Russian point of view prevailed. Annexation of the Polish eastern territories became a fact and my beloved town Vilna became Russian along with many others. Poland was compensated by lands in the west but ceased to enjoy democracy in the western sense of the word. She became an arena of political trials, the Communist-led government clamped down on protests, facts were distorted, General Anders along with others was deprived of Polish nationality and contacts with the West discouraged. In December 1943, at a dinner somewhere in Southern Italy, Harold Macmillan watched the Russian Deputy Commisar for Foreign Affairs, Vishinsky, who had a glass in his hand and "il fiasco del vino" in front of him, saying, "Democracy is like wine, it is all right if taken in moderation." That way the Russian expressed his version of democracy, and it was the overstatement of the year. In reality Vishinsky must have felt that freedom of expression displayed by democracies was as distasteful as adultery . . .

The heroism of the Russians was freshly in people's minds and no one wished to breathe a word against them, or even against Communist Poland. Poles in exile were disillusioned. In 1945 the Polish Government in London ceased to be recognized by Great Britain, the Polish army was not invited to take part in the Victory Parade, which took place in London in June 1946, and at the London funeral of General Bor Komorowski no representatives of the British Government or Services were present; the spokesman for the Ministry of Defence announced that the decision had been taken "after very careful consideration". All this was strange as the war was fought and won as much by the courage of the soldiers as by the integrity and intellect of their generals, politicians and scientists.*

Doctors, too, contributed to the victory – apart from tending to the wounded and caring for the fitness of the troops – they had always aided the leading men, all under terrible stress. Behind Emperor Nero was Andromachus; behind Emperor Marcus Aurelius – Galen; behind Napoleon – Dr. Maingault; behind President Roosevelt – Dr. McIntire; behind Premier Churchill – Lord Moran; behind Mussolini –

* Following the capture of a complex German cipher machine for coded radio signals by the Polish Secret Service, a British "Brains Trust" cracked the secrets in 1940, using electronic and computer methods.

Castellani; behind Hitler – Professor Morell* who acted more as a quack than a doctor; behind Himmler – Professor Gebhardt, a man who carried out experimental operations on Polish girls in the concentration camp at Auschwitz and who was made President of the German Red Cross.

Stalin and his lieutenants must have also relied on the medical profession as the dictator accused doctors of attempting to poison them. Their responsibility is great. Illnesses of famous people tend to affect the history of nations, even that of the whole world. The severe illness of the Roman Emperor Caligula brought tyranny and savagery. Tsarevitch Alexis' haemophilia hastened the Russian Revolution. The physical collapse of the American President Thomas Woodrow Wilson caused defeat of his ideas which aimed at a world government that would prevent future wars and secure just and lasting peace. Much happened to Poland after her dictator, Pilsudski, died of cancer. The last illness of another American President, Franklin Roosevelt, and the liver disease of the British Prime Minister, Anthony Eden, made an imprint on history, to name only a few.

The ingenuity and constant improvement of weapons like the artificial harbour "Mulberry", Bailey bridges, the radar,** barrage balloons, the Hurricanes, Spitfires, Mosquitoes, Beaufighters, the Wellingtons, Halifaxes and Lancasters, the Sunderland flying boats, the blind navigation and bombing aids, the Barnes Wallis bombs, and eventually the atomic bomb which was first exploded successfully at Almagordo, New Mexico, with the aid of fundamental British research, all these played an essential role. Of course, other nations were as inventive as the British, Allies and enemy alike. The Germans had their flying bombs and long-range rockets. The man behind them – Dr. Wernher von Braun – directed much of America's space programme after the war; as early as December 1934 his team designed a rocket which soared 7,000 feet. The achieved peace did not end the production of weapons which were becoming more sophisticated, more accurate, more deadly and automated. The "humanitarian" dynamite and gunpowder were out. The television-guided bombs capable of achieving great accuracy from a height of 30,000 feet and Napalm B (it sticks to the skin and burns the victim to death) were in; the latter

* Morell claimed to be the true discoverer of penicillin whose secret was supposed to be stolen by the British Secret Service.

· ** The name conveys what it means – the principle of echo; it can be spelt forward or backward.

155

underwent "improvement" since being used against Tokyo in 1945. It is a sobering thought to realize that at present as many people are being maimed and killed due to local wars and unrest from day to day as during World War II. And so it is pleasing to know that the Spring of 1967 was the only occasion in which the British decided to use Napalm bombs. These bombs were directed against . . . pollution of the sea with crude oil from the damaged tanker the "Torrey Canyon". She went aground off the Cornish coast en route to Wales.

Many scientists were parties to destruction by unwittingly misapplying science. Nobel, the inventor of dynamite, realized rather late its implications and remorsefully turned into a philanthropist instituting five yearly prizes – for peace, medicine, literature, physics and chemistry. Caro, a Polish Jew, who received the Nobel prize for chemistry, helped the German war effort in World War I by inventing a process for manufacturing potassium nitrogen. Haber, a German Jew and also a Nobel prize winner, was engaged in research on artificial fertilizers and helped unintentionally the production of explosives. By manufacturing poison gas as an insecticide he, again unwittingly, aided criminal elements which turned it against humanity. Einstein, who expounded nuclear-physics, contributed to the birth of the atom bomb, which saddened him in later years. The French physicist Joliot and his wife Irene,* the joint Nobel prize winners of 1935 for their discovery of artificial radioactivity, were pacifists at heart. Hitler gave them no option and they joined the scientific struggle against Germany. Andrei Sakharov who established the theoretical laws of controlled nuclear fisson and was named "the father of the Soviet hydrogen bomb", felt pangs of conscience and besides becoming the leading Soviet dissident, gave away the large fortune he amassed to cancer research. Patrick Blackett (later Lord Blackett), the 1948 Nobel prize-winning physicist, felt compelled to write a book: "Military and Political Consequences of Atomic Energy".

Lord Rutherford, a New Zealander, showed the way to release atomic energy and his pupils helped in the initial stages of the development of the atomic bomb by tackling the problem of atomic chain reactions. But it was Sir Joseph John Thomson, a Cavendish Professor and the Nobel prize winner for physics in 1906, who paved the way for the study of atomic physics – he was the discoverer of the electron. A

* The daughter of Marie Sklodowska Curie, the discoverer of polonium, which she named after her native country, and radium.

156

race started between the Allies and Germany to secure the catastrophic weapon. "Heavy water"* was needed to make it. A large supply was brought to France just before the German invasion from the Norsk Hydro Plant in Norway, at Joliot's request. Soon his collaborators, Halban and Kowarski, escaped to England and were given facilities at the Cavendish Laboratory, Cambridge. The British assisted them in getting the important liquid into England. The Metropolitan-Vickers Electrical Co. Ltd., and Imperial Chemical Industries Ltd., joined in research and construction. Action was also taken against the Germans' main source of the "heavy water" produced in Norway. The Norwegian Professor of physical chemistry, Leif Tronstad, one of the commandos, lost his life with a number of others. The Allies won the race and the atom bomb was finally made by the United States.

We were "fortunate" the enemy had no such weapons and thousands of Polish soldiers who survived Russian captivity and death on the battlefields, the so called Anders' Army, were now leaving Italy for hospitable Britain. The disenchanted Poles were apprehensive of their future. They longed for the war to end, but when it did they were unable to return to their country and families; they won the war and lost peace. One could easily understand the uneasiness of the Poles. They had, however, great ability for survival and adaptation, a quality partly ingrained and partly acquired through experience.

They began to make plans. I met a soldier who, on leaving for "rainy England", put all his savings into the buying of umbrellas before departing from Italy. It was a wonderful idea but it turned out to be a poor investment – umbrellas were cheaper in Britain. Various people had various plans. Some wished to emigrate to Canada, some to Australia, others to S. Africa, Puerto Rico, Argentina and the U.S.A.; in the end some 100,000 left for overseas. I had no such problems, I wished to stay in Britain. Many of my countrymen had the same idea – about 60,000 Polish ex-servicemen settled there. Later on refugees from Communist Poland chose exile in various European and far away countries. No wonder I found the knowledge of the Polish language very helpful in my various post-war travels.

I arrived in Liverpool with the rest of the Field Ambulance in the autumn of 1946, an English-Polish dictionary being among my most coveted possessions. From that moment my love–hate relationship with England began.

I was drafted to Atcham, near Shrewsbury, where Polish soldiers

* Containing hydrogen of double the usual mass.

who decided to return to their country, waited repatriation at the Transit Camp; by April 1946 some 23,000 had applied. I opened a medical post and a small infirmary in what was previously an American base. The building was well constructed and centrally heated. This was a blessing as the winter of 1946 was a severe one. In January 1947 I had an inspection by a Polish officer of advanced rank and age. He told me he had visited several camps and found life there disorganized because of frozen pipes. He was surprised to hear that this was not the case with us – the central heating saved us. He asked to see the lavatories and pulled the chain in each one. On hearing the noise of the cascading water a bright smile lit up his face; he listened as though he were a pupil of a conservatorium listening to Rachmaninov's Second Piano Concerto. "It is like music" he said, "I have not heard it for some weeks". He was sorry when the "tune" ceased. The place was dull and the atmosphere depressive, the weather did not improve matters.

I spent most of my spare time in the company of a patient who knew that he would soon die of a fatal disease of bone marrow – multiple myeloma, diagnosed some eight months previously. He was 49 and resigned to his fate, wishing to die among his family and in his own country. To-day the prospect of recovery from this disease is not so hopeless. I was tucked away from civilization pondering, on my short walks to Atcham's 18th century bridge, what the future had in store for me.

I spent my short leave in London and saw Professor Dible's first assistant in the Institute of Pathology at Hammersmith Hospital. I realized that for my future advancement in medicine I would have to pass the examination for Membership, but long before that I would have to master English. It was now universally spoken. In the early 20th century a citizen of Warsaw by the name of Zamenhof invented Esperanto hoping it would become a popular international language, but he did not quite succeed. The vast increase in communication between nations brought a great need for a common language, all the more so since Latin went out of existence (these days even from the doctor's vocabulary). Only the proprietary drugs are still bestowed with Latin names – their meanings are very promising – "Safe Aspirin", "Without equal", "Good sleep" . . . One wonders if Latin is used to hide such promises from the public.

My first stay in London was not exactly a qualified success – the metropolis was too big to be easily absorbed, everyone was a stranger, powdered eggs and soya sausages replaced spaghetti and pasta. Britain continued rationing longer than any other country, Germany included.* To see a film I had to freeze in a long queue outside the cinema. I went to Selfridges Departmental Store to purchase a percolator but by mistake asked for a perambulator and got annoyed when directed to the "wrong" department. The only thing in London familiar to me was its fog. It descended mercilessly at the end of a tiring day, making my eyes and throat sore and causing me to lose the way to my lodgings – just what I expected of London, having heard and read about its fog and having seen it on numerous drawings and photographs. Some years later I read of an American firm which was selling authentic fog samples as a souvenir from London. The Spring changed all this.

I admired the beauty of the countryside with its blossoms of various colours and the loveliness of spring flowers. There were many interesting places to visit. I liked Shrewsbury, a County town near Atcham with its old timbered houses, a dignified 17th century Guildhall, quaintly named streets and easy-going Salopians. In front of the library I noticed a bronze statue of Darwin – a native of Shrewsbury. I called on my friend Gustav who was in Chester. This is another County town with more timbered houses and well-preserved city walls of red stone, both medieval in character. Chester is the size of Shrewsbury but even more attractive. Here I saw many Roman remains, among them some columns, remnants of a fort tower and an amphitheatre with room for 9,000 spectators dated 100 A.D. I learned later that in the Roman settlement Aquae Sulis, now known as Bath, the Romans established an elaborate system of baths in 54 A.D. No doubt the Romans were vigorous, enterprising people. To-day the hot mineral springs are used for bathing and drinking by sufferers of rheumatism, gout, digestive disorders, victims of poliomyelitis and others anxious to restore their health and muscles. Returning to Chester, I was told that the place called Infirmary Field, situated not far from the Royal Infirmary, harbours many bodies of people who died of the plague when it ravaged the town in the old days.

In the meantime, the British Government ordered the formation of the Polish Resettlement Corps preparatory to demobilization of our Forces. Consequently I was granted temporary registration in the Medical Register and accepted a full-time post as Medical Officer in the Tuberculosis Unit of Polish General Hospital with 460 beds. Apart

* Rationing in Britain ended in 1954.

from soldiers, we had refugees, men and women, who flocked to the Corps from Poland, Germany and France.

The hospital had some fifteen doctors who had to pass the examination for the lower certificate in English. We went to Birmingham by train, all nervous of the approaching event. It was interesting to see the head of my department with the same worried look as mine. Only one man towered over all of us; his command of English was excellent and he was well conversant with English literature. He felt it was beneath his dignity to sit for the lower certificate, so he applied for the higher one and passed with flying colours. Dr. K. was a bright boy, and I was not in the least surprised when some years later he became a consultant of a teaching hospital and author of important medical papers.

To obtain the lower certificate in English of the University of Cambridge, I had to do dictation, reading, conversation, English composition and translation from and into English, for which a set time was given. All went smoothly until, in translation from Polish into English, I came across the word "step-mother". For the life of me I could not remember it and helplessly cursed all step-mothers on this earth, in Polish of course! I glanced at my watch and decided on the nearest description. I wrote: "Second-hand mother", in haste. The examiner understood, I passed, but my battle with the language was not yet over. Why say "kernel" when it is spelt colonel? How does one pronounce polish your Polish? How appalling to think that we have too many Poles, when one means *polls*. Was it her hare or hair? I knew what was new but could not spell it! And there was the weather, whether you liked it or not. How does one interpret on hearing that a Pole fought with a pole? No wonder my countrymen coined a new phrase – "The wooden wedding" – meaning two Poles got married . . .

In the train on the way back, all worried looks gone, we were singing with the head of our department joining in. We soon returned to our arduous duties and dealt with severe, distressing and some hopeless cases like those of tuberculous laryngitis in advanced stages. We had a good X-ray department with facilities for tomography, and we screened patients regularly. The majority of them developed the disease through deprivation and stresses which led to diminished resistance. Here they were provided with rest and good food in the hope of arresting their fevers and until now irrepressible coughs. As always, rest was the most promising weapon in our armament. Should this fail, there was the collapse therapy of various grades. In the second half of the nineteenth century Carlo Forlanini showed how to immobilize the diseased lung by injecting gas into the pleural cavity – we call it artificial pneumothorax. Such treatment was very useful, but it was not always free of complications, and it still required supportive measures – *REST* and good food.

In cases of failure, we resorted to other measures. In 1931 Banyai, whilst attempting artificial pneumothorax, introduced air into the abdomen due to a faulty technique. He was amazed to find that this brought improvement in the patient's condition. A new method of lung collapse was discovered – artificial pneumoperitoneum, and we in hospital took full advantage of it; during the three years I was there 199 patients were so treated. Another ray of hope appeared and pregnancy among the tuberculous patients was made just that much safer. These were only minor relaxation measures and less successful cases had to undergo some form of surgery. It could be a minor procedure or removal of portions of some seven to ten ribs to obtain a permanent collapse – so called thoracoplasty.

People under our care were all chronic patients who came to us to stay and who formed a close fraternity. Subconsciously they avoided the healthy population, somehow showing resentment towards them, but at the same time enjoying their privileged status. Among themselves they were very class conscious – patients who underwent thoracoplasty looked with condescension upon friends treated by minor procedures. Their attitude resembled that of the Russians with long sentences against the minor offenders. Women tried to look their best; slim figures, luminous eyes under long lashes and flushed cheeks accentuated their beauty. Being domesticated they made the hospital wards their home more readily than men. They kept themselves occupied by making toy-animals for bed-side companionship. I recollect memorable fêtes with parades of wheelchairs cleverly decorated with flowers into a boutique, gondola, rickshaw, vintage motor-car or perambulator, occupied by smiling patients in national costumes.

Older residents treated new-comers as an established convict would an inexperienced beginner. They greeted them with "Welcome to our midst" and initiated them to their new life which, in fact, amounted to intimidation. The poor souls were told that they would have to start with pneumothorax and end with the full thoracoplasty. A picture of abysmal gloom was painted and the new-arrival was heartbroken before he could exchange a word with a doctor. It took the staff several days to put things right and to gain the patient's confidence. His "colleagues", however, thought it was great fun.

In fact, tuberculosis was still a plague killing many people. One morning I was asked by Dr. B., a bacteriologist, to look through his microscope. Nonchalantly I commented: "Just ordinary tuberculous bacilli". Robert Koch discovered them in the early eighteen eighties, later named after him. They cause tuberculosis in man and many animals – birds, fowl, cattle, fish; since my student years I had seen thousands of them attacking any organ in the body they had chosen. Dr. B., shaking his head, said: "You are wrong, you know, these are not ordinary bacilli, they are *mine*". He pondered that more important people, some younger than he, died from the scourge – Spinoza, Keats, Chopin, Chekhov, Kafka, David Herbert Lawrence, Modigliani . . . The bacilli were Dr. B's. death warrant. I did not know that he was troubled by a cough and discomfort deep in his throat which led him to suspect sinister happenings. He suffered from laryngeal tuberculosis which he contracted in the course of his duties – as in any industry doctors are exposed to occupational hazards. Dr. B. changed his status to a patient, and a very ill one at that.

Fortunately a new drug was discovered and used in 1945 for the first time on a tuberculous patient – streptomycin. It got a terrific amount of publicity; papers reported wonderful cures by the "magic" drug. Such accounts brought a festive atmosphere into our wards and we observed happy faces full of hope. People were planning to pack their bags, ready for departure after a miraculous cure. But it was not to be. One day I saw a patient in his late thirties sitting in bed with tears streaming down his cheeks, a morning paper in his hands. On the front page was an article with the heading: "Streptomycin – not a magic drug." It listed serious side-effects, the problem of resistant strains, the short duration of the "cure". The patient was heart-broken and his mood was soon to be reflected by the rest. They were deceived by extravagant claims, and yet the drug was a life-saver.

In 1949 I treated with excellent results two children suffering from tuberculous meningitis by spinal injections of streptomycin. Up until then it was a fatal disease and I witnessed several deaths from it in the past. Soon we had PAS* and shortly after, Isoniazid which, in combination with streptomycin, were able to deal with all kinds of tuberculosis.

The full scale attack on this scourge had started in earnest. All forms of collapse therapy could be abandoned, the only surgical procedure sometimes applied being removal of the lesion itself or the attacked

* Para-aminosalicylic acid.

162

organ such as a kidney or a joint, with little risk and good results. Nowadays patients are satisfactorily treated at home with few restrictions on their activities. In consequence hospital wards for tuberculous patients were closed and the village at Papworth and that near Maidstone, both of which aimed at rehabilitation of such patients, switched their interests elsewhere. Swiss sanatoria, which for many decades had provided rest in the mountain air, were transformed into sports hotels.

The "invincible" disease was conquered and tuberculomania – a morbid belief that one is affected with tuberculosis – gave way to cancerophobia – the fear of cancer, a disease on the increase. I remember a patient admitted to our hospital with lung cancer, not for treatment but in order to spend the remaining months of his life in less distress. In 1950 I sent a patient with such a disease to Brompton Hospital in London where one of his lungs was removed. He made an excellent recovery and was never informed of the true nature of his disease. Twenty-four years later he is still doing well but complaining that he should not have had the operation as he couldn't hurry now as much as he did in the past. He was lucky though, for in spite of improved prognosis, lung cancer continues to carry a high mortality. The chest hospitals are still very much in existence, this time for patients with cancer, chronic bronchitis and heart diseases.

16

MD in Scotland – TB in England

> Life can only be understood backwards, but it must be
> lived forwards. *Sören Kierkegaard*

I had learned a great deal in the last few years, but to advance my status I knew I would have to aim for higher qualifications. From Durham University I received acknowledgement of my letter informing me that only persons who were Medical Graduates of the University could be admitted to the Degree of M.D. I heard that in March 1941 the University of Edinburgh founded the Polish School of Medicine, the only academic institution the Poles had at that tragic time when the ruthless Nazi terror was turning their country into an intellectual desert. In the past they struggled successfully against Russification by the Tsars and Germanization by the strong Chancellor Bismarck, but those rules were paradise compared to Hitler's régime. The idea of the Polish Faculty was conceived by Professor Crew of Edinburgh University and executed with the whole-hearted support of the Principal Sir Thomas Holland, the Dean Professor Sydney Smith, Professor Davidson and other members of the Faculty. They resolved to rescue the culture of a nation which produced Copernicus, Chopin, Paderewski, Wieniawski, Szymanowski, Joseph Conrad Korzeniowski, Sienkiewicz and Madame Curie. British people helped the Polish Forces to land on their shores after the collapse of France, and now the Scots were offering their sympathy, friendship and hospitality. Poles received generous gifts from the British Council, the Graduates Association of Edinburgh University, the publishers Livingstone and private individuals; it was an amazing gesture as they themselves were in peril. Clinics, hospital wards, laboratories, lecture rooms, etc., were provided. Chairs which could not be filled by Polish professors were taken over by their Scottish colleagues, and special courses in the English language were organized. It was another example of people

164

knowing hardship being more responsive to the sufferings of others. A similar reception greeted Poles in Edinburgh in 1831, after their unsuccessful rising, but the British were not at war then.

Besides, the Scottish people were returning Polish hospitality. In the sixteenth and seventeenth centuries, "golden age" of Poland, many Scots settled there driven either by religious persecution or the urge for adventure. When Spain, Germany, France and England witnessed religious strife, Poland guaranteed religious tolerance by a law passed in 1573. Some were soldiers of fortune,* some merchants, churchmen, doctors and diplomats "living industriously and honestly among foreigners". Larger cities had well-organized Scottish communities of some 30,000 families, and their national solidarity and care for the poor and ailing was proverbial. One member of such a community, an 18th century merchant by the name of Robert Brown, left a fund in his will to educate in Edinburgh two students from Poland of the Protestant religion and it is still functioning to this very day. Another Scot – Alexander Chalmers** – was four times Mayor of Warsaw, and John Stuart became the Chamberlain of Stanislav August Poniatowski, the last King of Poland. His son Geoffrey defended the monastery fortress of Czestochowa against the Austrians in 1809 and ten years later was promoted General. Dr. William Davidson was Senior Surgeon to John Casimir, the King of Poland; he published a number of works "amid the roar of cannon, the tumult of advancing and retreating armies and all miseries and dangers of war".

Many Scots were ennobled and the Polish nobility (Czartoryski, Poniatowski, Sobieski) married into the Scottish aristocracy. And so Scotland was an obvious choice for Polish exiles in 1831. Even earlier Dr. Andrew Sniadecki chose Edinburgh, famous for her Medical School, for postgraduate studies. Influenced by renowned Alexander Monro, James Gregory and Andrew Duncan, remembering the household name of John Cheyne, he returned to Poland and organized medical studies at my University of Vilna. A later graduate of that University, Lach-Szyrma, stayed several years in Edinburgh and on his return, impressed and in gratitude, he gave a beautiful picture of life in Scotland and of its customs and peculiarities. He described Sir Walter Scott and her other great men. Lach-Szyrma subsequently be-

* Prince Radziwill had special Scottish units in his private forces at the Court in Kieydany, and in the battle of Chocim in 1621 Scottish, English and Irish soldiers fought on the Polish side against the Turks.

** His tombstone in the Warsaw Cathedral perished with the destruction of the city in the Warsaw rising of 1944.

came a political exile in London. An exile by the name of Gregorowicz graduated at the Medical Faculty, Edinburgh, then dominated by Charles Bell and James Syme, and practised there. His obituary in "The Scotsman" of June 6, 1838 read: "His death was occasioned by the generous and fearless discharge of his duties for a poor family afflicted with typhus fever in the land which gave him asylum". Nine years later the already well-known Edinburgh professor of obstetrics, James Young Simpson, achieved painless delivery by means of chloroform. Much has been achieved since 1505 in which Surgeons and Barbers of Edinburgh were formed into a Corporation, receiving the monopoly of the sale of whisky. Many illustrious teachers appeared in the Edinburgh Medical School, among them Joseph Lister, and a host of its pupils became world-famous, like Addison, Bright, Graves, Stokes, Colles, Corrigan, Hodgkins, Leishman and Conan Doyle.

Polish fighters for freedom arrived again in Britain and the hospitable Scottish people opened the University to them, enabling the exiles to continue their intellectual life which had been interrupted. Poland's 7 universities and 21 academic schools were closed by the Germans who commented that "The Poles, as slave people, do not need education". In 1941 a great number of intellectuals were sent to the infamous concentration camp at Auschwitz (Oswiecim), among them the outstanding actor Stefan Jaracz and the notable stage director Leon Schiller. The "new order" was taking shape.

The atmosphere of Edinburgh had something which I had already experienced in Vilna. Students from various parts of the world added to the Scottish culture and folklore. I remember when I saw a Scotsman in a kilt for the first time; he was photographing a Papal Guard in Rome and I was most intrigued and undecided to whom my attention should go first. And here they were parading in various kilts, adorned by a sporran and skian dhu tucked under the colourful hose, speaking in their lilting accent. I heard of their Highland Games – a toss of the caber and throw of the hammer – listened to their bagpipes, a Scottish counterpart of a Polish kobza, tasted their porridge and haggis. It was not surprising that the Poles joined in their social activities, and girl students in national costumes performed folk dances. Poles were not in strange surroundings after all. Edinburgh behaved not as a stepmother to them, but as a *first*-hand mother. She adopted the orphaned youths with warmth and generosity, gave them a helping hand, shelter, food, cared for their intellectual needs, guided them, displayed unfailing kindness, understanding, consideration, forbearance,

166

interest in their welfare and taught them to speak, like any good mother would. She restored their faith in people and their own future, inspired and encouraged them to love again. It was just like coming home, only the language difficulty and the example shown to them changed Poles from good talkers to good doers ... In 1946 I met a Scottish family who gave a home to a Polish officer who was a friend for some years, and was now dying of tuberculosis. I escorted him from our hospital to their home in Stonehaven and witnessed a touching reunion.

On March 22, 1941, the inauguration ceremony of the Polish School of Medicine took place in the McEvan Hall. This hall symbolized a tradition of alma mater (some 400 years old), which has been engaged in a major Scottish industry – education. The ceremony began with the opening speech of Sir Thomas Holland – who reminded the audience that history repeated itself – some 800 years ago the schools of the Roman Empire were swept away by other Teutonic savages. He quoted words used in Napoleonic times by the younger William Pitt: "It is our just exultation, that we provide not only for our own safety, but hold out a prospect to nations now bending under the iron yoke of tyranny ... at least in this corner of the world, the name of liberty is still revered, cherished and sanctified". In turn Professor Sydney Smith, on behalf of the University, offered the place in which to work – freely, with complete sympathy, understanding and co-operation.

The School continued until 1949 and produced 227 medical graduates, many of whom were still able to soldier on. A hundred settled in Britain,* others went out all over the world. Years later at a reunion, one graduate proudly announced that he served with the Polish destroyer "Piorun" (Thunder), which engaged with the world's biggest German battleship "Bismarck" (45,000 tons) before the British brought an end to her. I was one of the nineteen who obtained the M.D. degree, guided by Senior Lecturer Tomaszewski. After acceptance of my thesis and examinations by Professor Cameron, who held the Chair in tuberculosis, and Professor Rostowski, the popular Dean of the Polish School of Medicine from 1946 until its closure, (his subject was neurology), I received my diploma. I was addressed in Latin by my Promotor, Professor Sir Stanley Davidson, wearing cap and gown. I listened to his pronunciation, so different from what I had

* The Medical Practitioners and Pharmacists Act 1947 allowed graduates of the Polish School to register as medical practitioners in the United Kingdom.

heard in Poland, but who is to say what the Roman language sounded like when we have only the written word to be guided by?

In June 1966, the University of Edinburgh conferred the Honorary Degree of Doctor of Law upon Professor Rostowski; in 1909 a similar honour fell on Madame Sklodowska-Curie – twice Nobel Prize winner who gave radium to mankind. In the quadrangle of the Medical Buildings in Edinburgh a plaque commemorates the Polish School of Medicine.

Back in the hospital where I worked, a man from the "Prudential Assurance Company" approached me asking: "What are your plans?" "To stay in Britain", I replied. "Then," he said with a smug smile and expression of a man who knows, "Then," he repeated, "you must take out a policy". He produced some figures showing how much I could get in 25 years on simple monthly payments – even better, a lump sum, should I lose a limb or an eye, or if I had the good fortune to drop dead. "Endowment should be your choice", he declared. With my past in mind, I settled for a 15-year-policy. I had faith in "The Prudential". I remembered their imposing offices in pre-war Warsaw – its first skyscraper – and I was confident that the present destruction of it would not alter the Company's financial status. One day we had a visitor from the Ministry in Poland. He hoped to enrol some doctors for work in their native country, but failed – no one applied. We all celebrated May 3 – Poland's Independence Day – as usual far from our land. I carried on screening the hollow-chested men with drooping shoulders who continued to file into the X-ray department. I was pushing air into their tummies, tapping fluids, rescuing the unfortunate ones from tension pneumothorax, taking care of those who recently underwent thoracoplasty, chasing tubercle bacilli . . . A Psychiatric Wing was attached to the hospital, with an additional team of doctors. I decided to visit an old colleague of mine who had been detained there some time ago. I had known him from our Cadet School days, then a cheerful promising pupil. I found the meeting very depressing. I hardly recognized in this pale, thin, vacant-looking, restless man the chubby, rosy-cheeked colleague of the old days. He could not register who I was. In the locked-up ward were many more such cases, the war had taken its toll.

Shortly afterwards I received the following letter from The War Office,
"Sir,
I am directed to inform you that, in view of your absorption into in-

dustry, you will relinquish your commission in the Polish Resettlement Corps with effect from March 16, 1948". The letter was signed on behalf of the Military Secretary who was a Lieutenant-General. I felt highly honoured to be addressed as "Sir", and that the letter ended with "I am, Sir,

Your obedient Servant".

It was a good start to my civilian life. I rejoiced, I was not made for a uniform. Subconsciously I hummed an old army song:

> "When I get my civvy clothes on
> Oh how happy I shall be.
> When I get my civvy clothes on —
> No more soldiering for me."

Shortly after obtaining the permanent registration with the General Medical Council* I started work in a British sanatorium where patients were treated with rest on open verandas, nourishing food, minor collapse therapy, Streptomycin and PAS. I found them more disciplined than the Polish patients. Here I completed an article which was subsequently published in the British Journal of Tuberculosis (July 1949).** Earlier, I had approached various Universities and Institutes in the U.S.A., France, Italy, Germany and Russia (as shown in my "References") for scientific information. I received helpful data from every one except the Soviet Union. The authorities there did not trouble to apologize, give an excuse or even the customary acknowledgement. The "iron curtain" was truly down.

Soon I was on the move again, this time as a Medical Registrar in a hospital in the London region which specialized in chest diseases. It had many facilities and was administered by a kindly man. The patients there, like most tuberculous patients all over the world, felt very much at home. On my first round on the wards, when I asked a bedridden patient how he felt, he answered with an expressionless face: "Bob's your uncle". "Very well", I said, being completely lost. At the first opportunity I asked the ward sister who accompanied me what he meant. "He probably did not wish to say O.K., not being in favour of American slang". In the next ward there was a patient whose time was running out, and he was too weak to speak. I stopped at the bottom of his bed and in small talk said some consoling words. He managed to

---

* By the Medical Act of 1858 doctors who wish to practise within the British Isles have to be on the Medical Register controlled by the General Medical Council.

** Cavities of the lower lobe in pulmonary tuberculosis. Pathology and treatment, with special reference to pneumoperitoneum.

give me a faint smile, and motioned me to come closer. On coming nearer I heard him whisper: "Doctor, I have good news for you, I can't be any worse . . ." Three days later he was dead. Some people have guts!

I began to study for Membership but found it heavy going; I was far from being happy.

Only now did I realize the full implications of the happenings in Poland. Contact with my country, now behind the "iron curtain", was very scanty, but eventually I was able to get in touch with an old friend who remained in Warsaw and survived. She wrote to me and enclosed a letter from my mother. It had the mark of the Red Cross and the words "Not known" stamped on the envelope. I had to gather all my courage to open it and many minutes passed before I was ready for it. It read: "My dear Bronek, I hope that this will find you in good health and spirits. I am glad to say I keep reasonably well and wait for the time of our reunion. Be brave, we are all at the mercy of God. Your loving Mother". "A million thanks, dear mother", I said to myself. The letter was dated September, 1943. My friend explained that the letter had been returned to the flat she shared with my then widowed mother, and she kept it in the hope of it reaching me one day. "Your mother", she continued, "was shot dead in the street the following spring during an exchange of fire". She was 65 and unable to run fast enough.

"There will be no reunion; where is God's mercy?" I cried. I felt blasphemous. Acting like the all mighty God, who is He to stay away from it all, trying to rule the greedy, aggressive, predatory, sinful, wicked mob from His glorious throne in Heaven where no prayer could reach Him? Infallible as the Pope! I heard myself mutter. All the good things told about Him – the "Loving God" seemed like a fable to me – there could not be a grain of truth in it. Our Creator?, Deliverer?, Creator and deliverer of what? If there ever was a Kingdom of God, it was turned into a bloody dictatorship. Life was as bad as death. God, possibly frustrated with His own creation, washed his hands of the whole business, leaving it to low-minded amateurs, ambitious egoists and advocates of violence, thus behaving like any deserter. He connived with the world's brutal forces and good, gentle people were not given a chance. Or was He duped? Did He age and get weary of mankind? Why did He let loose sorrow and death? Could it be that He began to hate his creation and was trying to destroy it? Did He attempt to bring the Fear of God into us as an ageing tyrant does? Perhaps He

170

fell into a long sleep whilst I was very much awake – mine were no dreams of Hell but reality. The best I could think of Him was that He did not exist at all. Was it then the Devil who made the world? Has the word "God" no meaning whatsoever? The question WHY remained.

Days passed and I heard of more and more horrors. An aunt of mine who remained in Warsaw with her two daughters heard German soldiers kicking on her gate one day and banging with their rifle butts. She opened her window and heard them shouting "Aufmachen!" (Open!). It was the day of the funeral of the SS Brigade-Fuehrer Kutschera, the hated commander of the SS and German Police, "the murderer of Warsaw", assassinated by the Polish underground on February 1, 1944. On the day of the funeral the Nazis drove the civilian population away from the houses along the route of the procession. Time stood still for my aunt, gripped with fear. Suddenly her nerve snapped; struck by the thought that the Nazis had come to take them away, she threw herself out of the window and landed on the pavement. One of her daughters followed her. They both died in agony a few hours later.

My cousin Jerzy (George) Gelbard, a well-known architect before the war, also stayed in Warsaw. He was a talented artist who exhibited his paintings in the French and Polish capitals. His wife Bela was very "arty" and liked to write articles for papers on various subjects, mainly stories about pet animals. She liked a Bohemian life and spent a lot of time among interesting people – writers, artists, singers, musicians – all brainy and having a zest for life, but penniless. They used to gather in the "Ziemianska" coffee-house in Mazowiecka Street. I vividly remember the day when I was invited to a big reception at my aunt's house. It was held in the same flat from which she later threw herself to the pavement. The large extended table in the dining room was laden with good things – large cakes, doughnuts, various pastries, sweets, nuts, dates, figs, grapes, apples . . . It was a feast to be . . . Bela arrived first, I soon followed her, and she let me into her conspiracy. In the yard several hungry artists had already gathered, invited by Bela. I watched and abetted her in lowering the wonderful cakes and fruit down, in a basket on a string. When the guests arrived, they found the reception rather disappointing . . . My aunt nearly had a fit when she realized what had happened, and was not on speaking terms with Bela for some time because of this prank. The light-hearted amusing incident took place six years before the war.

In 1940 Bela found herself in the Warsaw Ghetto. She was determined to survive, possessed by the desire to find out what the future would bring and to be able to tell the truth to people. It would be a thrill to tell someone afterwards: "You behaved like a swine, and no doubt you have not changed!" Living most of her life in fantasy, she talked of snow falling in the ghetto streets in August – she meant feathers dropping down from the eiderdowns ripped up by greedy SS men looking for hidden valuables. Her husband George bribed an SS man, who smuggled her to the nearby Otwock where she later witnessed Adele Tuwim, the mother of a Polish poet, being thrown out of a window by a Nazi thug, and the liquidation of the ghetto there. She escaped and found shelter with a poor village blacksmith who lacked both education and religious devotion. Neither the well-to-do people nor the ardent practitioners of prayers wished to have anything to do with her, since they were all afraid of reprisals. The blacksmith endowed her with his sister's name – Czajka (lapwing) which she kept for good. Bela herself began to loath the word "Jew". Now she hoped to be safe and the smell of manure from the cowshed was heaven to her. Heaven? Does it exist? For a while she thought it did. Christmas came and George managed to join her; she watched him painting, humming Parisien songs and laughing. However, in January, the daughter of the blacksmith brought George bad news from Warsaw – his best friends, a Jewish woman and her daughter he had left in a hide-out, were threatened by a blackmailer who hoped to extort a large sum of money from them for his silence. Without hesitation he left for Warsaw hoping to return with them, but the Gestapo arrested all three. George, who had forged papers, was kept in the Paviak prison for nearly nine months and tortured; he never returned.

One night Bela was awakened by the familiar noise of rifle butt blows, strong searchlights and shouts of "Aufmachen, Sicherheits polizei." It was like a scene from Dante's "Inferno". "This must be the end, I have lived forty-one troubled years, it will be a relief", she thought in a flash. Instinctively she looked in her mirror and saw her pale, wrinkled face, with bags under her eyes – the face of an old woman. The events of the last years brought her to near insanity, but in the face of sure death she was sane enough to fake it; miraculously her life was saved once more. She lay very still for a long time imagining she *must* be dead and was afraid to disturb the executioners who would kill her *again*. And so Bela survived this nightmare, saved from the jaws of death not for the first time. Later she wrote several books. In one of them: "I was saved by a blacksmith" she gave an account of her experiences under the German occupation – this time it was not fiction but human drama. She greeted the Soviet Army with open arms. Bela did not need to be converted, like another dying patient she muttered: "I can't be any worse".

For the rest of her countrymen the Soviets turned on their perfected propaganda. I was told of a conversation between a Soviet and a Polish citizen which took place in September 1939, soon after the Russians entered Poland. The Russian, knowing how difficult it was to obtain shoes in his own country, asked if similar difficulties were encountered in Poland. "Not at all", said the Pole, "You could buy one, two or even three pairs of shoes at the same time". "Really?" asked his companion, full of incredulity. "Do you mean to tell me that if I wished to purchase four pairs at once, I could have them?" "In that case", said the Pole, "they would be delivered to your house". "You amaze me", said the Russian, "I always thought that our propaganda was the best in the world, but I now see that yours is much better . . ."

Life in Poland had to go on. The Germans killed over five million Polish citizens, 3,200,000 of them were Jews.* Those the Gestapo could not trace, they lured, promising them expatriation as foreigners. Through their agents the Gestapo sold passports of Latin American countries and the tricked Jews were taken out of the towns to . . . extermination camps. Yet some hundred thousand of Jews survived thanks to people like Bela's blacksmith and to those who provided them with documents, hide-outs, food, clothes and medicines. Some prominent people were rescued that way.

Professor Ludwik Hirszfeld, a serologist and blood-group specialist of international repute, was found walking among the ruins of Warsaw, dazed and looking like a tramp, after the Germans fled the city. Arnold Szyfman, the long-time director of the Polish Theatre, was another survivor, sheltered by the playwright Morstin. It was not the first time that Poles who found themselves in a similar situation as the Jews showed understanding for their sufferings. After an unsuccessful rising in 1863 against Russian rule Polish sentiment towards down-trodden people was reflected by their famous writer Kraszewski – the author of "The Jew". A great number of the "chosen people" left for the "promised land"; only a tiny minority lives in Poland as Jews enjoying their "Historical Institute", the "Jewish State Theatre" and their own press. Many integrated with the Poles and retained their adopted names; the past was better forgotten. After all what is in a name? I met a heartless Miss Heart, an honest Mr. Fiddler, a solemn

* Out of 3,500,000 who lived in Poland before the war.

Mrs. Giggle, a placid Mrs. Jump, a white Mr. Black, a pale Miss Peach and a rosy cheeked Mrs. Pale, also a Mr. French who did not know a word of French and a Mr. Szczydlowski, born in London, who does not speak Polish. Examples are numerous. The common Jewish name Gitler, the Russian pronunciation for Hitler, would not do either.

The sufferings of the inhabitants of Poland were enormous. There was the case of Kazimierz Junosza Stepowski, an outstanding dramatic actor of pre-war years, who was shot by the resistance in 1943. He was a patriot all his life and trusted by the underground. His wife being addicted to morphia, craved for it and the distraught Junosza wishing to obtain the drug for his wife was forced to pass information, not of any great importance, to the Germans; it cost him his life. Obviously my own war time experiences were a paradise compared to life in Poland. When will the impulse to repay in kind cease! When will "An eye for an eye" policy stop, as it must in a civilized world! "Let's pack up hating each other", I thought.

After all this was over I felt miserable, drained of will, doubtful if I would ever sit for Membership and uncertain of my future. A delayed reaction, I suppose. I had little time to see my Polish friends and even less opportunity to make close liaison with the English. I went to buy flowers for a friend who was ill. In the shop I picked out some tulips myself. Another customer – a man with a reddish complexion, grey clipped moustache, impassive look, wearing a bowler hat and sporting a red carnation and the inevitable umbrella – an old Etonian type, stood beside me watching me closely. In my foreign accent I thanked the manager and on leaving heard the bowler-hatted man say to the florist in a superior manner and King's English: "And for me also two bunches of tulips of *your* choice", stressing the word "your". I went on my way downhearted and deflated, realizing that I was still the odd man out, a thousand-fold stranger. The same day I absentmindedly entered in my hospital notes "fleebites" instead of "phlebitis". It was not my day. The following morning I asked a patient for his date of birth, 1912 came the answer. "What day and month", I enquired. "Charles Dickens birthday", he proudly replied without a smile. I was lost, I still did not know. There was a lot to learn.

At this difficult time, as I was taking my first steps in a foreign land and needed someone to lean on, a terrible thing happened to me – my best friend Gustav died of acute leukaemia after a short illness. I was at the end of my tether and sank into a hopeless gloom, my senses became morbidly torpid, everything seemed discoloured, dark and dull. I was sick of life which was one hard incessant struggle, full of savageness, drudgery and wretchedness. I felt unable to fight my way through it any longer. I was aggrieved by the loss of people I loved and by the wasted years. I abhorred the rapacious, vagrant, miserable life studded with privations, indignities and humiliations, a life difficult to endure. There was no love left in this world, wild beasts were better than people, I thought. The anguish and emotional disturbance were worse than the worst pain. I felt my spirit was completely broken; if only I could pray. I was now forty years old and had little prospect of quick advancement, even should I be successful with examinations for Membership, my attempts seemed futile. Damn the advancement! I had enough of nomadic life, having no chance to make roots and friends, chasing jobs in various parts of the country, facing with trepidation the Honourable Members of the Regional Hospital Boards who threw intimate questions at me — "When did you start to learn English?", "What do you intend to do?", "Have you a family?", "Where are your friends?", "What are your hobbies?". I meant to say on more than one occasion: "Mind your own business", but I did not. It was all so worrying. I noticed that my trousers were getting looser and thought I was losing weight fast. To my relief I soon realized it was not me, only my trousers — the elastic had perished! "For heaven's sake, pull yourself together", I muttered. Gradually, my strength and confidence returned and I began to carve my way through the dark passage of life, still full of thorns. It struck me that love and illness, no matter if a joint phenomenon or two separate events, are part of life, and life without either is no life at all. I began to understand my malady and myself, and felt able to battle with life again.

I learned from a friend that a doctor in a busy practice in Greater London had suddenly lost his partner from a coronary thrombosis. I decided to take the plunge. I got the job, starting as an assistant and laboured for the next two-and-a-half years. It happened in October 1950 and it greatly changed my life. But times have changed and *change* was the order of the day for all people.

17

Is This Peace?

Why did Nature create man? Was it to show that she is big enough to make mistakes, or was it pure ignorance?

Holbrook Jackson

The end of the World War did not mean the end of the world's happenings. No Commonwealth country or Colony was lost by Britain in the War, only after it ended, and the sphere of her influence began to shrink. In August 1947 India turned into two independent states; Burma, Ceylon, Malaya and Iraq followed suit in 1948. Ireland ceased to be a Dominion, and the new state of Israel came into being the same year, giving impetus to the growing Arabism. British-educated African intelligentsia brought "wind of change" to their continent. In 1952 came the Cyprus crisis which lasted five years, and there was another upheaval in the summer of 1974. Racial policies swept through South Africa and Rhodesia. Immense changes were not confined to the British Commonwealth alone – there was chaos in the Belgian Congo, the French were at war against Indo-China and Algeria, Dutch India gained independence, Iceland broke away from Denmark, and several thrones were lost. For the first time in history the Pope left the Vatican for a world tour. Britain had to undergo the process of adaptation. Fortunately common sense replaced Commonwealth and the country was willing and able to adjust itself to the rapid changes around her. She prefers to forget the buccaneering days of the 16th century and has no desire of conquests and domination. Britain recognized the new states of Sudan, Cyprus, Ghana, Nigeria, Sierra Leone, Tanganyika, Kenya, Uganda, Malawi, Jamaica, Malaya, Malta and provides money and other aids to the underdeveloped new-comers, keeping the old ties with them even after they turned into Republics. It is a continuous process. In 1973 the nearly 300 year old British Colonial rule of the Bahamas Islands ended but good will remains. In 1974 Grenada, a volcanic island in the British West Indies, 21 miles long and 12 miles broad, followed suit.

176

Soon after the war the British people were full of praise and admiration for the brave Russians, and they saluted their twenty million dead. The two-and-a-half year siege of Leningrad at the cost of 700,000 lives was fresh in their minds. The politicians were more perceptive – they observed the Soviet expansion to the West through satellite Poland, East Germany, Rumania, Bulgaria, Hungary and in more recent years Czechoslovakia. They also observed the Russian threat to Berlin in 1948/9 and beyond, the Communist troops of North Korea attacking South Korea and a similar situation in Vietnam later on. They observed the actions of the Bolivian Army of National Liberation inspired by the revolutionary Che Guevara and those of the Uruguayan Tupamaros, the Philippine guerillas calling themselves the "New People's Army," the left-wing activists of the Middle East, the Marxist "People's Revolutionary Army" in Argentina with other threats of a Communist takeover. The Soviets had two names for the same happenings – the "Western imperialism" for their allies and the "liberation" for themselves: they call others fascists, a term which could be reserved for them. In 1949 the Russian scientists exploded an atom bomb which was believed to be stolen from the West. One of their physicists was Peter Kapitza, a former Cambridge student, Fellow of Trinity College, assistant director at the Cavendish Laboratory and director of the Mond Laboratory. In 1934 he was on a visit to Soviet Russia – at the time of the defection to the West of the young Russian mathematician Gom. Kapitza was detained by the Soviets in spite of the intervention of Lord Rutherford and subsequently became director of the Institute of Physical Problems in Moscow. The German born Klaus Fuchs, an atomic scientist who adopted Britain, turned traitor and passed vital secrets to the Russians; he was arrested in 1950.

In the Far East, China became a Communist country under Chairman Mao Tse Tung. On March 5, 1953, Stalin died and although the nightmare ended, Russian world policy remained unchanged as shown by the Cuban crisis of 1962, their continually increasing force on land, sea and in the air* and the continuous expansion of their influence which started with the October Revolution of 1917.

Kremlinology was still worth studying. Charles Bohlen, once the U.S.A. Ambassador to the U.S.S.R., confessed that the two most ridiculous statements he knew were: "Liquor doesn't affect me" and "I understand the Russians."

* Among her combat aircraft Russia has a twice-the-speed-of-sound bomber "Backfire" and her advanced surface to air guided missiles (SAMs) used in the Arab–Israeli war of 1973 surprised the West. 40% of Soviet national income goes to military needs.

In fact, the United States and Russia were at loggerheads and between these giants, Britain, remembering the last two wars, could not possibly feel secure. In 1952 Britain exploded an atom bomb, and three years later the hydrogen bomb. The bomb which destroyed Hiroshima was already obsolete. Soon after the explosion of the British atom bomb, the Americans exploded the hydrogen bomb, but in November 1952 its secrets were passed to the Soviets by the Rosenberg husband-and-wife-team. Later on France and China joined the "nuclear club." H stands for Hydrogen bomb and . . . Homo sapiens.

The wonders of modern science were not making life easier or safer, just the reverse – the powerful bombs, the spy-satellites forever increasing in size and number, electronic intelligence planes and electronic countermeasures (ECM) make life more complicated and defence more difficult. Fifteen thousand people marched from Aldermaston to Trafalgar Square in protest. Facing modern age and realities, Britain ended National Service and joined NATO, where all members contributed force to serve under a joint command in search of security and ultimate peace. It is easy to be afraid that history might repeat itself. There are many analogies. The United Nations Organization, founded to guard peace, reminds one of the League of Nations on which hopes were built before the second World War. The German Chancellor Herr Willy Brandt received the Nobel peace prize in 1971, as did another German Chancellor Stresemann who was so honoured in 1926. Could Brandt's* efforts be thwarted like those of Stresemann? Could there be another Hitler who would try to prove himself? Could nuclear weapons be home made and used by terrorists or criminals? Who knows? In spite of all this the United Nations Organization was a big step forward, and that it instituted the World Health Organization in 1948 was a good omen.

* Disillusioned, Brandt quit his office in May 1974.

18
The National Health Service is Born

I'm not denyin' the women are foolish. God Almighty made
'em to match the men.

Havelock Ellis

Prescriptions are shorter than arguments.

Richard Asher

The reason why worry kills more people than work is that
more people worry than work.

Robert Frost

Immediately after the war, power in Britain went to the Labour
Government under the Premiership of Mr. Attlee. In spite of difficulties in which the country found itself after the devastations, the
Government implemented the principles of a Welfare State with the
aim of giving opportunity to everyone. British people, undaunted by
years of war, were extending the Social Security measures and putting
faith in their future. Aneurin Bevan, then forty-seven years of age, was
made Minister of Health. A man of lucid mind and purpose, he pronounced that it is better to have a future than a past and that he came
to London to change the world. Like most colourful personalities he
had friends and enemies. The friends called him Nye and the enemies
called him "incorrigible rebel", "irresponsible bully", "arrogant
block-head", "Fuehrer" or just "a dangerous fellow".

His most bitter opponents were doctors, particularly the older ones.
They were afraid that he would destroy the tradition of their honoured profession, cause interference between doctor and patient, abol-
ish privacy, force them to treat ill people as numbers, violate the
principles of secrecy, encourage bureaucracy and introduce politics to
a non-political body; doctors' individualism would suffer and a more
casual relationship would ensue. They hurled abuse at him and dis-
paragingly called him Lord Thrombosis – a bloody clot in need of removal . . .

The B.M.A. declared itself against his proposals, and yet Aneurin
Bevan's plans were only the outcome of a gradual process which led

179

through Lloyd George's pre-War I implementation of the Health Insurance Scheme and the announcement of the Sir William Beveridge Report in 1942, accepted two years later. Bevan proposed a more even distribution of doctors and improvement of hospital facilities which the country lacked after the war. He wished to introduce a comprehensive administration to tackle the problem of the disabled, infirm and mentally sick, above all to make this service available to everyone – a unique undertaking. It was an effort to protect the health of the nation. Why then should they blame him for it?

It was a challenge which required time for reflection – a formidable organization with a new concept was proposed, and in the best tradition of the nation it was accepted by the doctors and patients alike, in spite of all the things which were said. It happened a bare three years after the war ended.

By July 5, 1948, the Appointed Day, three-quarters of the population had registered with the N.H.S. and two months later nearly 86% of General Practitioners had joined in.

I entered General Practice in October 1950. It was not a drift. I wished to embrace larger spheres of medicine, to see and treat patients at first-hand from start to finish, to know them better by establishing a more permanent relationship and to feel that they chose me. I looked forward to taking all responsibility on myself without interference and I welcomed the removal of the barrier of payment by the patients. It was comforting to know that I did not need to think of the client's pocket when prescribing treatment – an event gratifying to both parties. I heard a patient saying: "I was relieved to wake up from the anaesthetic without racking my brains how to foot the bill". Certainly no one went broke in Britain because of treatment one had received. Yet it was not exactly what I expected. The service was still in its infancy, far from running smoothly. I had more work than I could handle. Many who previously could not afford treatment were now taking advantage of the new service – they needed glasses, hearing aids, false teeth various investigations. Others were filling surgeries for trivialities, mostly laxatives – the penalty of civilization – all free of charge. The rest were attracted by the novelty or the wish to get something out of it, without actually being ill. A young man, a picture of health, weighing some thirteen stones, looked round my surgery as if he were in a "Delicatessen".

"What's wrong with you?" I asked.

"I am all right", he said, "but do you think you could prescribe some

180

cod liver oil for me?"

"Certainly not", I replied.

"Bad luck", he said with annoyance. "One has to be ill to get something . . ."

"No sign of ill health is the best sign I know," I commented. Perhaps I behaved as meanly as Nature which allows one to have only one whooping cough, one measles, one chickenpox in a life time . . .

The next "patient" was a woman with a little boy. She requested ear drops for him and was surprised that I looked into his ears. "There is nothing the matter with his ears," I said.

"But his chest, doctor," she continued, and was even more surprised that I wished to examine his chest.

"There is nothing wrong with his chest, either," I then pronounced.

With an air of disappointment, but still undeterred, she requested throat lozenges "which he likes so much . . ."

My patience exhausted, I told her: "Please do not waste our time in the future but go straight to the chemist. He will serve you with anything you choose". She departed offended and came off my list — it was my first casualty in general practice, without a pang of regret, however, on my part. In those early days, neither patients nor doctors were really settled. Some members of the venerable profession would try to attract clients by yielding to their demands and prescribing medicines and magic tonics uncalled for, or unwarranted large amounts of gauze, cotton wool and the like. There were doctors who spurned the new service, pursuing private patients and leaving the rest to their assistants, adding generously more risky calls which could have been a suspected smallpox and the like. It surprised me to meet patients who did not wish to be examined but were prepared to wait for hours just to see what they could get. After spending a lot of time with one, questioning and examining him, I would be accused of not giving proper attention should I omit the expected prescription. They came to the surgery with every little cold, leaving it with me and saying: "I prefer to see you, doctor, as you are a chest specialist. Some just came to assure themselves that they hadn't got a cold. Reassured they would say: "I also have *another smaller* complaint . . ."

A great number of patients, mostly women, often in the "change of life" when the production of female hormones begin to wane, fall to the strains and stresses of modern society, also loneliness. Left alone all day to their own devices, they anxiously await their husbands return. They were not well when they had their periods, and now they had lost them they didn't feel any better! Others had pre-examination, pre-marriage, pre-flying, pre-dental anxieties and the like! I treated patients for xenophobias, agoraphobias, claustrophobias, acrophobias, travelphobias, cancerophobias etcetera, etcetera, etcetera. I was able to reassure a patient that he didn't have lung cancer which he feared; it took a few sessions and I congratulated myself. He returned some weeks later greeting me with: "You did a good job, doctor, I know I have no lung cancer, but I worry about my wart, do you think it could be cancer?" Freeing the patient from one worry gave him the opportunity to invent another.

A very agitated woman came to me shaking and stammering: "I am going mad, I hear voices all the time." I was puzzled and gave her a sedative. She returned the same evening, all smiles, saying: "It is all right, it was only my neighbour who had a transistor in his garden". She lived up to her name, which was Jelly. All these people suffered from fear, through fear that they might suffer. Once an elderly spinster told me that in her case the miracle of creation was suppressed — she was going to see a proper doctor, meaning a psychiatrist. He later told me that she refused all medicines regarding them as poison; perhaps she had more sense than she was credited with!

To the few "never well" I made excuses, saying to myself: "Perhaps I tend to see the most miserable side of them when they visit me". I tried to help with drugs and friendly advice. I suggested to one woman that she bought a television set. She had a long history of neurosis and felt lonely because her husband, a busy executive, had to be away from home a great deal. It worked. Engrossed in musical programmes, she forgot the doctor. I was encouraged by this success and when another patient, a hard-working, down-to-earth woman, could not snap out of the depression caused by her husband's death and the loss of a life-long companion, I naturally made the same suggestion. I did not see her again for over a year and reckoned I had scored another success. One day she walked into my surgery with a minor skin complaint, well and happy. "I see my advice helped you a great deal", I said presumptuously, with a smile.

"Oh no, doctor, I watched the programmes for a while but the constant violence, sex, bad news, etc. made me cry. I feel much better though since I sold the set . . ."

I learned that there is seldom a place for a routine treatment in medicine and no one should wonder that doctors have to differ in their approach to patients. I remember a woman taking a lot of my time with most irrelevant details, when I had asked her to be brief. I heard her say with a voice betraying disappointment: "But my previous doctor insisted on my telling him *everything*!" I imagine he was not only her doctor and counsellor but confessor as well.

I once patiently listened to a long list of complaints of a "never well". She did not know my pain was worse than hers as I had cracked three ribs the previous night but had no one to whom I could complain! I found that the image of a doctor is such that he is a man apart who cannot possibly be ill, tired or suffer from any complaints reserved for his patients. "Fancy a doctor being ill!" He is also expected to have a supernatural memory. I was stopped in the street by a patient who asked me to write a prescription for "his pills". I was tempted to send him to Timbuktu but, not knowing at the time where it was, I asked with resignation: "Which ones?". "You surely must know, doctor, the white ones".

Doctors are also expected to remember the names of all their patients. I tried to keep up this image but not always with success. I once greeted a patient in the surgery, whom I had not seen for a few years, with "How are you Mr. Bishop?" He smiled and said: "You have promoted me, doctor, my name is Parson". I was not far off! In another instance, at the end of a busy surgery, I forgot the name of a woman who thought herself *the* most important patient in the practice. This horrified her and she came off my list the next day. But I remembered Mr. Fish well — he came with a swimmy head. There was something fishy about him . . .

People with backache posed a problem; often there was little one could do apart from advising them to rest and be patient. Nine out of ten are cured that way, but such advice was not always taken kindly.

"Doctor, I have backache and it keeps on and on," I heard.

"When did it start?" I enquired.

"Yesterday," came the answer.

One patient, already several weeks off work with backache, asked me for his *intimate* certificate, meaning an intermediate one. I saw a great number of such sufferers, many of them giving a history of some kind of strain. I wonder how many horses, camels and donkeys undergo such pain without being able to tell us about it. It is not always possible to diagnose such a complaint and, as among all human beings, there are honest and not-so-honest patients. How does one recognize a person with a genuine "lumbago" due to strain from a certificate-hunter putting it on, especially not knowing the patient well? No wonder firms now enquire if the prospective employee suffered from backache. Sometimes backache is an excuse to cover mental exhaustion and to refuse a medical certificate could only aggravate such a condition. A "lumbago" sufferer may aim subconsciously to prevent himself from standing up to the stresses of life. "Is it an unstable back or an unstable patient?" I asked myself. It could be a more serious complaint, in need of investigation, but the fact remains that very few such patients require manipulation and not more than one in a thousand will have an operation. I could never explain the rationale of the manipulative technique and used to compare it with the handling of my "Flying Standard", an old "banger" of post-war years which would only start after a mighty shake – I was moving *something* and it worked! And so my guiding principle always was to give the benefit of the doubt. There were limits of course. On examining a young man with a "bad stomach" who tried to assure me that he did not like to miss his work, I could find nothing, and asked him: "Are you feeling sick? Have you diarrhoea?" I got the reply "Not yet, doctor." I interposed "So in fact you are not *yet* ill!" Here the diagnosis was simple – a dodger.

People continued to stream to the surgeries. It happened yesterday, to-day and seemed that it would continue to-morrow and every-day. "I have a cough, doctor" – seeing her so often I just wrote the prescription. "And diarrhoea" – I added a Kaolin mixture. "Backache as well" – here came a pill. "And horrible itching" – the prescription swelled with another item. "Please do not forget my tablets for headache. I have many more complaints, I only mentioned the basic ones".

The next patient lodged a complaint that the ointment she was using did not make a scrap of difference. "Which ointment?", I asked, not remembering having prescribed one. "The one in the tube." I was still puzzled, but she explained: "The one you prescribed for my Aunt, it did her a lot of good, so she gave it to me". Doctors are not the only people patients get medical advice from! She was followed by a man who greeted me with "It is the winkles, doctor, I always get a stomach-ache from them". "Why do you eat them? I asked. "You don't know until you eat them!" I did not lose my patience. I remained cheerful and said to a worried woman patient: "What a beautiful day, it must make you feel better." "On the contrary, I worry in case we have to pay for it later."

An office girl was sent to me by her employer for a tonic because she fainted at work. I found that her two colleagues were on leave and their boss left all the work for her to do. I wrote to him that the best tonic for this girl would be to give her a few days off. . . .

A patient whom I sent to a surgeon with a large fatty tumour came back to report on her visit. Apparently the Consultant was more interested in her inguinal hernia repaired by Mr. Wakely some thirty-eight years ago. He told her, with a smile, that he was failed in his examination for the Fellowship by Mr. Wakeley on the very subject. An exacting day for me was drawing to an end. I had particularly busy surgeries after T.V. programmes on cancer which often ended with the advice: "If you think you might have similar symptoms, do contact your doctor."

Many visitors from abroad took advantage of the National Health Service. Some arrived in Britain for the sole purpose of being confined, tourists asked for spectacles . . . A few people practically lived in the surgery. When they did not appear for two or three weeks, I knew they must be on holiday. They would come as soon as they returned with "Nice to be back, it is a long time since I saw you, doctor." One such "regular" even sent his deputy to the surgery during the time he was on holiday, telling him that as many people were away, this would be the best time to see the doctor. Day and night various casualties, mostly children, arrived on my doorstep as I was more conveniently placed for them than the hospital.

Some patients were disarming. I asked a man if he ever had jaundice. The answer came: "Yes, I was born with it." A woman, questioned if she had any *children*, replied: "No . . . only two grown up sons." A layabout, out of work for many months, wished to know if there was anything he shouldn't do. A man who worked in a quarry thanked me for syringing his ears with "You blasted it out of me, doctor," and another one who had it done for the first time commented: "It was like brain-washing." A mother whose son had a barking cough enquired if it was because he loved his dog. When someone requested a powerful linctus, saying that he had left his wife in a state of near-collapse from lack of sleep, I commiserated with him and said: "Her cough must be very bad indeed." He shook his head. "Oh no, doctor, it is my cough which keeps her awake."

A patient who recently returned from a mental hospital told me she did not care for the place as it was full of neurotics. I heard a man saying "I do not know how my wife has the courage to stand all her pain," but in fact she was frightened to have her gallstones removed.

185

When a patient was told by the doctor: "You are only troubled by gas," he said this was an impossibility as his household was on electricity.

"You are coughing badly, let me listen to you," I said to a young man. He started to produce the best staccato-crescendo cough he could manage, without any sign of undressing. Seeing his effort, I did not wish to be impolite by interrupting him but in the end I was forced to say: "It's your chest I wish to listen to, not your cough."

Some patients were thorough. Enquiring the height of a woman patient, I was told with preciseness – 5 ft. 1 in. in stockings. Mrs. S. asked me if she could have her baby in hospital on a 48 hour stay: "I did not know you were expecting," I remarked. "Oh no, I'm not, I am only making enquiries."

Some were casual. "You must rest," I advised a patient. "Yes, doctor, thank you," and a minute later the same patient: "Doctor, can I go swimming?"

Some displayed ignorance in various ways. A man with a left sciatica enquired if the nerve ran only on that side, another if his finger was truly broken or just fractured, yet another for how long he should insert a suppository. When I looked at a young girl's foot, informing her it had a wart, she was disappointed with the diagnosis. She had hoped it would be a verruca – it sounded better.

Some were vain. A woman requested slimming pills without the need for them. To avoid argument I relented. "When do I take them, before or after meals?" she enquired. "Neither," I replied shrugging my shoulders.

In my university days I was taught by my pundits how to obtain the history of a patient, but I have since learned it is not always an easy task.

"What is your occupation?"

"Office work."

"What kind of office work?"

"Cleaning."

"What is your trouble?"

"I have a tummy ache, doctor."

"How long for?"

"For ages."

"Are your bowels open?"

"Not quite."

"What do you mean by that?"

"They do and they don't."

186

"You mean you are constipated?"

"I wouldn't know, I haven't been for four days."

She then began to be longwinded about her flatulence and I had to cut her short.

But yet I did not give up.

"You also told me you are coughing, what kind of cough is it?"

"A nasty one."

Undeterred, I probed further.

"What is your phlegm like?"

"I haven't looked yet."

"Do you smoke?"

"Yes and no."

"And when yes, how many?" I continued.

"It depends."

"On what?"

"On the thickness, anyway I smoke only one at a time."

"Do you sleep well?" I continued.

"Not very well, but soundly."

I was beaten, I had to give up, yet I could not refrain from the remark:

"It is not the world inside you, you should be interested in, but the one outside."

Once I enquired of an elderly lady when she had her ring inserted.

"A year after I had my new glasses," she answered after some meditation.

Yet medical history taking is an important part of an examination which helps to make a correct diagnosis. I was called to a fifty-seven year old woman who took to bed with a "terrible" stomach pain. Examination revealed nothing. "Is anything else the matter with you?" I asked. "I also have horrible migraine." This put me on my guard, I began to look for a nervous upset. In the end the patient revealed that the previous night her husband insisted on making love. "He still wants sex, I don't know what for" she said with resignation. On another occasion a hypochondriac developed an acute pain in the abdomen after some annoyance and rushed in a taxi late at night to the nearest hospital. His performance was so convincing that they removed the appendix right away; it was perfectly normal. If only he had consulted me I could have saved his appendix − he tried to fool me many times before by his hysterical behaviour.

These were functional disorders caused by stress in individuals prone to bizarre behaviour.

I learned to make a diagnoses that no one had taught me – "Stability in unstable behaviour," "Neurotic disability," "Compensation neurosis," "Work shy," "Trivia," "Defies classification . . ."

Patients' occupations and personalities could often be guessed by the notes they wrote to the doctor or from the way their samples arrived at the surgery. The requests for visits by a pianoforte teacher were written on her music notes, the water of some ladies was presented in perfume containers, of some gentlemen in whisky bottles. Once, around Christmas time, an expectant mother arrived at my antenatal session with an apology for not having her sample – "I carried it in a sherry bottle which was pinched whilst shopping." No wonder it took a doctor to create the famous detective character – Sherlock Holmes.

At the end of morning surgery I read my post – "Dear Doctor, you gave me 50 sleeping tablets. I have used them quite quickly as we had five visitors staying with us and we all shared them. Please may I have some more, also some tablets for headache? Thank you very much, Yours faithfully." "Dear Doctor, my hand and arm are very sore, I thought you might think of something that would ease it, Yours truly." "Dear Doctor, would you sign at once the enclosed certificate for coal as it is very important – they have a long waiting list. Please, doctor, address it yourself as they will take notice of your writing and not of mine." The next letter, crammed on two pages, almost illegible, which took me quite a time to decipher, ended with "I thought I would write to you instead of 'phoning to save your precious time . . ."

During the period in which one was restricted to £50 for foreign travel, I was approached by an elderly patient with a long history of depressive illness. He asked me to sign a blank declaration for an additional allowance to cover treatment by a specialist in Italy. I did it willingly; he was known to a number of psychiatrists in the area and I knew they did not wish to know him. A fortnight later I received a post-card from him, posted at an Italian beauty spot, in which he thanked me for my understanding attitude and said that he had made substantial progress. To consolidate the result he proposed extending his therapeutic stay for another fourteen days. Would I therefore contact his bank and instruct them to release more money. I replied by return, sending him a card with a nice view of London, and expressing my delight at his obvious recovery. "Your management of affairs proves you have now sufficiently recovered and are no more in need of costly treatment. I look forward to your return." It was interesting to see him in my surgery a week later, sun-tanned and smiling. He was wise enough not to mention our correspondence.

I enjoyed letters from consultants who were a great help to us, G.Ps', after all we cannot know everything. The letters were written in a most polite manner like: "I *beg* to refer you to my previous letter." "I discharge this patient into your capable hands." "Many thanks for referring him" etc. etc. They were also informative and very much to the point. "Since this man became redundant and his family left him, he seems very much happier and now has no complaints." "I saw this boy to-day, though really it was his mother who was the patient. I could find nothing wrong with the boy. I feel sure his mother will be hunting until she finds someone to agree with her that there is something the matter with the boy, and as you know, if she is assiduous enough she is bound to obtain that opinion in time from some hospital or other". "I arranged for Mrs. B. to have suitable therapy. However, she tells me she does not believe in electrical treatment and indeed does not think it necessary as her house is full of electrical appliances." "I understand that this young man recently got married and this will account for his back strain. I have suggested to him that he goes to bed by himself for the next four days." Another letter from a gynaecologist began: "I agree with you about her tenseness, I nearly lost my fingers!" Yet another letter assessed a patient well, saying, "He likes to be seen by different people, thinking that he might get a diagnosis confirmed or rejected.".

In those early days doctors were inundated with calls — usually at the most inconvenient times — when one was having a meal, or a bath, or in the middle of the night. Our receptionist heard a little boy at the other end of the telephone saying: "Will doctor please call on Mrs. W?"

"What address?" she enquired.

"I don't know," said the boy, "I don't know Mrs. W., I was promised a bob-a-job if I rang the doctor."

It was midnight when an agitated voice requested over the telephone an urgent visit to his wife. "She has a heart attack, I can't find her pulse." I jumped out of bed and just as I was leaving the house the telephone rang again. I heard the same voice: "It's all right, Doc, I found her pulse, I thought I would save you the call." I thanked him.

One night a neighbour called me to an old couple who lived alone as the man had complained of pain across the chest for several hours. I met his wife, an old darling, boiling a kettle downstairs in the kitchen.

189

She asked me to see to her husband whom she left ten minutes previously up in the bedroom. I found the patient dead and was unable to revive him. With uneasiness, I climbed down the stairs to find the old lady pouring tea for three. I had no heart to tell her the truth and called the neighbour. I persuaded the new widow to take a powerful sedative. I watched her become somewhat drowsy and gently came out with the truth, realising that she would be unable to grasp the full implication of it.

Another day I was called to a man who had developed a severe chest pain an hour previously and I thought he might be suffering from a coronary. One school of thought advised not to move such a patient in an early stage, another preferred immediate transfer to hospital should resuscitation be required suddenly. I decided to follow the first one and called on the patient again the next morning. I was rather worried when his wife opened the door with a sad, worn-out look and failed to answer my "Good morning" greeting. "How are things?" I asked with trepidation. "Not at all well, I'm afraid," and after a pause which seemed to me never ending, "I have nothing cheerful to report to you, doctor, sadly I must tell you . . . *I* have been sick". I sighed with relief.

I was called to a patient the very evening he had returned from hospital where he had been under observation. He continued to request visits from me the next day, the day after and practically every day. His wife told me he should go back to hospital as he would spoil her Christmas. A week later I received a communication from the hospital stating that in spite of many investigations there was nothing to be found and they were able to reassure him . . .

At 4 o-clock one morning the excited voice of a woman shouted through the earphone: "Please come at once, my husband has gone completely mad, he may set the house on fire or injure himself. Please hurry." I left my warm bed for a rainy, cold and windy morning and arrived in no time at her house. A man, approaching sixty, opened the door and greeted me with the usual opening: "So sorry, doctor, that my wife called you at this hour," followed by: "Good thing you are here, she is off her rocker." It transpired that her name was Sweet Daisy – she obviously did not live up to her parents' expectations . . . I guessed they had a quarrel and it took me three cups of tea – one with the wife, another with the husband, and the third with them both together to bring harmony to the house. I arrived home at seven o-clock, in time for my morning cup of tea.

It did not puzzle me that all patients continued to come back,

190

whether they received good or bad treatment, (although one would expect that they should stay away from me in either case). The fact is that an easy access to doctors and medicines prevents nature from doing its job. It is common knowledge that warts tend to disappear spontaneously but curetting them impairs autoimmunity. In endemic areas of oriental sore,* by experience, a custom was brought into being of witholding treatment directed against the parasite in the initial stages of the disease, in this way assuring the development of immunity against reinfection. In the mid 16th century Thomas Phaire expressed the opinion that "The best and sure help is not to meddle with any kind of medicines, but to let nature work her operation." I wish doctors and patients alike would remember it to-day.

Increased work load brought inevitable waiting and I once heard a witty remark from a patient with a thorn under his nail, that "it had grown larger since he entered the waiting room." I asked him why he did not attend Casualty. He shrugged his shoulders and said: "I went there once but the Casualty Officer was very casual." Patients coming to obtain trivialities for themselves, their relatives or even their neighbours, were the ones most indignant if kept waiting because someone in front of them needed a more thorough examination. But when their turn came they took up a heck of a lot of my time, starting with: "I will be very brief, I only want to ask you four things . . ." It is a pity I was taught how to start an interview with a patient and not how to end it! For the benefit of such patients I displayed a notice quoting a sage: "*Success* is getting what you want, *happiness* is wanting what you get, *unhappiness* is not knowing what you want and killing yourself to get it!"

It was lucky that a number of patients were of a seasonal brand. I got used to seeing a man who was troubled with twitching of the eyes and headache whenever he was unoccupied. A manager of a swimming pool, jolly and hard-working, was invariably apprehensive and in need of tranquillizers during the slack winter months; I observed that work often diverted patients from their mental anguish (Jerome K. Jerome wrote – It is impossible to enjoy idling thoroughly unless one has plenty of work to do – and the broadcaster David Franklin listed his recreation in "Who's Who" as work, which has been more fun than not working).

Another patient who required similar medication at specific times was the mother of a boy on vacation from college where he was learning

* Cutaneous Leishmaniasis.

191

pianoforte and was in need of practice. Hay fever, sunburn, and insect bites were seasonal, but so were football injuries at the week-end and headaches and indigestion immediately after Christmas. Backaches were prevalent with the start of the gardening season and the inevitable "lead swingers" on Mondays, which prompted me to give friendly advice to a patient with a record of numerous Monday calls to go on working, disregarding week-ends, as his condition could only be compared to that of my first car – once it stopped it needed a great effort to re-start!

Christmas activities bring an increased number of heart attacks in older people. Advice given to the profession by the eminent British Physician – Sir William Osler, a late Professor of Oxford – proved very useful. He pointed out that when a young man complains of his heart, one should look at his stomach, and when an old man complains of his stomach, one is obliged to look at his heart. Only summer diarrhoeas stopped being seasonal, turning into a popular event all the year round – a perennial illness. It might be caused by viruses, but also by modern living – poisonous chemicals used on farms and gardens, irregular hurried meals, deep freezing, pre-packing, nutrient supplements, preservatives, artificial colouring, synthetic flavouring, and of course laxatives. The World Health Organization announced allergic reaction from some drug colourants, and in 1969 cyclamates were banned from food products because of their possible harmful effect. It is a strange thing that gallons of preparations containing anti-biotics should be used against such diarrhoeas, as they are useless; the result of powerful advertising, I suppose. What is really needed is a guide towards better digestion and a powerful warning such as: "Do not dig your own grave with your own fork."

I am tempted to divide the population into two groups – people with malfunctioning bowel and those with normal habits. The first group needs subdivision – the venerable members of the community who are inconvenienced by constipation and those with looseness of the bowels. The first group is far more important as it comprises children, expectant and nursing mothers, executives chained to their office chairs and the elderly.

Medical Practitioners were so over-loaded with the filling of forms and influx of patients that some only had time to ask for their names and addresses before writing a prescription, without further questioning and the usual niceties. In the late autumn of 1952 a very thick fog descended on London and did not lift for several days – it was a mixture of fog and pollution; a new term "smog" was coined. Doctors were rushed off their feet and hospitals packed to overflowing with new arrivals. I remember sending a chronic bronchitic as an emergency to a hospital which he had attended regularly for several years, because of his sudden shortness of breath and heavy breathing. On admission he received treatment as a matter of urgency for the obvious cause – exacerbation of chronic bronchitis. After his death, a postmortem revealed a recent heart attack – there are no foregone conclusions, particularly in medicine. Not all patients were genuine. Medical men had to contend with parents anxious to deprive their children of tonsils and foreskins on the slightest provocation, and with adults eager to have all their teeth removed. It was a mad rush for the wrong things. A number of doctors exploded with wrath and left the country. It was estimated that an average of 400 doctors emigrated each year, five times the rate of the 1930's.*

I remember working in isolation, left to my own devices, carrying full responsibility twenty-four hours a day, day in, day out, my colleagues too busy with private patients or N.H.S. practice to be able to spare time for professional contacts, and the hospital doctors looking upon General Practitioners with condescension, seeing them engaged in a low-status occupation. Besides, hospitals had their own problems – a growing shortage of doctors necessitated their recruitment from abroad, many buildings were obsolete, there was a shortage of beds and nursing staff. It was succintly described as "A pretty ghastly, awful picture." A thirty-one-year-old patient of mine with advanced disseminated sclerosis, badly in need of hospitalization, was eventually admitted, after prolonged efforts, to a geriatric hospital – the only place where this chronic invalid, in full possession of his mental faculties, could be accommodated. There he lay helpless in a crowded ward among demented people, no one able to come to his assistance, save for the rare appearances of a nurse, too few of them for too many patients. It was a merciful release when he died after two years of misery in such an environment. This crippling disease affects some fifty thousand people in the United Kingdom alone. Virus is blamed for some but in fact neither the real cause nor cure has yet been discovered.

Obviously we lacked the kind of health service that William Beveridge envisaged and yet, surprisingly enough, it worked. Only a minority was unappreciative and demanding, and abuses were neither great nor typical; the wrong-doings were caused rather by lack of

* British Medical Journal, 4 July 1956, 1.

193

thought than through intention. There were worriers and warriors among the patients, but I learned that beside frivolous complaints there was appreciation, beside acrimony, good manners, beside intolerance, patience, beside lack of reliance, loyalty, beside ignorance, understanding, beside laziness, diligence, beside malice, goodwill, beside cowardice, courage, beside weakness, strength. A patient who had already waited five months to have his prostate removed, after receiving a note from the hospital informing him of a further delay due to renovations, sent a letter to the Management: "It is extremely nice of you to write, but you shouldn't go to all this trouble for me." I remember a rare visitor to the surgery who came to have his ears syringed. I saw him in a happy mood whistling like a boy. He stopped with "How are you, doctor?" At eighty-seven he still travelled each day to the solicitor's office in the City as he had done all his working life. I had deaf and dumb patients and those who were blind leading a normal life, working, raising families and seldom availing themselves of my services. I remember being called on New Year's Day by a blind couple to their daughter. I hoped this would be an occasion to wish them a Happy New Year. The house was spotlessly clean, everything was in the right place so that it could be easily found. On the floor I noticed a letter dropped through their letter-box. They asked me to read it thinking it came from a well-wisher. It read: "From the Housing Department – Notice of increase in rent by £8 per quarter is given herewith."

I remember another patient who had become totally blind some twenty years earlier through an explosion at school, and who obtained a University degree, got married and held a secure, responsible position with a local authority, his dog his constant companion.

I had a double above-knee amputee who was able to keep his job as an electrician; he was the breadwinner for a family of five, whom he liked to drive abroad, and who worked long hours seldom taking time off. Another case with a damaged spine, walking very unsteadily with the help of elbow crutches, was a hard and valued worker.

I watched a courageous young couple who had two children affected by the horrid infantile muscular atrophy – an inherited, progressive disease with a one in four risk for further pregnancies. The parents were fit and well, the condition being passed to their children from one of the ancestors. Before the disease could be diagnosed in the first baby, its mother was far advanced in her second pregnancy. It turned out that the second child was similarly affected. These unfortunate children were very intelligent, pretty, with bright, sparkling eyes and friendly dispositions. They could not raise their heads, stand, sit or even roll, and had to be turned over in bed, their limbs and trunk muscles being profoundly weak. Yet the parents coped remarkably well with the situation and managed to keep the children reasonably fit and happy.

I remember a client who seldom asked for my help calling me in one evening and apologising because of the late hour. He was used to the pain from his peptic ulcer which he earlier declined to have operated on. "I tried to ease it for the last twenty-four hours with my usual medicines, doctor, but this time they did not work." I was not surprised, he had a burst ulcer; fortunately the skilled hands of a surgeon and streptomycin saved his life.

A manual worker had not missed a single day from work since his complete gastrectomy for cancer of the stomach performed ten months previously. He arrived in my surgery, a year after his operation, with swollen legs and the spread of cancer into various parts of his body. "You must rest," I said, "I am giving you a medical certificate for twenty-eight days." "I do not wish to stay away from work that long," he answered quite categorically; he died ten weeks later. Another patient with incurable cancer said to his wife: "I told my doctor that I know of my condition and it shook him. Doctors have to face up to it!"

In 1974 the book "Despite Disability" appeared in Britain, in which disabled people tell how they go about their work leading normal lives.

Those were very courageous people following the example of famous patients such as Lord Nelson who, in spite of the loss of the right eye and arm, carried on his duties and inspired the men under his command, or Beethoven, whose deafness in the last period of his life did not put an end to composing great works, or Edison – the "father" of 20th century mechanical civilization and the inventor of the phonograph, deaf for a large part of his life. Sarah Bernhardt's leg amputation did not end her stage career, Bader continued flying after the loss of both legs and Richard Wood – who lost both legs in the Western Desert during the Second World War – was able to discharge great responsibilities as Minister of Pensions and National Insurance. The pianist Ungar – who won the international Chopin piano competition in Warsaw before the war – was blind, the Irish novelist Brown, crippled since birth with cerebral palsy, and the indomitable Michael Flanders – a well-known British entertainer, a victim of poliomyelitis confined to a wheelchair – lead normal useful lives. Jack Hawkins, the

195

actor, continued his career after being struck by cancer of the throat which robbed him of his voice. He developed a new "voice" using stomach muscles and diaphragm, and when it proved disappointing, he mimed and was dubbed by friends. He carried on his battle with the infliction submitting to an operation for an artificial voice box, still in an experimental stage, but succumbed.* Beethoven spoke for all of them when he pronounced: "I will take Fate by the throat, it shall not bend or break me!"

Poor health did not rob the painters Goya, Reynolds and Lautrec, the poets Pope and Burns, the writer and journalist Samuel Johnson, the television pioneer John Baird, the politician Franklin Roosevelt and many others of fame. One's own disabilities spur one to action, as in the case of John Dalton, who, affected by colour blindness, conducted important investigations into the nature of this handicap. A surgeon, Percival Pott, sustained a compound fracture of his leg in 1765 when he was thrown from his horse. His valuable observation became world-wide known as Pott's fracture.** Robert Schumann, once a pianist, turned into a renowned composer after he had sustained a permanent injury to his right hand. Marlene Dietrich was trained as a pianist but owing to an injured wrist took up acting and achieved success. David Franklin, Principal Bass at the Royal Opera House, Covent Garden, turned into a celebrated broadcaster when a throat operation damaged the top of his voice. One's disabilities are not necessarily a handicap. In the case of El Greco – a 16th century Graeco-Spanish painter – his foreshortened or strangely elongated figures with intense dramatic effect are attributed to the artist's astigmatism, and the long nose of Jimmy Durante brought this entertainer success (he was given the nickname of Schnozzola). An ugly appearance has helped many entertainers to reach the top of their profession.

I found great satisfaction in dealing with children. Most of my little patients were acute and very observant. Some stood on their dignity. I once watched a six-year-old boy who annoyed his mother by not wishing to undress prior to my examination. "Mummy," he said in a self-respecting voice, "I do not like to be shouted at." They knew their own minds too. When I asked a girl of eight if she had made any New Year's resolutions, I got a prompt answer: "Yes, – never to speak to my best

* Since then scientists at St. Bartholomews Hospital have succeeded in making an improved version.

** Similarly observation on himself and others by Thomas Sydenham – a celebrated 17th century physician and gout sufferer – provided a classic account of this disease in his treatise "The Treatment of Gout."

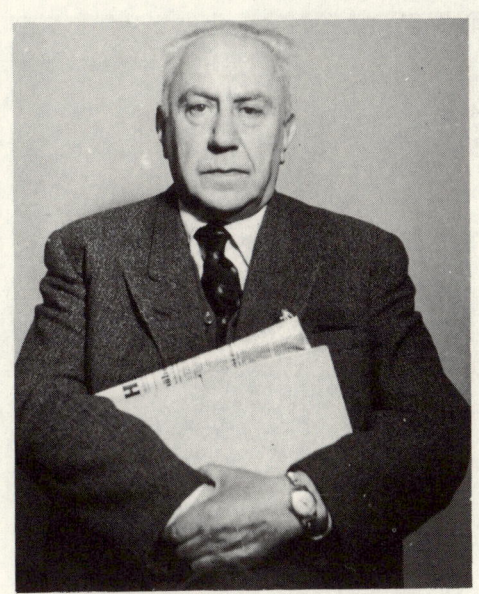

Professor Ludwik Hirszfeld

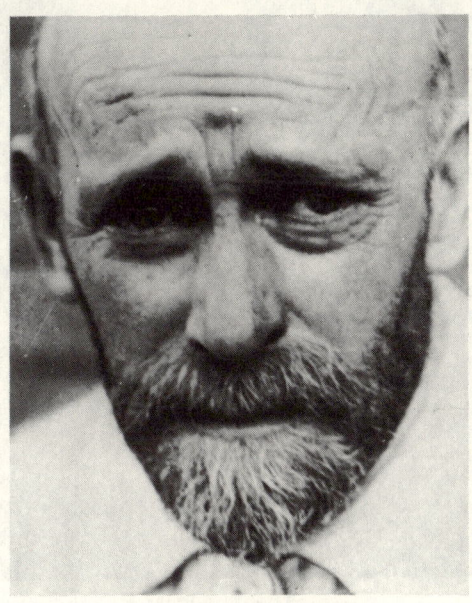

Doctor Janusz Korczak

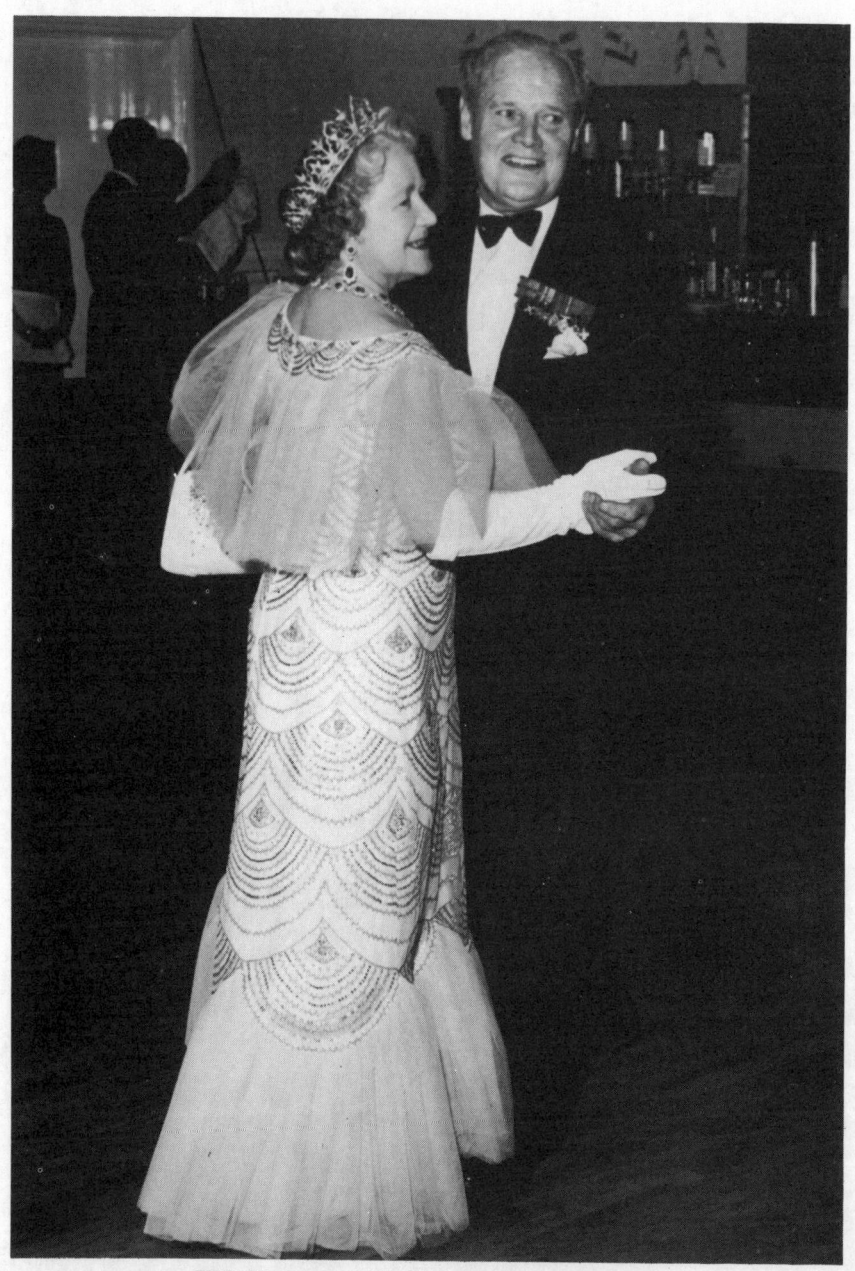

H.R.H. Queen Elizabeth the Queen Mother
dancing with Douglas Bader, August 1974

friend again, she is my worst *friend* now . . ." I remember a miserable looking nine-year-old brought to the surgery by his concerned mother. "What's the trouble?" "It's the pocket money, I don't get enough", I heard the boy say. Treating them as equals, showing patience and leniency were the prerequisites for building their confidence, that way winning half the battle. It was with regret that I sometimes had to look into a child's throat, a procedure they loathed, on my first encounter. I found it important to allay the mother's anxieties, as they were often transmitted to the child. I tried to discourage impatient, worried mothers from administering laxatives and sedatives on the slightest provocation, or to cultivate bad or unsocial habits. I saw a mother who put a pram in front of a flickering television and explained: "The baby cries for company, but in front of the set she is happy; if it is switched off or I am not about she whimpers." In another house I saw two television sets placed on opposite sides of a room with different programmes on. They were installed for the benefit of two young brothers to stop them quarrelling. I was sorry for the little innocents who were truly disarming. A woman who had a baby two weeks previously explained to her four-year-old daughter that the little sister she saw in the cot would be able to sit and eventually walk. A week later the four-year-old looked into the cot and said with disappointment: "Can't she sit up yet, mummy?" One little girl who had recently returned home from hospital, having an argument with her father, said in tears: "I am going back to hospital, they all love me there."

Children were excellent subjects for dental anaesthesia which has become safer since doctors learned to avoid hypoxia.* I usually tried to find childrens' inclinations, asking what he or she would like to be, then suggesting that they will turn into a racing driver, flyer, nurse or such like, usually with excellent results; afterwards the little patient would describe the car or outfit and its colour as implied by me.

Once I was amazed at the power of suggestion when I heard the comment of a piano teacher on my skilful whistling; when administering gas I remarked jokingly: "I will whistle the Hungarian Rhapsody to you," not giving any more thought to it

I once visited a three-year-old child on whom a diagnosis of acute leukaemia was made the previous week. The mother, who was yet unable to grasp the implications, told me: "The child is very shy, but in time she will get used to you, doctor." There will be no time for it, I thought with great sadness.

* Deficiency of oxygen in the inspired air.

Since then various new drugs have been used with some success and many cases reported which have survived more than five years from the beginning of this disease – a marked contrast to the old experience. This progress started in 1947 with the discovery that an antagonist of a particular vitamin – the folic acid – was quite effective against leukaemia. The research for new, more specific and less toxic agents in this disease continues.

Perhaps sub-consciously I identified myself with children. Like them I still had language difficulties and a scanty vocabulary. How is it, I pondered, that when an Englishman pronounces the word "wonder" it sounds like wunder, and when he means "wander" he says "wonder", that the same word "row" has two different meanings and pronunciations, yet the same spelling. I began to understand why almost every British household has an Oxford Dictionary. I had heard of Hamlet, the Danish Prince, but not in connection with a small village. I listened to a patient who talked of high fever when he meant hay fever. A man complained of poor expansion – I thought he meant his lungs, but he was talking of his business. I once thought a patient was stammering when I heard him saying: "I have the right to write to the right people." I wondered why a Scotsman was telling me about Spain (it turned out he complained of his spine), and why an Irishman stressed importance when he meant a lack of sexual power. I horrified a well-educated English lady when she heard me saying: "I had great difficulties with sex when on holiday in France," meaning gender, and upset a lady-doctor, back from her holiday, by my greeting: "I trust you had a good period." I infuriated my English friends when in response to their conventional "How are you?" I went into details about my health. Refusing an offer I would say "Thank you," as is customary in my native land, omitting the important "No". "I have been living for donkey's years in Twekesbury Avenue", said a patient in reply to my question. I raised my eyebrows. Why donkey's years and not elephant's, or better still why not tortoise's years – they surely live longer – and why miserable little streets without a single tree are called avenues!

I visited the London museums, galleries and theatres to widen my horizon. The metropolis grew on me, and when I knew it better I began to love it. I visited Dicken's "Old Curiosity Shop", saw plaques commemorating the stay of famous people in London like those of Sun-Yat-Sen, the founder of the Chinese Republic, Bizet, the French musician and composer, Marconi, the pioneer of wireless, Freud, the originator of psychoanalysis and others. I saw the Austrian actor Anton Wohlbruck* (Walbrook), who was adopted by Britain, in "Call Me Madam" and I watched with interest the musical "Carousel" which I saw as a straight play by the name of "Lilliom" with Hans Albers in Berlin in 1931. I enjoyed rides on the big double-decker buses, watching the bustle of the big city from the top deck. At the underground booking office a smiling blonde clerk threw the question "Single?" at me. "I am," said I returning her smile. I looked with curiosity at the London "Bobby" in his characteristic helmet. They proved to be all I had heard about them – well-informed, courteous, good-humoured and unarmed.

December 15, 1952 was a memorable day for me – I was granted naturalization and became a citizen of the United Kingdom and Colonies. The first visible sign of my new status was the right to sign passports and other important documents for my patients, most of them unknown to Ministers of Religion. My bedside manners improved and became more sophisticated. I now greeted my patients with "How nice to see you," and to find their age I asked elderly ladies how *young* they were. I set my surgery scales 4 lbs below weight, observing the happy faces of my overweight patients as they stepped off the scales. (Afterwards I entered their weights into my notes, discreetly adding on the missing pounds.)

Over a period of time I visited various parts of the country. On the way to beautiful North Devon I explored Exeter. I was interested to find that its Roman Wall was still in existence. About 50 A.D. this place was subdued by the Roman General Vespasian who later became Emperor. I was impressed with Exeter's ancient buildings and above all with its Cathedral whose Norman Towers are some 800 years old. I admired the ornate front wall with its many statues, the harmonious interior, and the elegance of the Cathedral. The magnificent Gothic vaulting supported on marble pillars and elaborate wooden carvings enhanced the beauty of the place. I noticed that some of the windows had plain glass – the result of German bombing. In May 1942 Exeter suffered a number of severe air raids and the Cathedral did not escape damage; after the war repairs costing some £80,000 were carried out. In 1971 major excavations were started, and the following year a large structure near the Cathedral was identified as part of a Roman Baths complex, probably used by the Legion of Vespasian. Mosaic fragments were found and the decorative roof of tiles with grotesque masks of

* Famed for his part in the film "The Warsaw Concerto".

women shows that the complex was lavishly appointed, possibly to impress the local people with the power and wealth of Rome.

On my first visit to the Cathedral I found its doors half closed. I had just arrived in Exeter, wearing a Tyrol scull cap and a cine camera slung over my shoulder. I looked round the door and was confronted by an usher in morning dress who cast a glance at me and putting his fingers to his lips, led me quietly to a seat near the front of the crowded Cathedral. Only then did I realise I was a gate-crasher at a big society wedding. I was taken for a foreign reporter – I had not yet acquired the look of a British subject! My integration was a long, drawn-out process . . .

19
Medicine Explodes

Change is inevitable. In a progressive country change is constant.
Benjamin Disraeli

What we anticipate seldom occurs; what we least expect generally
happens.   *Benjamin Disraeli*

Back home I continued my daily routine and noticed that as the years
passed by, conditions of work were steadily improving. Occasionally I
still came across an odd conversation when I asked a chronic bronchitic if the suppositories he requested were meant for breathing, I got
the answer: "No, they are for my back passage," or the odd letter: "I
have a slight twinge in my left lung, could you let me have a course of
penicillin *or* antibiotics, please?" A heavy smoker, who recently gave
up this vice, complained of discomfort in his chest and wondered if the
smoke was still coming out. A patient told me: "You hear some stories,
doctor, you could write a book." I just smiled. However, these were
soon by-gone days. The wireless, the television, the press, the advertising brought knowledge home to people; it was a knowledge one had
to reckon with. Town criers became superfluous!

The old art of medicine was acquired by practice and observation.
For example, seamen learnt that the addition of fresh fruit to their diet
would save them from scurvy long before science was able to explain
that this disease was due to a deficiency of Vitamin C discovered by
Szent Györgyi, and well before Hopkins won the Nobel prize for eluci-
dating the role of vitamins in the maintenance of health. Similarly, the
disease beri-beri (which leads to heart failure) was correctly attributed
to a diet limited to rice from which the vitamin-bearing husk had been
removed by "polishing", long before a Pole, Funk, (who incidentally
first proposed the term "vitamin") succeeded in extracting the life
saving Vit. B1 from the polishings.

The explosion of science in the post-war years changed the old art
into a scientific one based on experimentation and research. Rapid
technological advances underline the scientific trend and make doctors
and patients alike aware of the transformation. Not all is progress
though. The gross over-reliance of modern man on sleeping drugs,
tranquillizers, purgatives and such like is widely regarded as shame to
our time. One in six women and one in nine men enter hospital with

some mental illness in their life time.

Perhaps what people really need is not more leisure and prosperity – they have both, and it was the English who gave the world the "weekend" – but a more positive and less boring entertainment which requires participation and initiative. Perhaps we need less robots and less tedious jobs, yet more work which should be satisfying, even enjoyable. We will then have less patients who are determined not to get better. Here is something for the planners of our lives to think about.

But the scientific trend continues and the rate of progress is getting greater every day since it started to gain momentum. It was nearly three hundred years ago that a Dutchman from Delft by the name of Leeuwenhoek bestowed the microscope to the world and was the first man to see microbes. (However, the invention of the compound microscope was credited to the Dutch spectacles maker Zacharias Jansen and dated 1590.) Soon an Italian, Marcello Malpighi, was studying details of kidney, spleen and heart and an Englishman, Robert Hooke,* saw single cells in plants, looking like little boxes, of which living organisms are built. Constant improvement of microscopes and other instruments led to more and more details and better understanding of life. It was possible to see a cell as a semi-liquid, known as cytoplasm, with a dense centre called the nucleus, and enclosed by a membrane. In 1869 a Swiss by the name of Friedrich Miescher isolated from cell nuclei the nucleic acid, known as DNA.** DNA is the fundamental material of every living cell, responsible for the continuity of life, in other words – for heredity. The role of the nucleus in the life of the cell began to be understood. It needed the development of an electron microscope with high power of magnification, initiated in Germany in 1932 by Knoll and Ruska, and the more recent scanning one, before more minute details could be obtained and some vital biological phenomena explained. With the help of chromatographic analysis,*** X-ray crystallography etc. minute structures and complicated processes within the living cells have been studied. Since 1971 an electron microscope, 26 tons in weight, with a column 12 feet high, has been in

* In his "Micrographia" of 1664 he not only described a cell but also mentioned the possibility of man-made fibre, so foreseeing the discovery by the Englishmen Cross, Bevan and Beadle, made in 1892.

** Deoxyribonucleic acid.

*** A method discovered by the Russian botanist Tsvett in the early 1900's and adopted by scientists in 1939. In 1941 two Englishmen, Drs. Martin and Synge, modified it when studying the composition of protein. Their work brought them a Nobel prize.

operation in Toulouse, France. The instrument was assembled in a new building four storeys high, especially constructed for it, and at the cost of £2 million. A similar microscope was installed at Osaka University, Japan. It is feasible that one day the structure of DNA could be directly observed with a microscope.

In 1956 scientists counted twenty-three pairs of chromosomes in nucleus, a constant number in each typical human* cell. They are long strands of DNA composed of a succession of genes,** the hereditary elements. These days it is possible to detect abnormal chromosomes in yet unborn children. In the fourth month of pregnancy foetal cells can be obtained from the bag of waters which encompasses the child in the womb. We know that abnormal chromosomes are responsible for physical and mental defects such as mongolism, and possibly for criminal behaviour in some instances. One day, possibly in the not too distant future, a prenatal test could be a routine procedure, similar to blood grouping, with the aim of preventing abnormalities in the next generation.

Sub-germs, called viruses, one of the simplest forms of life, smaller than the cell itself, were discovered. They are responsible for influenza, the common cold, many upper respiratory tract infections, poliomyelitis, smallpox, measles, mumps, German measles and more, some still obscure.

In 1951 the naturalized American of Polish descent, Ludwik Gross, obtained a virus from the parotid gland of a mouse which induces leukaemia in this and other species. Statistics suggest that children born of mothers with a history of influenza in early pregnancy could be more vulnerable to leukaemia than others.

In 1969 a severe viral condition – Lassa fever – was first described and named after the place of its outbreak in Nigeria. Viruses behave in a mischievous way, therefore it is not surprising that they are blamed each day for something else. Studies on mice point to viruses as one of the possible causes of leukaemia*** and rheumatoid arthritis.****

New viruses are constantly being discovered. They attack indiscriminately – man as much as animal, plant and micro-organism. Made

* The cells of mongol children contain an extra chromosome.

** It was proved in 1934 by Painter of Texas; hence the term "genetics" for the studies concerned with the causes of similarities and differences between individuals and their ancestors.

*** Uncontrolled cancer-like growth of white blood cells.

**** Penicillamine, a useful drug in rheumatoid arthritis, has potent anti-viral properties.

only of protein and nucleic acid, these structures are too simple to have their own biological processes necessary for the release of energy, and to be able to live they invade the cell, using the processes of their host. It is all take and no give. They are parasites, better described as hijackers. The host cell is compelled to manufacture the essentials for the rapidly multiplying viruses – a kind of cellular take-over which can be watched in an electron microscope and photographed. This is why doctors have a big problem in defeating viruses – an attack on them means an attack on their host, in fact the patient. The viruses are aware of this impunity and even dare to attack bacteria, thus changing their names to bacteriophages, meaning "bacteria eaters". The viral protein contains an enzyme* which produces an erosion in the cell wall through which the bacteriophage core, consisting of nucleic acid, enters to take command directed exclusively towards production of new bacteriophage particles; the virus is only interested in its own perpetuation. Soon a complete dissolution of the cell wall is achieved and the new formed virus released. In 1969 Max Delbrueck, Alfred Hershey and Salvador Luria who work in the United States received a Nobel prize "for their discoveries concerning the replication mechanism and the genetic structure of viruses". To further our knowledge in this field virus laboratories were founded; in one of them, opened by Glaxo in 1950, the first British anti-polio vaccine, Polivirin, was developed.

In 1962 Watson and Crick, workers at the Cavendish laboratory in Cambridge, won the Nobel prize for the deduction of a twin spiral staircase-like structure of DNA particle** which they named "double helix". They solved one of the most fundamental problems of biology – how the genes, made of DNA, replicate. This structure was later confirmed by visual evidence provided by Griffiths in California. DNA particles are a thirteen millionth of an inch across. They provide instructions for the living cell to build a variety of proteins from twenty different kinds of amino acids by ordering them to link together in a specific sequence. The genetic information in DNA is transferred

---

*Enzymes are substances, usually protein in nature, which vary the rate of chemical reactions without being altered themselves. Life and death depend on succession of enzyme reactions which control biochemical processes. Many abnormalities have been traced to the fault in a particular enzyme; phenylketonuria, for instance, is caused by deficiency of the enzyme phenylalanine, and galactosaemia, in which the body is unable to utilize lactose, by deficiency of another specific enzyme.

**In the scientific world particle is called "molecule". Cells consist of such molecules and in turn form an organism.

from the nucleus to strands of RNA* in the cytoplasm by means of an enzyme known as messenger RNA; genes, in fact, control the synthesis of enzymes. The code of the protein-starting mechanism was deciphered unravelling the puzzle of protein construction. The knowledge of its architecture grew. This is of vital importance as the formation of a variety of proteins is the first step in the creation of an organism. If the DNA structure of the "parent cell" is changed in some way, the genetic code is changed too and a different protein pattern will result in the "daughter cells". Already scientists are able to transplant genes into micro-organisms.**

In 1970 the first laboratory synthesis of a protein,*** was announced. The same year the structure of another protein vital to human life**** was clarified, after Professor Dorothy Hodgkin of Oxford University succeeded in working out its three dimensional crystallographic structure. No wonder that scientists reflecting on the origin of life pause at a crystal as their possible ancestor – a link between non-living and living forms.

Proteins and nucleic acid are characteristic of living things, and light was thrown on cell activities such as synthesis of DNA, RNA and protein, the energy metabolism, the selective permeability function of cellular membranes etc. It was recognized that when a cell divides each daughter cell receives an exact copy of the parental hereditary material – the genes; its chemical structure was revealed. Genes determine the nature and number of enzymes within the living cell which in turn control all the reactions necessary for its functioning and engage in the synthesis of other proteins. For work in this field French scientists François Jacob, André Lwoff and Jacques Monod received a Nobel prize in 1965. Hereditary disorders such as colour blindness, albinism, light sensitivity, mongolism and other phenomena were elucidated. Nucleic acids are responsible for our inherited traits as each one directs

* *Ribonucleic acid.*
** Fear was expressed that such genetic manipulation might create a super-bug.
*** The enzyme ribonuclease.
**** Insulin, responsible for sugar regulation in the body. Until 1922 diabetic patients were threatened by death. That year Banting and Best discovered how to obtain insulin from animals – they knew its location but not its structure. The chemical structure was established by Sanger at Cambridge in 1960, and four years later Katsoyannis of New York synthesized human insulin. It is a complex protein and processing it is as yet too cumbersome and expensive for routine therapy. Professor Hodgkin's work may change this. Present day knowledge has already led to the commercial manufacture of synthetic "meat", known as Kesp, from soya beans. Several British companies are researching in this field, some using protein from fungus. A large-scale pilot plant is producing synthetic protein at the rate of two tons a week. Protein can even be made from natural gas.

the synthesis of a particular protein. The translation from nucleic acid to protein proceeds, as we already know, according to a systematic code. Enzymes are the watchdog which correct an erroneous synthesis, should it happen. The precision of protein synthesis, although of the highest order, is not entirely fool-proof and the error in translation may lead to mutation – a permanent transmissible change in the characteristics of an offspring from those of its parents. And so the nature of living cell is determined by the proteins it contains. Each has thousands of them and they perform chemical reactions required for normal life. Some of them are "suicidal" proteins which get destroyed in their functional process, others like transferin, which picks and binds iron, and other transport proteins repeat their performances again and again. Deficiency or absence of specific antihaemophilic globulin fraction of plasma causes haemophilia, and faulty protein synthesis may lead to thalassaemia – chronic anaemia usually observed in people from countries bordering on the Mediterranean Sea. Some cases of emphysema* are genetically determined. Several hereditary diseases are associated with enzymatic and therefore specific protein deficiencies. This may lead to phenylketonuria, a diminished thyroid activity or the impairment of growth in children. We began to understand the mechanism of inheritance despite its tremendous complexity.

Doctors offered a new service to the public – the "genetic counselling". Because they have learned genetic implications and can make the prenatal diagnosis of chromosome defects in foetus and determine its sex, doctors may be able to protect future generations from disastrous abnormalities. Chondroplastic dwarfs, congenital deafness, spina bifida, cleft palate, muscular dystrophy and the like may disappear for ever. It is estimated that there are 20–30,000 haemophiliacs in Great Britain. They are "bleeders" due to the defect of blood coagulation. The disease affects males and is transmitted by females. It is difficult to visualize who would advise Queen Victoria, should she live in present times, not to pass the inactive gene to the Tsarevitch Alexis, to Alfonso XIII and to the Battenberg family. Her youngest son died of it. In 1965 the American Judith Pool succeeded in condensing the clotting constituent of normal blood deficient in haemophiliacs. "Cryo", as the manufactured product is known, stops bleeding episodes and averts damage, even death. King George III suffered from severe mental disturbance, now attributed to acute porphyria – a rare metabolic disorder. He died in 1820, but the disease he was supposed to have suffered from was described only in 1911.

* Distension of the lungs.

206

Leslie Orgel, a Cambridge biochemist, had an interesting thought that defects occurring in enzymes required for biosynthesis, could cause ageing.

Joan Kaplan of Harvard Medical School and her associates found an enzyme which could be responsible for merging viral DNA and the DNA of the normal cell – a process critical to the production of cancer cells. Evidence has been mounting that certain types of virus by changing the structure of DNA can transform a normal cell into a tumour cell. There is not one cancer but many, of various types and sites, each one having its own characteristics, temperament, different virulence and growth. But they have one thing in common – they are all criminals! The cancer cells behave worse than hi-jackers. They do not content themselves to live off their host but act like the worst of Nazis. They multiply as fast as they can, only to fight cruelly for living space. They kill indiscriminately any life which stands in their path – adults and children alike; a slaughter on the same scale. Cancer cells become lawless and disorderly – every cell for itself so to speak – they enter blood vessels, lymph channels and lodge in distant organs. When they multiply and the growth flourishes, the unfortunate host emaciates; the fast multiplying cancer cells require a great deal of food. We saw such happenings in the Nazi-occupied countries. And so they have to be resisted with all possible force – knife, radiation or drugs – often several of them given simultaneously since they act during different phases of cell reproduction.

Firstly, one has to strive to locate, identify and assess the force of the attacker as soon as possible. A "wait and see" attitude is unjustifiable. If a therapy has to be efficient, a correct and early diagnosis is of the utmost importance. This is not always possible, especially in a deep-seated cancer. New, sophisticated methods, however, are constantly devised. Early breast cancer, for instance, can be detected by mammography and thermography and the smallest breast lump explored by means of simple needle aspiration or drill biopsy – well before a physical examination could be of any significant value (breast is the commonest site of cancer in women). No wonder doctors began to look for screening techniques and carcinodiagnostic agents. It would have been so much easier to defeat Hitler had he been counter-attacked in 1936 when reoccupying the Rhineland – a resolute stand then might have meant his downfall – nipping the "grand design" in the bud! In fact Marshal Pilsudski did propose to the Western Powers a preventive war against Hitler several years prior to the German assault, but was cold-shouldered. It is a sin to strike first, but it is seldom a mistake. To treat

207

a felon with honesty leads to dishonesty. To quote François Rabelais: "Keep running after a dog, and he will never bite you." Mass screenings take an important place in the fight against cancer, yet in some other situations they may cause confusion. What does one do when silent gallstones are discovered? A great number of us carry them happily, ignorant of it. Such knowledge would only worry the patient and doctor alike without necessity to interfere. I remember a spritely couple who were retiring to Spain and decided to undergo a complete screening. Laboratory tests detected some abnormality, possibly of no consequence, but such disclosure far from reassuring caused unwarranted anxiety.

It is no less important to assess the strength, the attitude and the resources of the attacked. In the uneven struggle between cancer and patient, the latter almost completely lacks the necessary defence mechanism which medical men call autoimmunity. It was indeed detected in cancer patients but appears to be very meagre, unlike most other diseases where autoimmunity plays an important role. As always, exceptions can be found. Miraculous cures brought by spontaneous regressions of cancer had been reported. Here the cancer patient showed stamina and ability to fight his own battle to health. For the same reason the rate of growth of a cancer and the chances of survival among sufferers with a similar type of complaint vary from individual to individual. I once listened to a lecture by Sir Cecil Wakely, Ex-President of the Royal College of Surgeons and Chairman of the Council of Imperial Cancer Research Fund. He showed the audience photographs of his patient with extensive and inoperable breast cancer, taken fifteen years earlier, and later ones without any sign of the disease. The patient had not received any treatment, her immune forces alone were able to terminate the disease. By various means doctors attempt to encourage even the slightest sign of defence. Some are against prophylactic and post-operative radiotherapy as it would interfere with natural defences. It was realized that immune factors may influence the behaviour of cancer. Many of us carry minimal microscopic growths sometime during our life but in the normal way our defence mechanism holds them under control. We occasionally witness a body holding the manifest cancer down; when immunity fails the disease appears. Everson and Cole* quoted 216 cases of various

* "Spontaneous regression of cancer", Everson and Cole, W. B. Saunders Co. Philadelphia and London, 1966.

types of cancer which have shown regression in the absence of any significant treatment. Our increasing knowledge of physiology of the thymus gland opens new possibilities for future treatment of immunological deficiencies. Due to such deficiencies some people are more susceptible to infection than others. They develop malignancies and other diseases like rheumatoid arthritis, vasculitis and so forth more readily. One day doctors may succeed in stimulating appropriate forces to the extent that full control over such diseases, including cancer, would be achieved though I do not expect it to happen to-morrow.

At present other resources have to be mobilized, among them drugs able to slow down the rapid proliferation of cancer cells in the attacked body. For instance, selected antibiotics and some substances derived from plants are known to inhibit DNA and other vital synthesis. That way they interfere with cell growth and cell division and lead to its death. Their toxicity is tolerable as they act somewhat selectively against the cancer cells. We know that a foetus demands increased amounts of the folic acid for its rapid growth – maternal requirements for it increases some tenfold over those of the non-pregnant woman and it is customary to provide them with regular supplies of this vitamin. No wonder folic acid *antagonists* are able to control some types of acute leukaemia where there is an excessive proliferation of white blood cells. Gross reduction of leukaemic cells by several drugs, now at doctors' disposal, enables some patients finally to eliminate the disease by his or her own immune mechanism. The old saying: "Medicus curat, natura sanat" remains valid. The long term survival rate in this disease has increased in the last few years and every year brings more hopeful possibilities.

But the battle with cancer is still far from victory, and those who spoke of the all-out cure supposedly found by Dr. Issels of Germany, only raised false hopes. Cancer still claims over twenty per cent of total deaths. It is not a question of money or facilities. The mighty and famous die as easily as the humble and obscure. Lester Pearson, former Canadian Prime Minister and a Nobel prize winner for peace, succumbed to cancer in 1972, as did Francis Chichester, the daring British yachtsman known all over the world; early in 1974 it was the turn of the American Ambassador to the U.S.S.R., Charles Bohlen, whom I have mentioned earlier. In both religious and scientific terms man rises from dust and turns into dust. However, the search for more effective, less toxic anti-cancer agents continues. The concept that cancer is an incurable disease has changed, besides doctors have

209

learned to alleviate suffering. The cancer patients are not defenceless any more.

Lastly, one has to be vigilant that the enemy does not strike again – the maxim: "Prevention is better than cure" is most apt here. Publicity against smoking, reminding people that mortality from lung cancer in Britain exceeded 30,000 in 1970, campaign against unhygienic customs, pollution and radiation, popularization of screening techniques in high risk groups, dissemination of knowledge – all this is in doctors' daily armamentarium. Their research paves the way to more healthy living. The government recognizes the importance of all these problems and facilitates doctors' efforts by offering research grants and various other means.

New diagnostic techniques have made enormous progress in all branches of medicine – lymphangiography in malignant diseases, angiography in brain tumours and renal diseases, continuous electro-cardiographic monitoring, cardiac catheterization and angiocardiography in heart conditions, selective cinecoronary arteriography in coronary heart disease, continuous monitoring of blood pressure in hypertension, cholangiography in liver disorders, cine radiography, isotope scanning of various organs, xeroradiography, xonics electron radiography, electromyography, ultrasonic applications . . . Skills were developed which allowed observation of human chromosomes and their aberrations. Computers took care of medical records. No more clumsy instruments used by ferocious gastroenterologists to endoscope stomachs. Schindler's already flexible side-vision type of gastroscope has gained in flexibility and length with the passage of time. Eventually doctors were able to scrutinize a number of other deep seated organs under direct vision. We witnessed a vast increase in laboratory tests. For the first time an enzyme was used as a diagnostic tool; in 1954 Wroblewski found that "S.G.O.T." levels are raised in patients with myocardial infarction.* The same year Bodansky recorded elevated levels of another enzyme in patients with cancer. The field of modern clinical enzymology was opened. Thyroid function tests became more refined . . . and more complicated. A *laboratory* diagnosis found a place.

Improved diagnostic aids cut down the number of "neurotics." In many instances such diagnosis is a waste bin into which doctors choose to dump their failures. A patient of mine with persistent abdominal

---

* Destruction of a piece of heart muscle.

pain lived under the guise of a neurotic until improved radiological technique disclosed small stones in his biliary tract!

Hospital equipment has become very sophisticated. The blood testing machine, Coulter "S", is capable of carrying out seven various tests every twelve seconds; there is just not enough blood available for the hospital in my vicinity to feed the robot. A multi-chemistry analyser carries out twenty different tests and accommodates three hundred samples in one hour. These are costly wonders. A single blood testing machine is priced at over £50,000, and the one for chemistry exceeds £60,000. An Auto-Analyser for platelets with a turnover of sixty blood samples an hour costs £5,000. In a specialized hospital I admired a huge cyclotron – an electromagnetic machine possessing a gigantic magnet – used for generating a stream of neutrons in the treatment of cancer. It is priceless – it saves lives. X-ray equipment is being constantly improved with the aim of avoiding risks to the patient. Godfrey Hounsfield invented a new brain X-ray technique – the E.M.I. Scanner. There are only four or five of them in the whole of Britain as each costs some £200,000. Every day throughout the year over half a million people occupy beds in the United Kingdom and Eire and some sixty million visit out-patient clinics each year. The total expenditure on hospital services for the financial year 1972/3 was estimated at £1,693 million. It is therefore not surprising that the cost of a patient's stay in a modern hospital is calculated at £100 per week and as from 1st April, 1973 the charges for resident private patient accommodation were increased to £137.20.

In spite of all advances there is still some small risk attached to diagnostic X-rays. Statistical evidence shows that children who have been X-rayed when still in the womb, were nearly twice as likely to succumb to malignant diseases before their tenth birthday as other children.*

Doctors have been aware of this for quite a time, but I remember older days when expectant mothers were X-rayed routinely in the early stages of pregnancy – a technique in disrepute for some years. Perhaps we still have too many X-ray examinations, no difference being made between the very young and not so young, once a doctor decides to establish a diagnosis. Many patients put pressure on their doctors to have "a picture taken" and a refusal often causes dissension.

Prompted by easy availability of diagnostic aids and blinded by science, some younger doctors cold-shouldered the taking of careful medical history, their own powers of observation and use of their

* B.M.J. 26 August, 1972.

fingers, for which there will always be a place! Where an older doctor was guided by experience the younger one leaned on statistics and elaborate mechanical requisites. An art was being turned into technology, not always to the patient's advantage. A mechanical diagnosis has its limitations. A good example is epilepsy where clinical diagnosis is far superior to clever electro-encephalography. The same applies to disseminated sclerosis and anorexia nervosa* – no X-rays, no laboratory tests or any other diagnostic techniques can aid diagnosis. Observation needs very few tools, if any, and can be extremely effective. It was the observation that dairy-maids were escaping smallpox, rampant in the 18th century, which led to the epoch-making vaccination. Denis Burkitt's scientific achievements were due to his powers of observation. When working as a surgeon in Uganda he first described a form of cancer common in African children, now known as Burkitt's tumour. He further observed the geographical distribution of the disease which led him to think that it may be caused by a virus; later several viruses were isolated from the diseased tissues.** Professor Brotzu observed the marine life near a Sardini sewage outfall and this led him him to new antibiotics; he used the crude products for treating typhoid fever and brucellosis with some success, much before these antibiotics were identified by Florey at Oxford. In 1948 a Sister in the Colchester Hospital observed in babies with neonatal jaundice that parts of their bodies exposed to the sun regained normal texture much quicker. It led to phototherapy adopted by the medical profession for this condition.

Over-specialization with fragmented knowledge could also be a drawback. A young would-be specialist used all his enthusiasm on a patient of mine who had a frozen shoulder. The doctor was successful all right but I had to treat this patient for a strained heart afterwards. It was forgotten that she was seventy-three years of age. I found that consultants with first-hand knowledge of general practice offered the best service to patients. Even such a clear-cut case as mending a fracture requires profound knowledge and is in fact a *medico*-surgical endeavour. It is not the bone alone that matters as equal attention has to be paid to the cause, patient's general health, circulatory system, muscles, age . . . It should be remembered that an ill person is inclined to be introspective and looks as much for the doctor's skill as for his support and reassurance. A doctor or a nurse can instil optimism into the patient, but can the same be expected from a mechanical device?

* A serious nervous condition which leads to emaciation, even death.
** The controversy over the causation of Burkitt's tumour continues.

The therapeutic progress has been astonishing. One can hardly believe that the operation for appendicitis, which practically carries no mortality, had a risk of over 50% deaths when it was first introduced by the Berlin surgeon Eduard Sonnenburg less than one hundred years ago. A test bearing his name advises that if a patient with an attack of appendicitis does not show an increase of temperature after administering an oily purgative, the disease is sufficiently quiescent to justify operation. None would contemplate giving a purgative in acute appendicitis these days; besides we have much better tests than that. The operation for appendicitis, performed on Edward VII in 1902, was as much publicized then as a heart transplant is to-day. Walter Sutton – who invented the chromosome theory of heredity in 1903 – succumbed to it at the age of 39. In 1926 Rudolf Valentino, the great lover of the screen, met the same fate; he was 31.

In my younger days I watched the removal of the prostate gland – a relatively frequent operation. It was carried out in two stages, months apart, during which time the patient had to be content with a tube protruding from the lower abdomen. Substantial blood loss through crude technique and infection resulted in a high mortality rate. In the late 1930's this procedure was simplified for suitable cases as a one stage operation of comparative safety. In 1947 Terence Millin introduced an even safer method which obviates incision of the bladder. Additionally, surgical diathermy coagulates the bleeding vessels by high frequency electric currents, achieving bloodless division of tissues. Removal of the womb and caesarian section, major operations in older days, are viewed as comparatively minor "ops" to-day.

Surgery has continued to increase in safety and scope. The two world wars drew attention to treatment of shock and perfected the technique of blood transfusion. I was carrying it out during the Italian campaign and saw many lives saved. The British Transfusion Service is one of the best in the world and donations are entirely voluntary.

The advances in anaesthetics gave further impetus to surgery. Since the beginning of this century when the German surgeon Ferdinand Sauerbruch found a method for opening the chest without causing collapse of the lungs, chest surgery developed into a fine art. The whole lung or part of it is removed to specification, heart defects surgically corrected, defective valves replaced by artificial ones, blocked arteries substituted by tubes. Discovery of anti-clotting agents assists such endeavours. It is strange that one such drug, Warfarin, was used for a long time as a rat poison. Babies born with serious heart defects are often easily recognizable on account of a bluish appearance, but until some twenty years ago doctors were powerless and such children succumbed to serious complications after years of suffering. I remember a cousin of mine who was the same age as myself. She was a blue baby – a delicate girl, easily tired and breathless. She led a very restricted life and died at the age of ten. Her parents lived all those years under constant stress and my favourite aunt, with whom I made the memorable trip to the High Tatra, fell out with her husband. To-day my cousin's condition would possibly be amenable to surgery and corrected, and the marriage of her parents saved. Among modern methods of heart investigation is cardiac catheterization. It was conceived in 1929 by a German doctor, Werner Forssmann, whose courage and conviction, after successful experiments on cadavers, allowed him to pass a catheter into his own heart. "I observed the tip of the catheter in a mirror held in front of the illuminated screen by a nurse" – he recalled – it reached the right atrium. No harm resulted and he repeated this procedure eight more times. Forssmann who was a surgical registrar contacted the leading Berlin surgeon, Professor Sauerbruch, but was told that the Professor "ran a clinic – not a circus." The medical men were appalled by the innovator's unorthodoxy, and so he left hospital for general practice.

It took twelve more years before cardiac catheterization was established by Cournand and Richards who shared a Nobel prize with Forssmann. Heart surgery continues to give new hope. It is often successful in relieving severe pain in coronary artery disease by supplying blood to the starved heart muscle which cries for it. In 1936 Beck in the U.S.A. endeavoured to bring more blood to the heart by application of grafts, and the following year a pmising young surgeon, Lawrence O'Shaughnessy, was doing it in England using omentum (duplication of peritoneum in the abdominal cavity). The tragic war deprived mankind of its potential benefactor – he was killed in 1940 at Dunkirk. Not for the first time has mankind suffered such a blow owing to its stupidity. In the French Revolution Antoine Lavoisier,* the founder of modern chemistry, was guillotined after hearing that "the Republic does not need learned men". In 1943 the work of world-famous geneticists, Eugene and Elizabeth Wollmans, was sadly terminated when they were arrested in the Pasteur Institute, Paris, deported and sent to the gas chambers.

* He believed that respiration depends solely on the lungs. Otto Warburg later proved that it is the cells which actually respire.

The recent five year survey of patients with aorto-coronary by-pass graft was most encouraging. Those suffering from severe angina were able to walk without pain a few days after being operated on and have continued to feel well. The survival rate of them was better than in the control group. In February 1973, Benjamin Frankel, a composer described as one of the major English symphonists of our time, died in London of a massive heart attack after surviving an earlier one. I knew this softly spoken, gentle and modest man well. He had to take a large amount of glyceryl trinitrin tablets for anginal pain for several years. To-day patients with severe angina are operated on not only for the relief of pain, but also to prevent a possible heart attack. It is no more a desperate, dire thrust, but effective treatment. Ten years ago a patient of mine in his early fifties developed chest pain. X-rays revealed a progressive widening of the aorta which was causing the pressure symptoms. Fatal rupture of the aorta was inevitable, yet no one would attempt surgery then. To-day surgeons are able to correct such aortic lesion and save many patients. In 1962 Dr. Melrose of the Hammersmith Hospital, having the benefit of Professor Aird's encouragement, invented the heart-lung machine which facilitates heart surgery.

In December 1967 Professor Christiaan Barnard of Cape Town carried out the first heart transplant. Such operations have since been done in other parts of the world, a few of them in Britain. But the most promising transplant operation, besides grafting a cornea to the eye, proved to be a kidney transplant. A new breed of doctors came into existence – that of transplant surgeons. It began in 1960. Initially the donor was a parent sibling with a well-matched graft giving a good chance of acceptance by the patient's body. Since 1963 kidney transplants from cadavers have also been used. This became possible because of better techniques in graft-matching and availability of improved immunosuppressive agents. Such drugs are able to counteract the immunological process of rejection of the foreign organ by the receiving tissue – the normal defence mechanism of the man or animal against a foreign body, in which enzymes play the key role. In 1972 the results of fifty-five such cadaver grafts, performed between 1965/68, were reported with survival up to seven years, all in reasonably good health.* Transplant operation spared a number of them the continuous, cumbersome and costly artificial kidney which needs a special renal unit manned by medical, nursing and technical staff. Transplants cost only 10 per cent of the cost per year of keeping a patient on

* British Medical Journal 29th July, 1972.

a kidney machine. However, prior to transplantation they have to make use of it, in hospital or at home. It is applied to thousands of patients all over the world. Damaged kidneys are unable to prevent a build up of toxins in the blood, and this procedure, introduced in 1960, does the necessary cleansing, so enabling the patient to survive. Improved storage of the donor's kidney and expansion of informational communication and transport enhance the prospect of kidney transplantations. It became an established form of treatment of end-stage chronic renal failure and special centres have been developed throughout the country.

A patient of mine, now thirty years of age, had a successful cadaver kidney transplant which has been working well since 1966. He has been on immunosuppressive drugs all this time and probably will need to continue taking them indefinitely. To see this patient I had to visit his home late one evening. He works long hours and values his own time and that of the doctors. He is enthusiastic about his operation and life in general. I admired his power of adaptation. He hoped I would display a poster in my car encouraging people to part with their organs and was rather disappointed when I coyly declined. Soon such advertising became acceptable and, by encouragement of Health Authorities, notices: "Your kidneys could help others to live" began to appear in doctors' surgeries.

A dramatic achievement of modern surgery was successful separation of conjoined twins.*

In 1953 the Dutch sisters Folkje and Tjitska De Vries were successfully separated in the Municipal Hospital of Leeuwarden, in 1954 a similar operation was carried out in London by Professor Aird and his team, and in 1965 yet another separation was achieved on the Italian sisters by a team of 15 medical men in the Margherita Clinic at Turin. The operation took five-and-a-half hours. Both sets of twins remain well, and so does the surviving girl of Professor Aird. The Philippino conjoined twins, brothers Godino, were joined together by the sacrum in about the same way as the Italian sisters. A surgical separation was performed, but neither survived it – the year was 1936. And still earlier no attempt of this kind was even contemplated. Brothers Chang and Eng** lived to their 63rd year, and death of one brought the end to the other. The Indian sisters, Gangamma and Gouramma, died in

* Twins physically joined together.

** They were born in 1811, in Siam, and so conjoined twins are known as Siamese twins.

1952 at the age of 53. Both couples spent their lives in travelling all over the world as a circus attraction.

Many have cause to be grateful for the immense achievements in plastic surgery. The team of Sir Harold Gillies, Sir Archibald McIndoe and Rainsford Mowlem was able to restore burnt and mutilated servicemen back to health; they also corrected serious malformations like a cleft-lip and palate and made many people happy by re-shaping their ears, noses, breasts and faces. By carrying out innovations they put plastic surgery on the map. Their pupils made a name for themselves in various parts of the world, like the internationally known Millard of Miami, U.S.A. Yet the first chair in Plastic Surgery was created at the University of Berlin, back in 1918. It went to the son of a rabbi from Koenigsberg – Jacques Joseph. Earlier, he had to leave his post as an Assistant at the University Surgical Clinic for initiating the reshaping of ears and noses. Only World War I made Joseph a respectable figure by giving him the opportunity of facial reconstruction for war victims. "Cosmetic surgery" extended its scope. I watched a few of my patients in whom cosmetic surgery not only increased their comfort, but also their morale. It was not just a question of beautification. A man in his thirties lived in perpetual misery hiding his neck, as a line had been tattooed round his neck with the inscription "cut here". "I consented to it when I was a drunken sailor", he sadly told me. Plastic surgery restored his happiness. Modern techniques are employed for *repair* or *reconstruction* of the human body, therefore it is strange that such efforts should bear the name "plastic surgery." Moreover, in this age of plastics such a term is misleading to the public. The war is over and it is hoped that it will never happen again, yet the *reconstructive* surgery must remain in demand because of road, industrial and sport casualties, and those caused by violence.

Orthopaedic surgeons were not out-done. Alloys have been developed that could remain indefinitely in the body without corrosion and in 1935 Marius Smith-Peterson, an American, introduced a nail for fixing a fractured hip. Until then such a condition, frequently encountered in the elderly, put patients in peril. Smith-Peterson changed all this. In November 1972 Lady Churchill, 87 years of age, left Westminster Hospital "in the pink of condition" three weeks after breaking her hip. "Internal fixation" for various fractures scrapped the long periods in plaster. The modern treatment enables better restoration of function of the broken limbs and earlier return to activity. Introduction of metal and plastic hips and other joints, knees and fingers among them, opened a whole new avenue. A patient of mine had a very successful total replacement of the shoulder by an artificial joint. People disabled by rheumatoid arthritis undergo a series of operations to restore their mobility and above all to alleviate pain, thus attaining a more independent, satisfying and useful life. In fact the treatment of disabling rheumatoid arthritis became a combined medico-surgical endeavour. Several of my patients have benefited this way. Such advances are only possible through research and experimentation. I once listened to an exposition concerned with progress in the field of bone replacement. A lecturer demonstrated photographs of a dog which had a bone transplanted. The poor pet looked sadly at his master who was stroking his head. A close-up showed a healed scar on the dog's leg. The experimental animal was watched for some months after which it had to be destroyed to examine the implanted bone. I felt just as sad as the dog. It reminded me of the photographs of women inmates of the Ravensbrueck concentration camp showing their deep, long leg scars – the evidence of scientific experiments on those human guinea-pigs.

Another field of surgery was brought to prominence by sheer necessity – that of traumatic surgery. Towards the end of the last century an innocent moving toy appeared on the British Roads – the automobile. It claimed its first victim on August 17, 1896 when a pedestrian was killed at Crystal Palace, London, and two-and-a-half years later a driver lost his life at Grove Hill, Harrow, Middlesex. The speed limit was then eight miles per hour. With the passage of years the automobile became like a monster, getting bolder, dangerous, indispensible and ubiquitous, still retaining some good, pleasure-like qualities. A kind of Dr. Jekyll and Mr. Hyde, the latter holding roads to ransom. During 1972, 7,730 people, drivers and pedestrians alike, were killed and some 350,000 injured – the ever increasing figures matching the expanding traffic. Violence and suicide claimed many more victims. But I heard of one act of violence done "in good faith." A convict asked another inmate to do him a favour and to hit him on the head with a bottle so that he could change prison for hospital. His "friend" obliged and he succeeded in reaching it . . . dead.

Casualty departments, until recently the Cinderellas of medicine, were given fuller attention and their work was delegated to more experienced men than in the past. Prompt, skilful resuscitation and help from qualified anaesthetists enabled many more lives to be saved. Naturally, expert aftercare of high standards is a prerequisite for the success in all major surgical procedures.

Rehabilitation to the fullest physical and mental ability is aimed for, and teams comprising of doctors, physiotherapists, occupational psychologists, therapists, work supervisers, resettlement officers, social workers and so forth were formed. Patients' disabilities are dealt with in the context of their whole personalities and problems involved. Group therapy treatment for alcoholics, drug addicts, those who suffered a myocardial infarction and so forth is such an example. Modern rehabilitation tries to restore physique, mind and social status. Doctors of to-day are much better equipped to deal with complexities of medical situations than their predecessors. But it took two world wars to achieve it.

A vast pharmaceutical armamentarium became a powerful weapon. Sulphonamides were joined by antibiotics which, although themselves derived from various microbes, destroy others or inhibit their growth. They fight among themselves like the human race! Louis Pasteur, the great French scientist of the 19th century, observed that dangerous germs perish in a matter of hours when introduced into the soil. He concluded that they were killed by other germs with which the earth teems. It is a matter of living space and survival, a struggle which never stops. He noticed that a similar fight takes place in the air. Pasteur was one of the greatest microbe hunters of all time. No wonder man began to manipulate germs against those which were attacking him. By means of inoculations homo sapiens was able sapiently to turn microbes against their own kind to his own advantage. In other instances germs help to correct damage caused by other species. In 1917 Wagner-Jauregg, a Viennese psychiatrist, introduced with success treatment for paralytic dementia – a result of syphilitic infection, by injecting patients with malaria parasites. Even such vicious germs as haemolytic streptococci can do man a good turn. The enzyme streptokinase, formed during their growth, dissolves clots in blood vessels and may be used in coronary thrombosis. In 1901 the first effective antibiotic, pyocyanase, was isolated from a microbe but abandoned because of its hazards to the patient.

In 1928 Professor Alexander Fleming, a bacteriologist, noted in the laboratory at St. Mary's Hospital, London, a phenomenon which led him to the discovery of penicillin. It was a perishable, elusive substance from a mould. Eleven years later a team working in the Sir William Dunn School of Pathology at Oxford and headed by Howard Florey and Ernst Chain succeeded in extracting penicillin. Experiments soon proved that penicillin protects mice against many infections without causing toxic effects. Subsequently it was found that the drug affects microbes by interfering with their cell-wall formation. It was a case of one germ destroying another.

On February 12, 1941, a London Bobby, dangerously ill with blood poisoning, was injected with penicillin. The amount of the drug available was very small and this very first patient relapsed after initial dramatic improvement and soon died owing to insufficient dosage. (A man is 3,000 times the weight of a mouse). A little later, Florey had to give his entire supply of penicillin to St. Mary's Hospital to save Fleming's friend ill with meningitis. It worked. When more penicillin had been made available, a number of cures were obtained at the Radcliffe Infirmary, Oxford. With the help of an American company a large-scale production followed, and the output was devoted primarily to the war effort. During the 3rd year of the war, when Churchill was struck by pneumonia, penicillin saved his life. D-Day was faced with sufficient supplies to save thousands of casualties. Mass production of penicillin had to go to the U.S.A., outside the bombing range.

Since 1945 antibiotic fermentation plants have begun to emerge in Britain, the one at Ulverston in Lancashire being the biggest of its kind in Europe. With the passage of time and more widespread use of the drug many microbes learnt to defend themselves against penicillin. They produce enzymes, collectively called penicillinase, capable of decomposing the penicillin. Medical people call such artful germs the "penicillin-resistant" organisms. Scientists went to counter attack. They were able to determine the structure of penicillin molecule and isolate its nucleus. In the 1950's modifications of the penicillin molecule were achieved in the British Beecham Research Laboratories. A variety of semi-synthetic penicillins with increased range of activity against germs was achieved — in fact over 2,000 of them. Some have the ability to resist decomposition by penicillinase, and many are well absorbed when given by mouth, so obviating frequent painful injections. After 30 years of use, penicillin is still the drug of choice for a host of infections and the possibility of producing new varieties remains great. But we have learnt to treat penicillin with discretion, and the practice of using it, for instance, as a poultry feed supplement to stimulate the growth or to prolong food shelf-life has been restricted.

Penicillin was viewed as a wonder drug by many, but it was far from being a panacea. Serious diseases like smallpox, poliomyelitis, typhoid fever, typhus, dysentery and above all the scourge of tuberculosis were unaffected. In 1933 some 32,000 people under 65 died of tuberculosis in England and Wales alone. Professor Selman Waksman of Rutgers University, New Jersey, pondered about this and recollected Louis Pasteur's own perception. He observed that the tubercle bacillus was unable to live in the soil for any length of time and turned to it in search of a new antibiotic. The task of scouring the soil was a gigantic one, but Waksman found willing help from his assistants and students. Thousands of soil cultures were examined and in January 1944 he was able to announce the isolation of streptomycin, effective against the tubercle bacillus. Many more lives were saved, and in 1952 the bene-factor received a Nobel prize. He went a long way since he left the Ukraine in 1910 to avoid persecution of the Tsarist régime. More re-cently a semisynthetic derivate of the rifamycin group of antibiotics, rifampicin, was introduced and proved very effective against tubercu-losis and much better tolerated than streptomycin. It is fortunate that patients are able to obtain them through the National Health Service. A month's treatment with rifampicin alone costs more than £18 and has to be continued for a few years.

Higher standards of living consolidated the results and made tuber-culosis a near vanishing disease. *Near* vanishing only as a longer span of life today lets us look for it among the elderly, often debilitated and not-so-well-off citizens. The influx of people from the underdeveloped countries also carries a potential threat.

In 1947 a soil sample from Caracas, Venezuela, yielded organisms which produced chloromycetin – a brand name of chloramphenicol, isolated by Bartz. It is effective in typhoid fever and other diseases but was found to be a double-edged weapon as it might have a damaging effect on some organs.

A feverish attempt to wrest more antibiotics from the soil in the fight for yet unconquered diseases was under way – a hunt all over the globe. It was now Pfizer's turn. This American Pharmaceutical Com-pany paid some hundred pounds each to airline pilots to bring back soil samples from all over the world to its laboratories in Brooklyn. Ar-rangements were also made with many missionaries, explorers, trav-ellers and so forth. In 1949 a scoop of earth brought from Argentina yielded an important antibiotic, appropriately named Terramycin; "terra" is the Latin word for soil. Since then a number of closely re-lated substances, collectively called tetracyclines, have been used. They are known as "broad-spectrum" antibiotics, the range against germs being considerably wider than that of their predecessors. Like penicillins they are also employed for the increase of meat and poultry production, although mass produced vitamins are preferred for similar effect.

But scientists found that not only the earth yields desirable microbes. In 1945 Professor Brotzu, an Italian, took a mould from the sea off Sardinia which, at his request, was investigated by the Oxford team at the Sir William Dunn School of Pathology. From this mould several antibiotics have been obtained, among them cephalosporin C. Later the nucleus of cephalosporin C was isolated, so enabling the Glaxo scientists to develop an improved broad-spectrum semisynthetic antibiotic-cephaloridine. It did not happen in a flash – the year was 1964. In 1973 the second generation of cephalosporin family was introduced – cephradine, of a wider spectrum and quicker action due to better absorption. Along came Gentamicin, Kanamycin . . .

The broad-spectrum antibiotics attack a wide variety of microbes – those causing diseases as much as the sinless ones. A great many of them live in the large bowel, competing for available food supply, but nature sees to it that a well adjusted balance is preserved. Every day each of us witness harmony in the living world. The multiplying of worms in the soil gets restricted by competition among themselves for space and food, climatic conditions and by birds eating them etc. The propagation of birds in turn is controlled by similar means and the hunting man. Now, broad spectrum antibiotics disturb the delicate balance. Those microbes not affected by antibiotics multiply freely when the opposing organisms are suppressed. The once harmless microbes become a nuisance after reaching great numbers. All of us have seen "thrush" in an infant – whitish spots in the mouth caused by fungi. Such fungal infection often spreads to other parts of the body producing a number of unpleasant symptoms and is the penalty of treatment by antibiotics. Moreover, in the normal course of events, the harmless inhabitants of the intestinal lumen produce certain vitamins, especially those belonging to the B group, essential for the health of the body. As a result of antibiotic treatment, however, the abnormal bacterial flora robs the host of those vital substances causing nutritional deficiency. It is like going against nature. Again, the undaunted inventive mind of man was able to defend him – an antibiotic, nystatin, with a broad antifungal activity, was isolated by Hazen and Brown in 1949. Vitamin replacement is another safeguard.

In the late 1960's Hitchings of the United States discovered trimethoprim after twenty years of study; in the later stage he was helped by the British scientist Bushby. Trimethoprim inhibits an enzyme and causes cessation of bacterial DNA synthesis. By binding many thousand times more avdly than it does to the corresponding human enzyme, trimethoprim disrupts an essential biological process in certain bacteria without exerting a similar effect in the cells of human host. Sulphonamides, introduced by Domagk twenty-five years earlier, have a similar action. Each prevents the growth of many bacteria – we say the drug exerts a bacterio*static* action. By combining both drugs a smaller amount of each is required for bacteria*cidal* (destructive to bacteria) effect. A superior kind of chemotherapeutic agent was created, effective against various diseases including typhoid fever, urinary infections, bronchitis, gonorrhoea, brucellosis, etc.

Protective inoculations found an important place in the fight against germs. It all started at the turn of the 18th century when Edward Jenner protected a boy against smallpox by introducing the vaccinal virus into his arm. He obtained it from the finger of a dairy-maid infected by cowpox. Smallpox was a killer. It was so prevalent that the *absence* of pock-marks was used as a descriptive peculiarity enjoyed mostly by dairy-maids. Another Englishman – Almroth Wright – achieved protection against typhoid fever in volunteers bound for the Boer War by injecting dead typhoid bacilli into them. Albert Calmette and Alphonse Guerin, French bacteriologists, introduced vaccination of infants against tuberculosis by infecting them with tubercle bacillus deprived of its virulence. This procedure has since been applied to those teenagers who lack immunity against this germ. B.C.G.* vaccine protects them against tuberculosis. Afterwards scientists introduced many more vaccines – against tetanus, diphtheria, cholera, rabies, plague, typhus, yellow fever, poliomyelitis, influenza, measles, German measles, even mumps.

But not only germs kill human beings, and so scientists had to cast their eyes to other life-saving drugs besides chemotherapeutic agents and antibiotics. Several of them revolutionized treatment.

The era of corticosteroids started in 1949 when patients crippled with arthritis were given extract from the "cortex" – the outer wall of the adrenal glands situated above each kidney. In a short time joint pains and stiffness were dramatically relieved. A year later two Americans – Hench and Kendall – shared the Nobel prize with Reichstein, a Swiss. It was soon noticed that asthma, allergies and other inflammatory diseases, even the effects of stress and shock, were helped by

* Bacillus Calmette Guerin.

223

treatment with corticosteroids. 100 per cent mortality from pemphigus vulgaris was halved. Yet the treatment headed for disappointment because of its many harmful effects. Again, the fine balance existing in the body was disturbed. Less dangerous and much more potent synthetic analogues – "prednisone" and "prednisolone" – were introduced by the Schering Corporation in New Jersey in 1955. The drug found a wide use and is also employed for many skin diseases, treatment of which was previously neglected. Steroids, like antibiotics, help to fatten livestock. They have great potential in agriculture – steroids exist in plants and play an important role in their growth. Man is no exception. Steroid male hormones retard the breakdown of tissue and speed up cellular growth by promoting the synthesis of protein. In medical circles this is called the constructive *anabolic* metabolism. Several anabolic agents were created for use on underweight patients, debilitated by illness or advanced age. They can also help cancer victims where malignant cells take more than their share of nourishing substances from the host, upsetting his or her metabolism. Thousands of steroids are in existence, natural and synthetic, all having a basic common structure. Seven more scientists have been awarded Nobel prizes for work in this field.

Important sex hormones were elucidated well before the era of corticosteroids. "Hormone" means "urging on" in Greek. Such substances exert a specific effect on the activity of cells in various – even distant – parts of the body; they are in fact chemical messengers. As a means of communication between millions of cells they provide a regulatory system required for normal functioning of the body and are supreme integrators of events. Hormones imprint emotional behaviour, human personality and sex – in short – they shape us. The first pure sex hormone was isolated by Butenandt in 1929. It was a female hormone, an oestrogenic compound. Two years earlier Selmar Aschheim and Bernhardt Zondek, Berlin gynaecologists, discovered that the urine of pregnant women and mares is a fruitful source of hormone. They devised a test for pregnancy, injecting woman's urine into immature female mice. Their research laid the foundation of Butenandt's work, sponsored by a German pharmaceutical firm Schering. Soon replacement therapy for correcting deficiencies existing in menstrual disorders, miscarriages, and "change of life" was instituted but only on a very limited scale. The required hormones had first to be obtained from urine of pregnant women, to be later substituted by that of mares, and eventually produced synthetically.

Many hormones are related to steroids. By 1938 another Schering scientist, Inhoffen, synthesized ovarian hormone – Oestradiol – from cholesterol, upon which we must look as a pre-hormone. Cholesterol is a major body steroid, a fatty substance in our blood, whose structure was established in 1928 by Windaus and Wieland. It had to be obtained from animal sources such as the spinal cords of cattle and consequently its supply was restricted. Then came the breakthrough. Scientists succeeded in reproducing the pregnancy hormone, progesterone, from a plant* which grows in Mexico, following the successful attempt of Butenandt. This enabled mass production of progesterone by the Amn firm Syntex. The drug was given by injections. In 1951 an oral progestational agent was synthesized and led to the birth control pill which came on the market nine years later. The egg "ovum" develops into an infant only after leaving its depot – "ovary" and meeting a travelling male sperm. It is this fertilized single cell which gives rise to the body structure. Following liberation of the ovum, a process known as ovulation, a yellow mass called "yellow body" (the "corpus luteum") develops in the part of the ovary which the egg has vaated. It secretes progesterone responsible for subsequent changes in the womb. During pregnancy the female hormones – oestrogen and progesterone – prevent the egg from leaving the ovary so making further conception impossible.

Important early studies were carried out by Dr. Gregory Pincus at the Worcester Foundation, U.S.A. The "Pincus pill" combined a synthetic oestrogen** with progestational*** agent. By then the problem of world population explosion was widely recognized. Since 1956 poverty stricken Puerto Rican women with large families have acted as guinea pigs. At the end of the eighteenth century the Reverend Thomas Robert Malthus stressed the danger of population increase beyond the means of subsistence.**** In the struggle against over population he advocated late marriage and abstinence. It has not worked. The pill proved to be the most reliable method of blocking pregnancy, with an almost 100 per cent reliability if properly used. The cautious British waited until 1960 before releasing it to the public. The method is almost as effective as sterilization. As with most of the drugs, undesir-

* Sex hormones and adrenal cortical hormones are linked with ergosterol, a substance found in plants, and analogous to the cholesterol. It would explain the use of some herbs by old civilization with the hope of preventing conception.

** Mestranol, a synthetic modification of Inhoffen's oestradiol.

*** Norethindrone and Norethynodrel.

**** Essay on the Principle of Population.

able effects are unavoidable, but accumulation of knowledge enabled scientists to produce a safer pill. There are 29 brands on the market today and 2 million women take them in Britain alone. It has wider possibilities. The raisers of livestock proposed putting their cows and ewes on medicated "pill-like" feed for a certain time to bring the sexual period of their animals to a specific date by withdrawing such medication. That way a whole herd could be artificially inseminated simultaneously – a stock rising to order. It is possible that a similar medication could control the fertility of domestic animals and wild life. It was reported that in Brisbane, Australia, an attempt was made to reduce the cat population by giving them crushed contraceptive pills in their daily milk. It met with success as they had no more kittens. The observation was also made that tom cats became more ladylike.

It is of interest that research-chemists of several countries have been able to produce totally synthetic equivalents of all the naturally occuring steroid hormones.

In a personal sense infertility can be as big a problem as overfertility. Sterility caused by faulty ovaries drove a twenty-eight-year-old patient of mine to distraction. She clung to the hope of having a child when the new drug, clomiphene, capable of inducing ovulation in selected cases, was announced in 1966. In this case there was no happy ending. Intercourse should have been timed to coincide with the expected date of ovulation. The woman was instructed to explain this to the husband and in doing so passed her apprehension to him, so that the poor man was unable to oblige, a thing that had never happened to him before . . . Emotional factors do play tricks with sexual functions in both sexes. (I observed this phenomenon in the forced labour camps.) Unfortunately, the treatment could not be repeated, the drug being in very short supply. Perhaps it happened for the best. Doctors at that time had little knowledge of the dosage required and a number of multiple births caused by ovarian over-stimulation and reaching as many as six had occurred, posing hazards.

A great surge of research activity resulted in an increased amount of drugs. In 1935 "prostaglandin" was extracted from the prostate gland, hence the name. Its chemical identity was established in 1962 enabling manufacture of the drug. Fourteen varieties of prostaglandins are known already, with the potential of treating a wide range of diseases. A synthetic prostaglandin "Prostin E_2" can be used for termination of pregnancy and induction of labour.

226

Drugs* which combat the bone pain in Paget's disease were introduced — a feat which escaped us till now.

Psychiatric illness was not excluded from the breath-taking progress of medical science. Specific chemo-therapy for various mental disorders was introduced. For centuries such patients were considered to be possessed by a demon and were subjected to intolerable sufferings in the endeavour to drive the evil spirit out of them. They were kept in prison-like buildings, out of sight and ostracized for life. They were called "lunatics" — creatures from another planet. "Mad houses" were visited by many people in search of amusement and William Hogarth and Francisco Goya painted them as social documents which reveal the intense horrors. It was Bedlam.** The nurses acted as guards and frustrated doctors looked on helplessly at the irrational, violent patients, trying to restrain them and finding a straight-jacket the only successful remedy. Nurses immersed them for hours in water or wrapped them in wet sheets, calling it hydro-*therapy*. More human treatment of ailments with cold water came later, pioneered by the Germans — farmer Vincenz Priessnitz and priest Sebastian Kneipp — eventually to be turned into scientific hydrotherapy by physician Wilhelm Winternitz. The unfortunate mental patients were looked upon as ferocious animals and Draconian measures used on them. People who suffered from nervous conditions such as anxiety, tension, insomnia and maladjustments were able to find only partial help from valeriana, bromides, opiates, chloral, paraldehyde and barbiturates.

Perhaps the best of all remedies was the spoken word by a sympathetic doctor. Such conversation could be rewarding for both of them. I was once told by a schizophrenic confined to a mental institution because of hallucinations, that his hearing was so much better than those around him. "Why did they put you in here then?" I asked. "It is simple, a majority has power over a minority and likes to use it," he explained with a smile. Even a madman has his logic. The spoken word was often reinforced by a placebo, a make-believe medicine, in the hope of spontaneous cure. "Prescribing is the art of amusing the patient while nature effects a remedy", wrote Voltaire in the eighteenth century. He was right to some extent — a depressive illness, for instance, tends to resolve spontaneously.

* Calcitonin and mitramycin.

** "Bedlam" — Asylum for the insane in Bishopsgate, London, some four centuries back. The words "Bedlam" and "madhouse" were since extended to an uproar of any kind.

But the unexpected happened. Since 1933 seriously disturbed patients have been treated by insulin therapy and in 1937 the electro-convulsive therapy – ECT – was also introduced. 1935 saw the beginning of brain surgery – leucotomy. But it was the year 1952 which made an epoch in psychiatric treatment bringing peace to Bedlam.

In that year the first tranquillizing drug, chlorpromazine, appeared, able to mitigate aggressive moods and delusions. It proved effective in a number of psychotic illnesses and various other conditions. Many related compounds have been developed since, followed by a host of drugs able to relieve anxiety efficiently.

Scientists got glimpses of pharmacological events in the human brain. Neurochemistry and biological psychiatry came into being preceeded by molecular biology. Back in 1921 Ernst Kretschmer of Germany described the alleged relationship between certain mental illnesses and certain types of body build. Later mongolism and other abnormalities accompanied by a mental defect were traced to faults in chromosomes. Such faults are sometimes confined to a small strip of chromosome, a molecular entity. Deprivation of the body of vital substances, whatever the cause, also plays an important role. The brain cells, like other cells, require for their metabolism the presence of Vitamin B complex. We have already heard that such deprivation leads to mental confusion in beri-beri and pellagra (vitamin B.12 deficiency, on the other hand, can lead to degeneration of the spinal cord). Myxoedema – a disease caused by a large deficiency of thyroid activity – may lead to various flagrant psychosis. A patient of mine led a miserable existence after having a leucotomy performed many years ago when she was in her forties. At the time she suffered from a "hopeless" psychosis – was irrational, often violent, with ideas of persecution. Much later myxoedema was diagnosed in this patient. Richard Asher, a physician at the Central Middlesex Hospital in the fifties, introduced the phrase "Myxoedematous Madness". Excessive activity of the thyroid gland may cause a maniac condition. Doctors recognized that a mental illness can be the consequence of disease of other organs than the brain and the thyroid. Another patient, a hard-working business man, developed sudden hallucinations and tried to throw himself out of the window. He was taken to hospital and treated with sedation. On the day when he should have started electroconvulsive therapy, he developed a high fever and a full scale investigation commenced. The "psychotic" patient was found to be suffering from cancer of the pancreas.

Mental illness was at last recognized as a physical occurrence, one which should be treated and not spurned. Brain and the rest of the nervous system need a great deal of energy for the elaborate functions. It is provided by the metabolism of blood-borne glucose. An adequate blood supply is of paramount importance for delivery of this glucose and the essential oxygen to the cells. Everyone knows how sensitive the brain is to even small deprivation of such a supply, as witnessed in a simple faint and sclerosis of the cerebral vessels. Certain amines, serotonin among them, also play a significant role in the central nervous system. The enzyme involved in the metabolism of serotonin is monoamine oxidase. Increase of the amount of serotonin in the brain produces changes in behaviour and could be responsible for emotional reaction. The knowledge that serotonin is important in mood regulation helped to institute effective treatment for the until now unapproachable illness – depression – known in olden days as melancholy. It is not caused by invasion of the mythical "black bile" after all!

The first anti-depressive drug was introduced in 1957 and was a potent monoamine oxidase inhibitor, in short MAOI. Other MAO inhibitors followed. MAOI's, when combined with certain foods, are known to bring severe hypertension, and are also able to cause hazardous potentiation of other drugs.* Because of these dangers and their varied performance the early enthusiasm for MAOI's turned into mistrust. Some thought that the drug only blocks the uptake of body noradrenaline which stimulates the nervous system. However, seventeen years of its use brought a new understanding of the biochemical activity of the drug and of the chemical changes that occur in affective illness. By blocking oxidation of monoamines, it raises amine levels and this way influences depression. It became known that monoamine oxidase consists of several enzyme systems and the suggestion was made that differences in clinical response to the drug might be due to its *selective* inhibition. People with phobic anxieties, not uncommon today, are particularly helped by MAOI's. One day doctors may succeed in tailoring specific inhibitors for depressed patients with such accuracy as to enable them to achieve a predictable clinical response.

In 1958 another anti-depressive agent appeared by the name of imipramine. Unfortunately, amphetamines known as "pep pills" and massively used in the past for their stimulating effect on the central nervous system (they were used during World War II by the German

* The recent study of migraine points a finger at the deficiency of monoamine oxidase as a likely cause (this enzyme tends to destroy any excess of harmful amines introduced by some foods).

Panzer troops), had to be almost abandoned by the medical profession. They produce only transient elevation of mood, their effect soon wears off and depression is felt with a vengeance. Moreover, their abuse and dependence pose a major social problem, especially among younger people, and a number of internationally known sportsmen fell victim to such practices. In the last war amphetamines were widely used by Japan for her Forces and factory workers. It caused a real epidemic of stimulant-taking in the post-war years; they had to be banned.

Mania is in all probability a biochemical upset as it can be initiated by one drug and relieved by another; in 1949 lithium salts were introduced for this condition with good effect. Lysergic acid diethylamide known as LSD has a striking effect on the brain. A new science was born – the biochemistry of mental function. It is able to alter one's mind by modifying feelings, perception and behaviour.

We are living in times of a successful revolution. The ignorance was removed and treatment with mind-changing substances achieved making many psychiatric patients less restless, less destructive and enabling them to leave institutions for community life. It gave hope to those who until now lived without hope.

Yes, the last twenty years greatly improved the quality of life. Doctors are able to relieve tension and anxiety, to help to overcome spells of depression, to bring sounder sleep without untoward effects, to mitigate grief. Helped by therapeutic advances they modify the nature of emotional responses and behaviour in man.

We have moved a long way from Professor Rose's "cytoarchitectonic" studies of the brain, and the sole anatomical structure, or morphology, became an outdated scientific tool, the emphasis being changed to function. But a great deal of research has still to be done to improve control over human behaviour. Such research meets with special difficulties. Experimentation on humans is limited for obvious reasons, and it is not easy to judge various emotions in animals with predictive value in man. Was the dog hostile and aggressive because it was given amphetamine, or because it happened to be a dog? We are simply guessing. We should also remember that every disease when connected with pain or discomfort has certain mental aspects not directly related to pathology.

Mood swings should be wisely accepted. It is a true saying: "No one is perfect", and there is no such thing as normality. To try to change one's personality by constant swallowing of pills would be as irresponsible as to "correct" the slanting eyes of a Japanese. More

230

important, an anxiety even to a point of anguish often constitutes a normal positive response to everyday stresses with which we have to learn to live. They are a driving force in life expressed in terms of ambition, the desire to assert oneself, etc. Insight and self-criticism are vital ingredients of progress. Sensitiveness is an asset and modesty a virtue. There is nothing more dull and irritating than a self-satisfied unimpeachable "know it all" braggart. Thus Samuel Johnson would not be able to write his "Lives of English Poets", Ignaz Semmelweis to rescue mothers in childbirth from puerperal fever, Vincent Van Gogh and Edward Munch to paint as they did, Charles Darwin to become the "father" of the theory of evolution and Jeanne d'Arc, French patriot and saint, Jack London, novelist, Orde Wingate, soldier extraordinary, to find a place in posterity, were they well-balanced, contented people and not the soul-searching ones they really were. The French composer, Hector Berlioz, attempted suicide in the early years of his career and doctors of Professor Aird's stature and Richard Asher's ability succumbed to internal stresses.

Marie Curie was an example where misfortune was turned into a driving force. The discoverer of radium lost her beloved husband and dedicated partner in their scientific work at the age of thirty-eight; Pierre Curie was killed in a street accident in 1906. More work was the prescription for Marie's grief and in 1911 she was awarded the Nobel prize for chemistry. Pablo Picasso expressed tensions in his private life through the symbolism of a bull-fight, and his great canvas "Guernica" was conceived by the tragic passion over happenings in the Spanish Civil War. John Howard who lived in the second half of the 18th century lost his wife in childbirth when he was thirty-nine. Howard devoted the rest of his life to the reform of prisons and various institutions of the sick which included plague houses in Britain and abroad.* Yet another example was the Polish writer Gabriela Zapolska. After an unsuccessful marriage she devoted herself to writing and dealt with the position of women exposing the hypocrisy of middle- and upper-class morality.

Many of the intellectual achievements of Jewish people could be explained by the unhappy circumstances in which they lived. Baruch Spinoza, the 17th century Dutch philosopher, was born of Jewish émigré family from intolerant Spain. Sigmund Freud suffered humiliations because of his Jewish origin. The Lwoff family, like that of Waksman, the discoverer of streptomycin, left pogrom-happy Russia

* "Account of the Principal Lazarettos in Europe", 1789.

and settled in France. In 1965 their son André became a Nobel prize winner held in great esteem by the scientific world. Konrad Bloch who left Germany for the United States in 1936 because of racial discrimination received the Nobel prize in 1964 for untangling the mystery of biological formation and regulation of cholesterol. Dr. Kissinger, the American Secretary of State, was a refugee from Nazi Germany. All these people, and many more, like the Russian physicist Andrei Sakharov and the Nobel prize-winning author Alexander Solzhenitsyn achieved success, even if in a personal sense they were not always successful. Internal strife seldom leads to happiness, but it can produce a most valuable life. Healers should be on their guard when clashing with the course of nature.

The astonishing progress was not confined to the fields of surgery, antibiotics, hormones and mind-changing drugs alone. Diabetics, saved by insulin, were in many instances able to discard injections for tablets. A similar thing happened to patients with accumulation of fluid in their body (dropsy) who needed an increased output of urine. In olden days such unfortunate people were deprived of salt in their diet and even bread had to be free of it. They were given hazardous mercurial injections or large doses of horrible tasting urea by mouth. Their value was limited and they often failed to act. Paracentesis – mechanical removal of fluid from the chest or abdomen – had to be applied, and when this also failed, Southey's tubes were inserted into the swollen legs or multiple incisions made in the skin. Sepsis was a calculated risk, there were no antibiotics to eliminate such a hazard. Then came a long list of non-mercurial oral drugs able to increase the output of urine – effective, quite safe, convenient, without danger of causing damage to kidneys. They are used not only in patients with an excess of body fluids but also in management of high blood pressure. A galaxy of other drugs, achieving a similar effect, have also appeared. The treatment of hypertension has become less difficult, less troublesome and so it was possible to extend it to more moderate forms of the disease. By relieving high blood pressure, complications as serious as myocardial infarction, popularly called "coronary", are being prevented and life prolonged.

Knowledge of allergies has also made big strides. The term was coined by the Austrian Paediatrician – Clemens Freiherr von Pirquet – in 1897 and is now a common word. Everyone knows of hay-fever, incidentally already described in 1565 by Leonardo Botallo, of asthma and of sensitivity to drugs, cosmetics and the like. I am often disbe-

232

lieved by patients when I trace his or her complaint to the use of lacquer or cosmetics. "But I have been using the same brand for years, doctor," I hear again and again. The fact is that, as in hay-fever, a person becomes sensitized by initial contact without showing any reaction. Such sensitization, however, results in production of substances tending to neutralize the foreign, and therefore harmful, matter with which such a person came in contact. These substances were given the name of "antibodies". Further contacts with the same offender, which we then call allergen, give rise to symptoms. Reaction between an antibody and allergen induces toxic substances, among which is histamine. The name means "Tissue amin", it being a widespread substance, easily liberated from cells. When it is pointed out to patients that hay-fever sufferers are sensitized to pollen protein, foreign to them, in their early childhood and therefore develop symptoms several years later, they accept the explanation. Better understanding of the phenomenon of allergy enabled more effective treatment and sharing the knowledge with sufferers. Scores of symptom-relieving drugs are used along with desensitization and most of all – preventive measures – which aim at avoidance of offending causes. In 1937 Frenchmen, Bovet and Staub, working at the Pasteur Institute, Paris, introduced the first antihistamine. Although these compounds are helpful in relieving symptoms of hay-fever and other allergic responses, they are of little use in asthma where histamine is only one of several causative factors. In prevention of this condition the introduction of disodium cromoglycate in 1970 marked an important advance. Many patients requiring treatment with corticosteroids were able to reduce the dosage or even to stop the drug altogether. Disodium cromoglycate is a safe drug which inhibits the antigen induced release of toxic substances occasioned by reaction between antibody and allergen. It is used as inhalation of powdered material. A novel therapeutic approach to asthma came into being. The research project began in 1956. First, guinea pigs and rats were used, then dogs and monkeys, and fresh human lungs removed at surgery were also employed. The substance has been shown to be effective in preventing bronchial spasm – the allergic response in the lungs in sensitized patients. The drug affords good protection to many asthma sufferers for whom desensitization, corticosteroids and various ephedrine compounds can be reduced or dispensed with altogether. Disodium cromoglycate is not a placebo, but in a complaint such as asthma supportive measures may be required – education in breathing, sedatives, psychotherapy. It can be triggered off, besides

233

various allergies, by infection, exercise, emotion . . . Some fifteen years ago a patient of mine was showing a poor response to treatment of his asthma by orthodox methods. In desperation, I referred him to Dr. Maginet in London who practised hypnosis. The doctor traced the attacks to the shock the patient received some twenty years earlier on finding his friend lying in a garage full of exhaust fumes. When the significance of that episode was explained to him, his asthmatic attacks ceased completely. Here it is worth mentioning how much human reactions vary. The suicide of a young colleague witnessed by the German poet Goethe resulted in the famous novel: "The sufferings of the young Werther", written by him at the age of twenty-five.

New oral drugs* widen bronchi by selectively stimulating their musculature and this way effectively relieve symptoms of asthma; the heart is not affected. This was not possible in the olden days when adrenaline *had* to be injected for this condition. It stimulates the heart, raises blood pressure, causes restlessness. Often a number of these injections were needed to wear off the attack. The only possible alternative was ephedrine, given by mouth, which unfortunately produces similar side-effects. Steroids, which are still used for severe cases of asthma, are also frowned upon because of unwanted effects.

Another group of drugs** suppress certain of the actions of adrenaline and noradrenaline, both present in the body. They are used for calming hearts which thump in stressful situations; they take the heart out of one's mouth so to speak. But by damping down the heart, these new drugs slow the heart rate and lower the blood pressure. In this way they bring relief from anginal pain and are the best drugs available for this dreaded and not uncommon condition. Yet, despite all sophisticated modern drugs, the old treatment with glyceryl trinitrate, reassurance and patient's readjustment has stood the test of time. We continue to be guided by experiences of the 18th century physician from London – William Heberden – who first described angina (in Latin of course!) and attempted its treatment, also of Sir William Osler who made a study of it.

Pregnancy and labour are much more safe and less uncomfortable these days. Puerperal sepsis which killed thousands of women, among them Jane Seymour, the 3rd wife of King Henry VIII after she gave birth to Edward VI, disappeared a long time ago. Toxaemia of pregnancy is prevented or efficiently dealt with, complications of

* Beta-adrenergic stimulants.

** Beta-adrenergic blocking agents.

234

labour averted in time, delivery less painful and living up to its name – "natural childbirth". Even a caesarean section is a comparatively simple and safe procedure preferred by some women to the orthodox delivery. Life-threatening post-partum haemorrhage is almost unheard of. A continuous fall of death-rate through pregnancy in Britain has been recorded. And, unlike in the olden days, there is no fear that something might happen to the baby. In 1850 Charles West reported that "one child in five dies within a year after birth and one in three before the completion of the fifth year". Marshal Tito's parents had fifteen children of whom only seven survived infancy. These days pneumonia, osteomyelitis and other serious infections are prevented or arrested in time, besides we have resuscitators, ventilators, incubators . . .

Birth is a natural process. Patients get pregnant and have babies because, and in spite of, what we do for them. A heavy young woman arrived at my surgery with a sample of urine complaining of frequency. I had never seen her before – her husband registered the woman with me a few months earlier. The urine did not show any abnormality and I decided to examine the patient internally. She laid down on the couch without removing her skirt. To my amazement my stretched fingers touched the baby's head. "My dear," I said, "You will be having a baby very soon!" She did not believe me. "It's not possible, I can't be. I've been having regular periods, although . . .," she paused, "they have been much more scanty than in the past." I knew there was no more time for argument. "Well," I said, "I am sending you to hospital for a second opinion. . ." "All right," I heard, "I am only doing it to convince you, doctor, that you are wrong, this question of pregnancy is just preposterous." "Would you like me to call an ambulance or will you have a taxi?" I enquired regardless. "No thank you, I have to do some more shopping first, before I go to hospital." And out she went – slowly, reluctantly, carrying a large shopping bag with her. She was lucky, she reached the hospital an hour before her delivery. It went without a hitch. Her husband was at work, when he was informed that he had become a father. He cast his eyes on the calendar thinking it must be All Fool's Day. Each of us make mistakes sometimes, and doctors are not immune, but I was right that time! In retrospect the woman was impressed with my diagnosis, and although she moved some few miles away, she has remained my patient.

And so we see progress in every branch of medicine.

I have touched on many new drugs and remedies but left out the

235

most important two – oxygen and water. One fifth of the earth's atmosphere is oxygen. Doctors learnt its importance in general anaesthesia, myocardial infarction, pulmonary failure and various other conditions. The endotracheal tube and the peak flow meter (assesses the capacity of the lungs) are among their tools, and they are able to ventilate* patients. The British Oxygen Company is very much in business. Our awareness of the deficiency of oxygen in the inspired air and its dangers is another measure of safety among the medical profession.

Water is the cheapest medicine; 71 per cent of our planet is covered by it. Water combats dehydration in acute gastroenteritis and other conditions, dilutes and eliminates toxic substances, humidifies "croupy" throats, loosens inspissated sputum, gives daily comfort . . . Since over 60 per cent of our body is water, no wonder it is constantly in need of it. Besides, there is a saying, "Drinking water neither makes a man sick, nor in debt, nor his wife a widow."

Man should not forget another useful remedy – REST. We ought to rest our gut when it is out of order, and our heart, brain, eyes and muscles when they are tired.

Lastly, we must realize that despite all marvels in the field of surgery, it is only a crude method which usually takes over where physicians have failed. Drugs are to be preferred to chest surgery in tuberculosis, and to brain surgery in mental diseases. Gallstones, for instance, have to be removed surgically only because up until now doctors have failed to dissolve them efficiently and with safety. At the present time a trial** is going on at Hammersmith to achieve such a goal. The wise man, Benjamin Brodie, 19th century English surgeon, promoted conservative treatment of diseased joints and effected reduction in the number of amputations. The enthusiasm for surgery in arterial renal stenosis, to combat high blood pressure, has waned. This very day efforts are made to replace the crude and hazardous operation for slipped disc with injection of the enzyme chymopapain derived from the papaya plant into the offending place, which treatment is said to cause the disc to shrink and slip back into place. Scientists look for the possibility of replacing hypophysectomy – a major surgical procedure for advanced cancer – by selective *pharmacological* removal of pituitary hormone.

It is a pity that one "action" is altogether forgotten – *leaving well alone* so that nature could step in!

* Intermittent inflation of lungs with air in place of spontaneous respiration.

** With chenodeoxycholic acid, originating from bile.

However, I have witnessed an enormous increase in man's understanding of nature in my lifetime. The great advances in diagnostic procedure and treatment benefited many of my patients. It was little short of a miracle.

The discovery that an atom consists of a nucleus and some surrounding electrons was made just over sixty years ago. Since then knowledge of the structure of atoms has been extended to molecules that one finds in living organisms. The protein molecules and their special class – the "operational proteins", otherwise enzymes, were found to be of special importance. We learnt to understand the biomechanics of DNA by means of which organisms reproduce themselves. Our constantly increasing knowledge of enzymes and various aspects of cellular metabolism leads us to a better comprehension of the intricate functioning of living creatures from micro-organisms to human, in health and disease. The secrets of the biology of the cell began to open. It seems that the basis of all life on earth boils down to one fundamental happening – the communion of proteins with nucleic acids. Involved physical and mechanical processes constantly take place in the living body so that energy can be produced for various activities. Even in a state of complete rest a person uses energy for essential happenings such as beating of the heart, breathing and maintenance of body warmth. Such processes are known under the term of metabolism. In some instances energy is used to convert simple substances into more complex ones and we speak of *ana*bolism – "building up", in Greek. When complex substances are being changed to simpler ones, often with release of energy, we talk of *cat*abolism – "breaking down" process.

The progress went far beyond medical science and culminated in putting men on the moon for the second time. It was an American achievement, although the Russians succeeded in the soft landing of sensitive instruments with the object of obtaining important data. The Russians chose as the next target the planet Mars whose nearest approach, on 23 August, was some 35 million miles away, but their unmanned spacecraft may need to cover a voyage of over 200 million miles. Not to be outdone the Americans sent an unmanned spacecraft to the vicinity of the planet Jupiter and reckon that it will reach its target within two years. In 1974 they obtained photographs of Mercury, the smallest planet and closest to the sun, some 96 million miles away.

20

Some of our Benefactors

Life is a gift: from the few to the many; from those who know and
have to those who do not know and have not.

Amedeo Modigliani

All advances have not come to us by chance alone, but mainly by hard
work and the devotion of many. Biophysics, biochemistry, molecular
biology, genetics, immunology — all these sciences — helped by technology and engineering skill,* found practical applications to medicine. Electron microscopes, a variety of physical and chemical
techniques as well as automation were some of the tools helping to
solve medical problems. The forward-looking engineers were no less
important than the medical men. They assisted in solving mechanical
problems which have been hampering doctors — after all — the structure of bones and joints is a feet of engineering. Surgeons stopped
trying to save as much as possible of a damaged limb and paid more attention to the mechanics of function putting their trust in well-
designed prostheses. Easily controlled electronic aids were devised to
help severely disabled people in their rehabilitation. They are now able
to control their environment — to switch on lights, heaters, television,
use a telephone or a typewriter. Most of the time it is a team which
counts, not the labours of an old-type lonely wizard shut in four walls.

In the changing world Britain's military power and political influence were much reduced but not so her scientific achievements. Scientists engaged in the war effort were now able to focus their attention on
peaceful projects. Barnes Wallis, the inventor of the Dambuster's
bouncing bomb, developed the swing-wing plane. Professor Maurice
Wilkins, who worked on the atomic bomb, turned to molecular biology
and among other things we owe him early X-ray photographs of DNA.
Professor Alan Hodgkin, the war time worker on radar, switched his
interests to conduction of nerve impulses. Andrew Fielding Huxley
who researched in gunnery now joined him and developed microtome
for electron microscope sections. Radar was adopted for telecommuni-

---

* Philip Drinker, contemporary public health engineer in the U.S.A. devised an
apparatus for producing artificial respiration over long periods, which has saved many
lives.

238

cations and its principle was applied to the sonic torch for the blind and sonic aid foetal monitor which records the state of the unborn baby during its mother's labour. The system enabled air pollution studies by observing reflections of the laser beam from atmospheric particles. Nuclear energy was used in the fight against cancer. The submarine detection device used in World War II led to the echo sounder which determines the depth of the sea accurate to within six feet. It also led to echocardiography which safely delineates structure and motion of the heart and great vessels, to echoence phalography for investigation in strokes, to echorenogram in kidney investigation and echo-uterogram for womb investigation. Professor Solly Zuckerman,* who used goats to find out what effect bombs would have on humans (he was an adviser to Air Chief Marshal Tedder), turned to more peaceful studies. Wilkins, Hodgkin, and Huxley became Nobel prize winners and in all some fifty British scientists have been so honoured since the distinction was first set up by the Swedish inventor of dynamite in 1901. It was gratifying to know that sixteen of them had won it for work in medicine and physiology. In 1972 another Briton – Dr. Denis Burkitt – received an American distinction of international prestige for his work in cancer, and early in 1973 Dr. Michael Epstein of Bristol University and Dr. Michael Wright of the University of Southampton were presented with West Germany's highest award for outstanding work in medical research. This was in the best tradition of British science which achieved second place among many nations, surpassed only by the U.S.A. It has kept up the pace determined by such giants as Harvey, Newton, Dalton, Faraday, Joule, Kelvin, Thomson, Rutherford and many others. Five refugees from Nazi Germany contributed their own Nobel prizes.** Among them was Ernst Chain who, with the Oxford team, solved the problem of producing penicillin. The twenty-seven-year-old Jewish scientist, endangered by the Nazis, arrived in Britain in 1933. Many more foreign scientists settled in Britain, helped by the Academic Assistance Council. Bernard Katz left Germany in 1935 for racial reasons, and has held the post of Professor of Biophysics at University College, London, since 1952. A Nobel prize winner of 1970, he is much interested in studies of the physio-chemical mechanism of neuromuscular transmission – the release from the nerve of

* Now Baron Zuckerman, he was reviewing the state of the hospital scientific and technical services.

** In 1974 three more Nobel prizes were awarded to British scientists. One of them was the Austrian-born economist Friedrich von Hayek.

a specific chemical substance which subsequently acts on the muscle cell.

These people were paying their debt for Britain's hospitality and the freedom afforded to them – the treasure they had lost earlier. Such a debt was also paid by Chaim Weizmann, the man who became the first President of the State of Israel. He spent his childhood in Pinsk, a town on the Polish marshes, at the time when Poland and especially the Jews were oppressed by Imperial Russia. Barred as a Jew from Russian universities, Chaim Weizmann went to Germany to study chemistry. He came to Britain in 1904 to take a lectureship in chemistry at Manchester University. His wife was able to practise as a doctor, a rare career for a woman in those days. Britain was their friend and Dr. Weizmann repaid the friendship in two successive wars. In 1917 he solved the country's problem of a serious ammunition shortage. Britain needed acetone for manufacturing an explosive called cordite. The immigrant chemist provided the crucial substance by fermenting corn; he used a bacterial cousin of the tetanus germ. Thanks to his inventiveness the needed product was manufactured in bulk in sufficient quantities to save the armament industry. The by-product butanol was discarded. In the second world war Dr. Weizmann made another famous contribution. After the fall of Malaya in 1942, he showed how to develop a synthetic rubber on which Britain and the United States depended. He fermented butanol which was ultimately converted to butadiene – the starting material. Polish-born Jacob Bronowski, who came here in 1920 at the age of twelve, became a British scientist, lecturer and writer. In 1945 he participated in British Chiefs of Staff Mission to Japan. As director of the Council for Biology in Human Affairs he lectured about man and nature. Among his published works are: "The Common Sense of Science", "The Face of Violence", "Science and Human Values" and "The Identity of Man".

The second world war brought a number of refugees to Britain who showed their gratitude to the country as best they could. Dr. Guttman, later Sir Ludwig, C.B.E., came from Germany. He contributed greatly to the rehabilitation of war victims who were soon joined by people maimed by road accidents, industrial machines, even sport, violence also by those with strokes, disabling arthritis, poliomyelitis (many saved on Drinker respirators). It is estimated that there are some two million such people. The sports stadium for paralysed and other disabled at Stoke Mandeville was his brain child. He is the founder of the National Spinal Injuries Centre. It is he who organized the international sports competitions for paraplegics. Such ventures added interest, hope, fitness and greater integration with the community for the less fortunate, but courageous people. It was a success story and many more centres for paraplegics were founded in various parts of the country. Fittingly, a well-known contemporary Polish name to the British is that of a painter – Feliks Topolski. He served as a British war artist in World War II, portrayed the Coronation ceremonies and official state visits of the Queen, and also many famous people. Yet another immigrant, a doctor from Germany, became active in the psychiatric field. Dr. Max Glatt diverted his efforts towards problems of drug addiction and alcoholism. In St. Bernard's Hospital, Southall, I watched him handling such patients with skill and understanding. These are international diseases and a number of "junkies" and alcoholics arrived in the U.K. from various parts of the globe. Great Britain was not only sought after by refugees! Heroin, cocaine, "purple heart" and other pep pill addicts, LSD worshippers and "pot" (marijuana) smokers formed the junkie community which threatens our society. In some fifteen years they filled the almost empty British scene of the mid 1950's. I recollect a man who came to me with the story of having had a car accident a few weeks previously which resulted in his wife's miscarriage. It haunted him and he had to have pills from his doctor which pepped him up. He said he was now living in my area and gave me the necessary particulars not being able to produce the medical card. He asked me for "his" pill. It was a controlled drug, but I had no reason to disbelieve his story. A fortnight later another man presented himself to me complaining of being depressed and requested the same pill. I became suspicious and soon found that he had given me false particulars. His friend had told him how easy it was to obtain the drug. The man was arrested and a number of pills were found on him. He was charged with deception and unlawful possession of drugs. This was my first encounter with junkies.

Not all refugees were an asset to their adopted land. Like other countries they had black sheep among them. One such stray, by the name of Peter Rachman, enriched English vocabulary. A new word was coined in memory of him – "Rachmanism". It means extortion and unscrupulous behaviour.

We owe the discoveries and the enormous progress, witnessed by the last generation, to an intellectual group of scientists. Much of the work was achieved through hard work and perseverance. The syphilitic agent – spirocheta pallida – was discovered in 1905 by Schaudinn and Hoffmann, and Paul Ehrlich set out to defeat it. His anti-syphilitic preparation, arsphenamine, was synthesized in 1909, after six hundred and six trials, most of which were failures. His modesty led him to a statement that for seven years of misfortune he had one moment of good luck! Later on came Ehrlich's neoarsphenamine also known as neo-salvarson and by its number 914 . . . It was the standard treatment for syphilis until 1943, when penicillin took over. In the old days syphilis was a rampant disease. The expressive style of the renowned Polish sculptor Wit Stwosz, who worked in Cracow in the last three decades of the 15th century, portrayed the saddle noses and congenital stigmata of syphilis. Posterity remembers only the famous sufferers like Paul Gauguin, the great French painter, Robert Schuman, the German composer who tried to drown himself and died two years later in an asylum, Guy de Maupassant, French novelist who struggled with general paralysis of the insane (GPI) and succumbed to it at the age of forty-three. The painter, Francisco Goya, and Beethoven, the composer, are also reported to have been victims of syphilis.

The therapeutic value of sulphonamides was announced by Gerhard Domagk in 1935, only after he carried out numerous experiments and tried the drug on his own daughter. He won the Nobel prize in 1939, but was unable to receive it as it was on Hitler's prohibited list. He was temporarily arrested by the Gestapo, yet the Nazis were unable to break his spirit. In 1951 Domagk introduced isoniazid, an important anti-tuberculous drug, widely used to this very day. By 1952 psychic stimulation resulting in euphoria, even elation, was noticed in patients treated for tuberculosis with isoniazid or iproniazid. One of the more perceptive doctors used those drugs in the treatment of fatigued tuberculosis patients with psychiatric overtones. Iproniazid, a monoamine oxidase inhibitor, was a precursor of a number of similar drugs effective in depressive illness. In 1942 a doctor who attempted to treat typhoid fever with a sulphonamide derivate noticed that it lowered the level of sugar in the blood. It was, however, the year 1955 which went down in medical history. In that year two German doctors, Franke and a young houseman Fuchs, observed that another sulphonamide known as tolbutamide induced deficiency of sugar in the blood of a patient whom they treated for pneumonia, making him much worse. The ill man trembled and sweated profusely. Dr. Fuchs took the drug himself and developed identical symptoms. Thanks to a chance finding and the doctors' intelligent approach, an oral anti-diabetic agent was discovered.

Many more important discoveries owe at least some of their success to a lucky chance. One September day in 1928 Sir Alexander Fleming noticed, on return from holiday, accidental contamination of one of the culture plates he left in his laboratory. He observed the killing effect of penicillin mould on vicious germs* he had been studying. But mere chance was not enough to investigate such phenomenon – one had to have a scientific mind, as was the case with him. For thousands of years people watched apples falling off trees, but it needed Isaac Newton to explain the nature of gravity. Sir Alexander's discovery eventually revolutionized twentieth century medicine. The first idea of "the pill" crossed people's mind in 1944, when a technician of the pharmaceutical firm "Syntex" in Mexico City reported, to his annoyance, that rabbits tested for purity of the recently produced progesterone stopped multiplying. Another chance finding, already mentioned, was treatment of pulmonary tuberculosis with artificial pneumoperitoneum initiated in 1931 through a faulty technique of Dr. Banyai. He subsequently noticed that this improved patient's condition.

In 1958 Dr. Sones of Cleveland, Ohio, U.S.A. accidently put a catheter into the right coronary artery while performing an aortogram, but observed no ill effects. This stimulated deliberate selective catheterization of coronary arteries and led to selective cine coronary arteriography as a reasonably safe and valuable diagnostic procedure which determines with great precision the location and extent of coronary disease. The modern anti-cancer drugs, vincristine and vinblastin, the alkaloids from the Vinca plant, were also discovered accidentally in 1958 during a search for newer substances to control diabetes. It was noticed that animals who received these compounds were soon dead from blood-poisoning. Researchers showed that the drugs were causing gross reduction in the number of leucocytes (white corpuscles of blood. It will be remembered that leucocytes rally against the invasion of germs.) Clinical trials began in 1960 and led to the use of vinca alkaloids in acute leukaemia, lymphosarcoma, Hodgkin's disease, Burkitt's lymphoma** and allied conditions. Folic acid antagonist used for treatment of cancer showed itself beneficial

* Staphylococci.

** Only if another cytotoxic drug, cyclophosphamide, has failed.

for those patients who also had suffered from psoriasis. It provided a new therapeutic impetus in dealing with severe disabling psoriasis for which treatment has been very limited. A search for safer and more effective agents continues. Chlorpromazine, synthesized by Charpentier in 1950 in search of a suitable *antihistamine* drug, was later proved to have potent sedative activity and became the first and leading *tranquilliser*. Looking back to the 18th century we will recollect Dr. William Withering, the initiator of treatment with foxglove of cardiac patients. He accidentally met a sick old woman who benefited from a secret herbal tea and traced it to foxglove. And so a new term was formed – SERENDIPITY – the faculty of making happy and unexpected discoveries by accident.

We have seen that the British played their part in the scientific achievements and their inventiveness must be recorded. In 1958 Christopher Cockerell introduced the Hovercraft. It does not serve as a ferry alone. A hover-bed is used for patients with extensive burns. Such an air bed was suggested for expectant mothers in the last stages of pregnancy in the hope of reducing body strain, so making a mother-to-be virtually weightless. A hovercraft train is under consideration. Frank Whittle invented the first jet engine for an aircraft. Other examples are an efficient heart-lung machine, previously mentioned, and less dramatic but as important, the innovation of plastic boots at King's College Hospital, London. By automatic inflation and deflation they maintain blood circulation as a precaution against thrombosis. Further, a bonded carbon fibre of exceptional strength, the first vertical take-off aircraft, and the Anglo-French supersonic Concorde. British technologists designed a new jet engine which will cut noise by half. The "old country" has not grown old after all. No wonder its inventiveness marched with endurance and the spirit of adventure. Francis Chichester already had cancer when he sailed round the world in 1966 and attempted another big venture shortly before his death. In 1957 Dr. Vivian Fuchs led a party of twelve which accomplished the first crossing of the Antarctic continent, and during 1968/9 the first crossing of the entire Polar ice-cap was achieved by Wally Herbert and his team. Such exploits were in the old tradition of Drake, Raleigh, Cook, Livingstone, Burton, Speke, Stanley, Charles Sturt, Eyre, Giles and Scott. In 1974 a British team undertook the Zaire River expedition navigating its 2,718-mile, perilous stretch – so commemorating the centenary of Stanley's exploration.

* In 1974 British Shell showed the world how to produce protein from natural gas.

And so they helped to transform our lives along with other nations. It has been an all round transformation, but as a doctor I am only qualified to dwell on the medical aspect of it.

Blood letting and purges disappeared. I still remember leeches being put to patients' heads after strokes. I watched the slimy creatures engorge with human blood – their food. The medical leech, "hirudo medicinalis", was employed for a number of pathological conditions all over the world. This species was in such demand that it practically disappeared. I recollect the common saying: "Qui bene purgat, bene curat" (who purges well treats well), reflecting the attitude of doctors who had only very few drugs at their disposal. The list was headed by castor-oil calomel (a mercurial purgative), saline purgatives, vegetable purgatives, paraffin and salicylates. I must not forget mercury and arsenic, both anti-syphilitic remedies, the latter also used as a "tonic"! When, as a small boy, I developed a stomach upset I was forced to swallow obnoxious castor oil in black coffee, carrying the taste of it with me for the whole day. I preferred it though to soap enema! When I was well I had to take a daily dose of cod liver oil without a hope of getting the more refined Scott's Emulsion. Now the drugs have to look attractive and be to everyone's taste. Gone are anti-bacterial horse sera known to have caused death in susceptible persons and cupping glasses, as many as twenty of them applied to the trunk to draw blood to the surface. Tracheostomy tubes have practically disappeared. One does not see peg legs any more, neither extensive scars from radiation or pitted "pocks". Incision of the ear membrane, a procedure in which I became an expert, is hardly used, and mastoid operations are a rarity. I have not seen a Pott's hump caused by a diseased vertebra for thirty-five years, except when visiting a remote part of Morocco in 1964, and very rarely empyema (accumulation of pus in the chest). Collapse therapy, widely used for pulmonary tuberculosis, was dispensed with; voices are heard saying that some cases of lung cancer could be the result of previous treatment with artificial pneumothorax. Gone are tight corsets and damp dwellings deprived of light and with them numerous irritable ladies who suffered from "green sickness' – chlorosis. Local Authorities were no doubt to some extent responsible – the smaller the windows, the smaller the rates!

I remember debilitated children with scrophula – suppurating lymphatic glands due to tuberculosis. Milk from cows infected by it was often responsible for scrophulosis but the hygiene and antibiotic treatment of to-day have eliminated all that. I recollect children with legs

245

bent because of rickets. This last disease, caused by inadequate diet and lack of sunshine, was prevalent in the British Isles. I knew it in Poland under the name "English disease". The word "rickets" was apparently taken from the old English word "wrick" which means "to twist". Children ceased to die from meningitis. Isolation wards sheltering cases of diphtheria, scarlet fever and erysipelas were closed. Severe eye inflammation of the new-born brought through the mothers' gonorrhoea, syphilitic saddle noses, tabes dorsalis and general paralysis of the insane (GPI) are nightmares of the past. Doctors do not see many women suffering from pelvic inflammation. Lobar pneumonia, exophthalmic goiter, endocarditis, nephritis, amyloidosis, rheumatic fever, chorea (also known as St. Vitus Dance), and their serious consequences are a rarity. By understanding the nature of coeliac disease* its victims are saved. Pain was an accepted fact of life as being God's will, but it is no more. Scientists continue to find better treatment for disabling diseases. Levodopa, introduced in 1970, brought dramatic changes into the lives of many patients struck by Parkinson's Disease, completely changing its outlook. It proved to be the best drug we ever had for this disease, able to improve three quarters of such patients, and restore some to normality. The drug is able to relieve them of the distressing features such as stiffness, tremor, speech difficulties and dribbling of saliva. Levodopa was isolated by Guggenheim as far back as 1913 and waited all this time for its rightful place. To many eye-sight, the most cherished possession, has been restored. A corneal graft is most rewarding as it does not have any blood vessels and so rejection cannot take place. Detachment of the innermost coat of the eyeball – the retina – has been treatable since the 1930's, thus saving such patients from blindness. Children's squints and other abnormalities, as well as disfigurements, are removed which offers them a more happy life.

Today the accent is on prophylaxis. Epidemics are as much prevented as confined diseases. In 1664/65 thirty-two thousand Londoners died of bubonic plague out of half a million of the population. Eating bread made from rye and contaminated by a fungus known as ergot caused many outbreaks of ergotism. Women suffered from spontaneous abortions and people's fingers, toes, even whole limbs became

* A bowel disorder first described in 1889 by the London physician Samuel Gee. Only in 1957 its cause was found to be an inborn error of metabolism. Such patients show intolerance to the protein – gluten – found in cereals. Gluten-free diet keeps them alive and well.

shrivelled and black as if they had been charred. Ergotism was popularly known as St. Anthony's fire, as he himself suffered from this disease. Now they are no more.

Up to eighteen years ago people in the prime of life were often struck by infantile paralysis, commonly known as "polio". The disease killed some, in others it spread to nerves and muscles leaving them with disabilities for life. Now the terror of it is gone. It all started in 1949 when the American Enders showed how to breed the polio virus. In 1954 another American, Dr. Jonas Salk, introduced a vaccine from "dead" viruses, but a year later such vaccine caused paralysis in over two hundred children, eleven of whom died. Moreover, it was only partly effective, although able to cut down the rate of polio. It was very fortunate that Dr. Albert Sabin arrived on the American scene. He was of Russian origin and decided to take to Soviet Russia the live but weakened virus vaccine he produced. It proved to be a success and these days children all over the world swallow the Sabin's vaccine which equips them with immunity against infantile paralysis. In 1931 a similar fate met the BCG vaccine introduced for protection against tuberculosis. Seventy-one German children from Luebeck died of tuberculosis infection after being vaccinated with BCG. The disaster was caused by a laboratory error. Albert Calmette, the discoverer of BCG, and his vaccine were vindicated only after an exhaustive enquiry which shortened the scientist's life. Another disease, phenylketonuria, which causes mental defects, is preventable thanks to early detection. It is compulsory for a midwife to take a blood sample from each new born baby.

Doctors are alerted to the possibility of urinary infection in a very young child before any real damage is done to the kidneys. The whole range of diagnostic aids are at doctors' disposal — suprapubic aspiration of urine, culture media, intravenous pyelograms, imicturating cystograms etc. Early detection of a not-so-uncommon peculiarity of the ureteric reflux saves such children from developing high blood pressure in adult life or from events which can lead to kidney transplantation.

All of us know the expression "Mad as a hatter" but how many know how it came about? Well, I will tell you. At the turn of the last century hatters worked with fur and treated it with mercury. They eventually suffered from chronic mercurial poisoning. They looked pale, displayed tremor, sweating, foul breath, irritability, speech disturbance, loss of memory, sometimes mania. Prevention of industrial

247

diseases has made great strides since and is gaining momentum. Part-time factory doctors are in the process of transformation into Employment Medical Officers – a new breed specializing in prevention. It is a fact that silicosis (due to the inhalation of the dust of stone), asbestosis, begassosis (due to refuse products in sugar making), suberosis (due to cork dust), byssinosis (due to the inhalation of cotton dust in factories) and the like have practically disappeared. Mining and textile industries of the past were the main offenders. Such illnesses are preventable but not curable. Once the formation of fibrous tissue sets in the lungs, removal from an injurious exposure cannot stop the progress of the disease. If the number of such unfortunate patients is small today it is only because it invariably shortens their lives. I had the misfortune to watch two such patients sliding down the slippery slope, unresponsive to treatment, crippled and doomed. People like them do not pose a big problem any more, they have ceased to exist, and practical dust control along with other preventive measures afford comparative safety to their successors. I have seen the great care the "Kodak" factories in Britain have taken to enforce safety regulations, and the interest shown by the management for the welfare of their employees. Should, however, an injurious dust exposure occur, an *early* diagnosis by means of lung biopsy* prevents disaster.

The "Medic-alert" organization came into being and provides a bracelet with the appropriate medical warning of a patient's condition. Accidents can happen, a diabetic, a patient with failing kidneys or high blood pressure, is unable to tell of his or her condition or susceptibility to some drugs or other agents if found unconscious.

No wonder that institutions for bed-rest and nursing of hopeless cases have been transformed into sophisticated, modern establishments aiming at cures.

A success story?

No, not entirely. Bad housing conditions, bad nutrition, infectious and industrial diseases pose less of a problem today only to be superseded by increased stresses, elevated blood pressures, heart diseases, air pollution, excessive noise, smoking, drinking . . . New drugs brought new risks. The ever increasing consumption of drugs is frowned upon by the medical profession. The number of children admitted to hospital in Britain with accidental poisoning by medicines has doubled in the last ten years; often these were the "left-overs" of the hoarding parents.

* Examination of a piece of tissue removed from a living subject.

248

Doctors eliminated many diseases and learned to cure others, but they also discovered and created new ones. (Yet, it should be said that some diseases with a modern interest have in fact existed for a very long time. Paget's disease described by Sir James Paget in 1877 had been found in a skull of an ancient Egyptian, and also in medieval Anglo-Saxon specimens.) In 1957 it was brought to doctors' attention that a hiatus hernia, representing the protrusion of an abdominal organ into the chest cavity, can be acquired through pregnancy, wearing tight corsets, heavy lifting or through being involved in an accident, especially in middle-aged obese subjects. Since then *acquired* hiatus hernia, earlier unheard of, became a favourite diagnosis readily acknowledged at X-ray examination. Acute ischaemia of the gut, especially ischaemic colitis – a local and temporary deficiency of blood in that region – is another new entity which explains some abdominal pain in the elderly, unexplained before. Disc trouble has been discovered in Egyptian mummies, 5,000 years old, yet the common cause of backache and sciatica remained an enigma until 1937 when Glorieux of Bruges traced sciatica to the bulging of an intervertebral disc and, later on, James Cyriax of St. Thomas's Hospital, London, drew our attention to the same cause of "lumbago". Anaemia ceased to be a simple diagnosis and became a pointer to a variety of pathological conditions. Haematology, medical science concerned with blood, underwent great changes since the Oxford physiologist John Haldane and Hermann Sahli, the Berne physician, showed us at the beginning of the century how to estimate haemoglobin. In the late 1930's medical attention was drawn to puzzling pneumonias of unknown cause – they were named primary atypical pneumonias. Viruses were implicated, until it was established in 1961 that a new micro-organism – mycoplasma pneumoniae – was responsible for some respiratory infections of man. (It is the smallest free-living organism and, as it lacks a cell wall, it assumes many forms.) The knowledge that mycoplasma pneumoniae is resistant to penicillin has been of practical consequence.

Familiar remedies have been supplanted by more effective preparations but many of the drugs we use are two-faced. Treatment of Parkinson's disease can lead to anxiety, agitation and aggression. On the other hand tranquillers such as phenothiazines can cause "parkinsonism." Oral antidiabetic drugs *stimulate* secretion of insulin derived from the pancreas, but may *depress* the function of another important gland – the thyroid. Oral diuretics can lead to gout or potassium depletion, liquorice root extract, which helps to heal peptic ulcers, can

249

affect the heart and antituberculous drug Isoniazid – various nerves. Contraceptive pills sometimes cause thrombosis or depression. A very useful sedative – chlorpromazine – may affect the liver, a valuable antibiotic chloramphenicol sometimes leads to an abnormal state of the blood, and tetracyclines can cause renal failure in those prone to it. Chloraquine, used in the treatment of lupus and rheumatoid arthritis, can induce blindness, so can anticoagulants by causing haemorrhages. Thalidomide "epidemic", first noted in 1950, is, of course, known to everyone. Even the "innoxious" talcum powder can be harmful if not sufficiently purified. It is in fact magnesium silicate, obtained from the rocks, and as such can be contaminated by asbestos, a substance injurious to health. And so it is a vicious circle.

The introduction of natural gas significantly reduced carbon monoxide poisoning and notorious barbiturates were curbed by doctors. Yet, self-poisoning with new drugs, anti-depressants, a multitude of hypnotics or paracetamol among them, necessitate intense medical care, and so Poisoning Treatment Centres had to be opened.

A name added to the medical vocabulary is "retroperitoneal fibrosis," a chronic inflammation in the lower lumbar region, often of unknown cause, which can be iatrogenic, in other words produced by physicians. Attention has been focussed on diseases brought about by autoimmunity such as chronic inflammation of the thyroid, known also by the name of Hashimoto's* disease. Modern research points to the same cause for such enigmatic diseases as rheumatoid arthritis and systemic lupus erythematosus. The almost conquered pernicious anaemia appears to pose a similar problem. Chronic bronchitis and coronary artery diseases are on the increase. The term "English disease" remains on the agenda, it only changed its meaning being reserved for chronic bronchitis or rheumatism.

Industrial hazards, smoking and longevity increased the number of bladder tumours. The cause of non-specific urethritis, a common genital infection, remains uncertain and its treatment – unsatisfactory. We are in possession of efficient drugs for venereal diseases, yet they spread faster than ever before, and the incidence of diarrhoeas** remains undiminished in spite of hygienic preparation and the delivery

* Hakaru Hashimoto, contemporary Japanese surgeon.

** By means of electromicroscopy Parvoviruses ("parvus" means small), Orbiviruses and others have been identified as the causes of some outbreaks of acute enteritis in man. One day, no doubt, scientists will grow them in culture and produce specific vaccines.

250

of food wrapped in polythene and untouched by hand. We spend millions of pounds on research producing a galaxy of wonder drugs but the mechanism of many diseases, some very common, is still not well understood. Our knowledge of schizophrenia, migraine, disseminated sclerosis, rheumatoid arthritis, systemic lupus erythematosus (SLE), psoriasis, scleroderma, sarcoidosis, etc. has not advanced very much. The latter was described by Sir Jonathan Hutchinson in 1878, but its cause remains unknown. Why do parsons get migraine more often on Mondays – their day of rest? Faced with cerebral arteriosclerosis or generalised emphysema, we are ignorant and powerless. We have more luck with Hodgkin's disease as we are now able to treat it effectively, although we do not know its cause. We also treat acne with small doses of tetracyclines very successfully, not having a clue why this works. Many more efficacious measures cannot be scientifically explained. No one knows the mechanism by which dramatic relief of skeletal pain is achieved by radiation in metastatic cancer. We are puzzled by the irrational behaviour of warts. We know everything about impotence, yet are unable to treat the problem satisfactorily – albeit artificial insemination. We only begin to unravel the secrets of the thymus gland. The cure for viruses still eludes us. In 1970 the Registrar General's Office reported 6,091 deaths from influenza in Britain, in France 10,000 were reported the previous year. Virus killed the Leader of the Opposition, Hugh Gaitskell, at fifty-four, in a very short time. Water and rest is still the best treatment for the common cold, influenza, viral hepatitis, cholera, and salt and water (saline) are essential in the management of shock. We try to overcome our difficulties by protecting people against viruses and vaccinate them against these germs. To thwart man's efforts to protect himself from influenza virus the latter changes its tactics from year to year. For retinitis pigmentosa which produces blindness in middle age we can do precious little. Diabetic retinopathy is on the increase and we now have 8,000 diabetics, some only thirty years of age, who are registered as blind.

Dr. Christiaan Barnard showed us how one can outlive one's own heart, but not for long as there is no break-through yet in the problem of rejection. Out of 32 lung transplants there were only 3 survivors. There is an acute shortage of donor organs, besides, the cost of transplant operations is gigantic. We do not take "no" for an answer, and resuscitate people already dead by the grace of God, so assuming His power over life and death. I once paid a casual visit to a lonely widow in her seventy-second year. I have known her and her husband for twenty-two years. The woman has suffered from diabetes and severe angina, and various tablets she was taking, far from relieving suffering, were adding to her misery. I found that she had just taken a large overdose of sleeping tablets and rushed her to hospital. She was saved but never forgave me my interference and our good doctor-patient relationship came to an end. The concept of death became more complex. Yesterday it meant that the heart ceased functioning, to-day it means the brain, to-morrow it could be the cell. It is no longer a problem of being kept alive but of being able to die in peace. Cryonic Societies in the U.S.A., as well as one in Paris, keep dead bodies in a capsule filled with liquid nitrogen at − 196 degrees Centigrade, when all molecular movement ceases. They give the corpses the prospect of immortality in the hope that one day science may revive them! The price one has to pay to be kept alive at all costs may sometimes be too high. My University Professor, a religious man of high principles and intelligence who had undoubted regard for the sanctity of human life, committed suicide when confronted with cancer of the stomach. Many remain intolerant of death looking upon it as a very final event. It might not be. Must we shun our obvious responsibility as doctors and ignore a sufferer's most fervent plea? If the patient preserves full mental capacity, is tortured by a painful condition and knows that it is incurable, is it not cowardly, even merciless, not to relieve such a person from his burden?

We have a greater number of liver diseases today than ever before. Possibly a genetic predisposition is accentuated by certain drugs. Doctors' guilty conscience prompts them to do something about it. The most affected are offered a liver transplant − not the real answer but a worth while procedure; a five-year survival is on record.

With advancing years we observe more strokes, more diseases of the heart, arteries and bones, more cancer, more deafness and blindness, more dementia. Elderly patients account for nearly half the total mental hospital population. The treated hypertensives live longer only to die from a heart attack. I often feel we do too much. Heroic measures may produce "cabbages". Leucotomy of older days was one such example. It was an unhappy day when I noticed foetal heart irregularity on a routine ante-natal examination some twenty years ago. I rushed the woman to hospital where the baby was delivered prematurely by caesarian section. It proved to be a wrong baby. Tuberous sclerosis, yet another curious disease we do not know much about, was diagnosed. The child was mentally deficient, behaved like an animal,

252

suffered from convulsive seizures and brought misery to himself and the family for the whole of the eighteen years of his wretched life.

Doctors' efforts to thwart the scurge of tuberculosis were frustrated by another scourge – that of alcoholism.

Coronary artery disease is more threatening to-day than road accidents, drug taking and violence lumped together; many such victims are under forty. We teach prevention without much success. Smokeless zones are full of smoking people who are overweight because of overeating, love of alcohol and contempt for exercise. I did not witness a single heart attack among the many people of various ages I served in the Soviet sub-arctic labour camps. They lived in appalling weather conditions and otherwise, but were well exercised, not overfed and deprived of smoking and pollution. One might argue that they were dying just the same! Yet, in diseases of the arteries – the richer the man, the more likely a victim of heart attack or stroke. Israel has observed a considerable rise in the incidence of diabetes and deaths from coronary disease among the once primitive Sephardim (Jews from Asia and north Africa, as opposed to Ashkenazim who came from Europe) since their arrival there. Such are the effects of "westernization". Diverticulosis – pouches along the border of the large bowel – is brought on by bad habits such as taking food devoid of roughage and abuse of purgatives. I have a patient who consumes large amounts of beer which puts him off balance. He comes to me for medicines to settle his stomach. I told him to mend his ways, but he does not believe in prevention, only cure! Others are in the habit of swallowing aspirins and such like, only to go to the doctor for more pills in an effort to eliminate the discomfort they brought on themselves. Medical men have to treat allergies caused by oil of juniper with which gin is flavoured, by quinine contained in tonic-water or through other articles, either in the diet or by self-medication. Women are victims of mascaras, hair sprays, dyes, deodorants and such like. Most of these people are aware of their peculiar susceptibilities, yet cannot resist their own weaknesses. Doctors have to put right the patients' wrong doings. Yet, doctors are not entirely free of blame. They administer pills which impair vitamin absorption only to add more pills to counteract it! Patients are condemned to processing a multiplicity of drugs inside their bodies – an amateurish way of going on – the return to old mixtures with a variety of drugs. Some impatient doctors rush to administer various agents aimed at dissolving clots in the vessels and forget that blood has its own thrombolytic mechanism.

Many mental patients are turned back to community, but some commit acts of violence.

So much on the debit side, but we must not forget the large profits we accrued. People do live longer, they do lead more comfortable and interesting lives. Many blind people recover their eyesight, the near-deaf are helped by effective hearing aids and faulty hearts assisted by pacemakers. Examples are numerous. All the pros and cons should be weighed. Doctors ought to be courageous enough to retain useful drugs despite their side effects. Caution and familiarization, not unwarranted dismissal, should be the password. Timidity can kill as much as overconfidence. For instance, corticosteroids are a must in Addison's disease* and depriving a pemphigus sufferer of corticosteroids would condemn such a patient to death. In some ocular conditions high doses of this drug can be sight saving. A similar consideration applies to the cancer therapy and to suppression of immune reactions in transplantation surgery.

But, we must remember that a mild diabetes responds to simple dietary measures, as will peptic ulcers in many cases. So will a number of other ailments. Relief of stress and simple care focussed on a patient will often suffice. There is no need *always* to try to get to the bottom of things using very elaborate gadgets. All doctors have easy access to a stethoscope but only a very few to an echocardiograph and such like. Besides, good will and the power of suggestion go a long way. Miracles are performed with acupuncture which the Chinese have practised for more than 5,000 years. Some claim that such results are achieved because of correction of imbalance and restoration of equillibrium and harmony by "Chi", the life force. I have no knowledge of acupuncture and can only surmise that this is a kind of "mesmerism." The method claims successes in anaesthesia deaf-mutism, management of high blood pressure and a cure for a number of painful conditions, drug addiction, even impotence. There are numerous points for acupuncture along the channels of energy called "meridians" in connection with different parts of the body. Where do they stick needles for impotence, I wonder? . . .

I was once called in to an intelligent woman of seventy-six with a backache. I noticed some twenty corks in her bed placed near her feet. She explained she had been listening on the wireless to an Indian doctor who advocated corks for leg cramps from which she suffered. Such a cure was later "confirmed" in a daily paper, she told me. Ap-

---

* Adrenal insufficiency.

254

parently it is an old Indian "remedy." She swore it worked on her extremely well – the night cramps disappeared completely. She got so dependent on this treatment that each time a cork fell out of the bed, she would get out to retrieve it, being afraid of missing a single one! I advised her not to overdose herself . . . I wondered if this "remedy" was invented by ingenious licencees! Cork is certainly safer than quinine and it appears to be just as effective. An old physician would coin the phrase "suberose" treatment; I am simply saying – a corky one. But, the patient is not interested in a name, only in the cure. They are not helped by the diagnosis of "ankylosing spondylitis" also known under many other names – doctors who coined the terms have not a clue what it's all about! Doctors' views do change, sometimes as quickly and as radically as women's fashions, and like ladies' wear their treatment does go out of fashion. The old cry: "All tonsils out" has died, replaced by the standing order "Keep tonsils in"; they learned that given time mother nature brings their regression anyway. The old advice that butter and sugar are good for you was abandoned after doctors learned that such indulgence can lead to coronary heart disease. Widely used iodine, mercurials, borax, camphor and tartar were dropped from the medical armamentarium, gamma globulins are no longer favoured for the prevention of German measles and vaccination against smallpox ceased to be compulsory. Penicillamine, derived from penicillin, has been known for many years* and only recently generated greater interest in its use in rheumatoid arthritis. It certainly brings great relief to such sufferers, but no cure can be expected until scientists find the cause of the disease. Doctors, in desperation, resorted to gold injections, abandoned them because of their many side effects, and started them again.

Only aspirin – a salicylate – and placebos have never left the scene. Literally millions of pounds of aspirin are produced each year all over the world, with various firms competing in its presentation and safety. It was first synthesized by Von Gerdhardt in 1853 and introduced into medicine by the Bayer firm.

This came about because the chemist Felix Hoffman, employed by the firm, decided to research into salicylic compounds being moved by the plea of his rheumatic father. The commercial synthesis was much cheaper than the preparation from natural sources – the willow and poplar bark and oil of wintergreen – the ancient folk remedies for pain and fever. Since then we have witnessed a great many presentations of

* It was discovered in 1942 by Abraham from the William Dunn School in Oxford.

255

aspirin, constantly in use; as an effervescent drug in Alka-Seltzer, soluble, buffered or enteric-coated tablet, a microencapsulated form, an orange flavoured chewing gum . . . In 1973 yet another presentation of aspirin was made available and a liquid *stable* form is being developed. It is estimated that some six thousand million tablets of aspirin are being consumed in Britain alone. It is a pillar of self-medication used for mild fevers, headaches, toothache, muscle and skeletal pain, in menstruation or just as a "pick-me-up".* Doctors use it widely in rheumatoid arthritis and allied conditions. The strange thing is that, in spite of numerous investigations, no one understands to the present day *how* the drug works, apart from the fact that it has anti-inflammatory and analgesic action observed in millions of people. They can't all be wrong! Some surmise that the drug helps to control the defence mechanism of the body. There are many biochemical actions of the salicylates. It was postulated that they could transport copper liberated from the cells in rheumatic diseases back to its cells of origin. It is known that copper salts have an antipyretic** action and that drugs which bind copper produce symptoms of rheumatic disease in previously healthy people. Copper shows usually high levels in the blood tissues of patients with rheumatoid arthritis, and salicylates, similar to penicillamine, enhance copper excretion. Allegedly, aspirin decreases the production of prostaglandins and in this way mitigates various symptoms of diseases; a fever is one of them. We have advocates of aspirin for managing diarrhoea in cholera. Yet, aspirin is a two-faced drug. It may cause gastric irritation and severe bleeding, especially among the elderly. I had to rush such a patient to hospital for blood transfusion made necessary by such self-medication. This inexpensive drug is a temptation to many.

Patients on the whole are a strange breed. They expect to be helped solely by doctors' efforts and do not intend to exert themselves. A thermometer is seldom among their possessions, they call a doctor to take the temperature. Our advice against smoking, drinking, over-eating etc. usually goes overboard. A soft bed causes a bad back, a soft seat- stiff joints, soft water – heart disease, exhaust fumes in place of oxygen more heart diseases, soft food – bad teeth, constipation and piles. There is a high incidence of obesity and mild diabetes among the youth

* Jack Hawkins tells us how he developed a frightful nervous twitch everytime he went on the set in his early film career, and how he managed to control it by taking aspirin.

** Relieving fever.

256

of today. I watched with amazement parents taking children to and from near-by schools in their cars, knowing that they live only a few streets away. A short time ago I received a hospital report on a nine year-old saying: "Unfortunately school parties have proved too much for already overweight Joanne, and she gained two pounds in the last fortnight". It is a misplaced joy which zero-rating of Value Added Tax on sweets, ice cream, soft drinks, crisps and peanuts brought to British children.* It only aids dental decay, obesity, diabetes, and in later years, heart disease. Many diseases could be prevented, but patients elect to burden doctors by demanding treatment, only to go back to their old, harmful routine – some to driving, some to drinking, some to smoking, many to all three. More often than not it is the patient's job to improve one's resistance, to avoid stresses and to reduce fears. Investigation of public speakers, racing drivers and parachute jumpers proved that the expression "I was frightened to death" is not a meaningless saying. It is a wonder that by and large doctors succeed, and soon have the clergy back on their knees and the rest in their driving seats. They owe such quick rehabilitation to the car which everyone possesses these days. The patient does not need to walk too soon. He just sits among a deafening noise and traffic fumes on his return to society. No wonder that people caught in the whirlpool of modern living are worried. Despite more leisure, more hygiene, better economic and social conditions, and many other advantages, they remain as restless and unhappy as ever. Until now they were only bowel conscious, now they are also sleep-conscious. Our way of life affects children too. Some get nervous and frightened being shut away high up on the top floor of big blocks of flats. I know of children who developed bald patches on their scalps through twiddling their hair and pulling it out. It happens so often that a new medical term was coined – trichotillomania. Some boys and girls have been exposed to a hostile environment since birth; they had to face their restless parents and perhaps the "battered babies" phenomenon, a growing problem. Doctors do not approve of these trends, but they are not rebels and those of them who are able to withstand the way of life we live are willing to teach others to look on the brighter side; there is nothing else they can do.

In spite of it all, they were dynamic decades for medical science in which profits vastly exceeded debits, and the trend continues. In the summer of 1974 the first apparently healthy test-tube baby was announced in Britain; a five-day-old embryo, cultivated in a laboratory,

* The shortage of sugar during 1974 was good news.

257

was transplanted into the mother's womb eighteen months earlier. Much attention is given to the new discipline – gerentology – the study of ageing. Our elaborate methods soon seem crude and primitive, the conquest of viruses and various cancers is in sight, the dream of heart transplantation might become true and so forth. What one does and says today becomes outdated tomorrow and apart from speculation there is no way to stay ahead of the continuously growing knowledge. One prediction is a certainty – there is a future for the future! Ervin Page, who determined the structure of serotonin, put it in a nut shell: "When I say today, I mean tomorrow, because I am writing this yesterday." Yet it merits to utter a word of caution that in spite of all human cleverness so far nature holds the upper hand. We have more cures but not less illness. Man has no control over earthquakes, volcanic eruptions, landslides, floods, hurricanes, avalanches, droughts, neither is there a hope that he will ever eradicate all the diseases. It is significant that many illnesses and death rate bear relationship to climatic conditions. When man attempts to conquer nature, he must pay a price, no matter how modest was his success. DDT is one such example. This insect-killing powder which spelled doom to flees, mosquitoes and lice saving millions of lives from malaria and typhus, has also harmed all kind of creatures. This has disturbed the balance of nature, and DDT had to be put under tight control in Britain, and banned altogether from use in the U.S.A. In another instance scientists warn against the hazards of "genetic engineering" in which segments of DNA are isolated and rejoined. Such research, besides potential benefits, may bring disaster to man by unwittingly producing a germ of greatly enhanced virulence with increased incidence of cancer and other diseases. Thus it is not surprising that even in this age of science faith healers, Christian Scientists and pilgrimages to Lourdes are still sought by patients whom doctors have failed, that the fringe practitioners of medicine are kept busy and yoga and similar pursuits turn into a cult. What surprises me is that they sometimes succeed! But then unexplained things do happen, and given time diseases may vanish of their own accord. It has been known to us for a long time that our eyes receive tiny, *upside down* pictures, but how is it that we are able to perceive the world around us in a normal fashion? We know that there is a collaboration between eye and brain and it is understandable that should the "waveling" go off course, illusions or hallucinations would ensue. Yet it is amazing that this does not happen much more often. Besides, we cannot always rely on what the eye tells

258

us — we do suffer from optical illusions; even colours don't exist in reality. Much we see is a product of our imagination — one has only to watch a person in love — beauty is in the eye of the beholder. How sleep comes about remains a mystery, yet it is an activity on which about one-third of the human life is spent and insomnia, especially in the elderly, is one of the most common disorders. The static control of our bodies, in spite of continuous cell deaths and their replacement, is as impressive as it is puzzling. The surprising thing is not that some of our cells may overgrow regardless of the rest of them, as in cancer, but that a perfect balance is struck between these processes through our lives. Let's take body noradrenaline. It is continuously released, metabolized and synthesized, yet it maintains a remarkably constant level in tissues. We witness breathtaking perfection. Man, ape and monkey belong to the same order of primates. Darwin's theory of evolution traced man to ape. Modern scientists go much further and talk of crystal as our ancestor; atoms and molecules in living things were shown to be identical to the ones found in non-living things. But where do the crystal and atom come from? If life was synthesized from simple carbon compounds and minerals of the prebiotic earth, as John Haldane Junior suggested, the question — who created the earth — remains. Is life unique to earth? What is the purpose and the Force behind? Will we ever know? Following reason too far is unreasonable. Every being has to die and return to earth, reduced to basic chemical elements. No one can escape this destiny. It has been happening since the first living creature was born. After then what? Are there other shores for man after dissolution of his body? Man's questioning mind never rests and many deep thinkers found themselves in troubled waters — even when dealing with earthly matters — Socrates, Galileo, Voltaire, Semmelweis. . .Alchemy, palmistry, astrology and spiritualism have failed to bring people nearer the truth.

Confucius, the Chinese sage of the fifth century B.C., dealt only with mundane affairs and declared that the other world is beyond human comprehension. Such a pursuit would be unwise for homo sapiens. The ultimate wisdom must be the acceptance of the limits imposed on man by nature. Besides, to live with the unknown has its charm. The ending of a mystery and the crumbling of a make-believe-world of a child does not make it more happy. And so it is not such a bad thing that many questions remain unsolved, and not surprising that the occult and black magic and exorcism exist to this very day.

Advancement and dissemination of knowledge brought an inevitable crisis in religious beliefs, yet only to a point. An astute scientist is humbled by the miracle of creation and turns his efforts towards *practical* religion – the love of his fellow men. In my youth I knew devotees who used to talk to God many times during the course of a day, yet had nothing to say to people nearby. Those people waited impatiently to depart from the earth they hated. Others call on God only when threatened by danger. I prefer Padre Borrelli, the "father" of urchins in Naples, and Mother Teresa, of Calcutta, the founder of the Order of Missionaries of Charity, who turned their beliefs into practice. Perhaps Finley Dunne, an American humorist, is right when he says: "If Christian Scientists had more science and doctors more Christianity, it wouldn't make any difference which you called in – if you had a good nurse."

21
Reflections on Women, the Young and the Medical Profession

Women are wiser than men because they know less and understand more.

James Stephens

You teach your daughters the diameters of the planets, and wonder what you have done that they do not delight in your company.

Samuel Johnson

Give me chastity and self-restraint, but do not give it yet.

Saint Augustine

Profound political and scientific changes have altered the social and economic pattern of life beyond recognition. If a tiny minority can still throw money around, there are only a few who are near starving. The distinction which existed between manual and "white collar" workers has become much less pronounced. The lower and upper-middle classes merged with the middle class and prosperity is shared more equally. They were given greater opportunities for training, education, employment and leisure. Grants were taken for granted. The number of qualified teachers rose substantially. One person in four is now a student at school, college, polytechnic or university. The school leaving age was raised to sixteen. The blind, the deaf, the mentally handicapped received schooling and training to ease their burden. Public libraries sprang up all over the country, paperback books appeared in ever increasing numbers finding eager readers; sketch clubs, horticultural societies, cookery classes and the like gained popularity. More people own their own houses. Luxuries became necessities. A car and television are general possessions. For those who can't afford a big car and colour television, there is a mini car, a mini set or hire purchase, a mini trip or a package tour and a mini steak. There is just not enough time to absorb all the amenities. Frequently changing fashions caused people to substitute made-to-measure suits and dresses, once meant to last, for ready-made garments. A holiday abroad, often to far away

261

countries, is a common event. People go there and experience bad sanitation, the wrong food, rare diseases, and they blister in the sun. They *flock* to beaches in search of *solitude*. A brief exotic holiday often starts with the doubtful pleasure of various immunizations and pill-swallowing, forecasting doubtful enjoyment. Hardly anyone goes hungry on this island; the reverse is true – people tend to overeat. Eating habits have changed, both in quantity and quality. Supermarkets provide quick and varied purchases. Trips abroad give people a taste for unusual, imaginative, national and often exotic dishes, fruit and alcoholic beverages. They are helped by numerous cookery recipes and aided by delicatessens. Television programmes widen their culinary knowledge. Buttermilk, a liquid left after churning and discarded in the old days, is now saved for connoisseurs. People who do not go abroad still meet foreigners – the tourists, au pair girls, waiters, etc. The world has shrunk a great deal – the channel can be crossed in just over half an hour by hovercraft and we may soon have trains travelling at 150 miles per hour. In September 1973 Concorde flew from Washington to Paris in $3\frac{1}{2}$ hours, at an average speed of 954 mph and in June 1974 it did the 12,000-mile trip from Paris to Rio and back in less than 12 flying hours. No wonder foreign restaurants are patronized by British people more than ever before. They drink as much coffee as tea today, but I still prefer English tea to English coffee. British tourists to Spain, France and Italy were often wooed by advertisements: "English tea", with prices matching the imported goods. Now the traditional English tea with scones and jam or toasted buns is a dying custom, going the way of the world-famous British breakfast of "bacon and egg". It was uplifting to read that "the average Englishman still drinks at least 2,400 cups a year." Jobs became less dangerous due to safety devices. Adding machines, computers and other technological advances made work easier, quicker, more accurate, not so strenuous and often less dull. A great many people enjoy a five-day working week. Not so long ago the 56-hour week was standard. These days it is not possible to discern the social class to which a man belongs by his affluence, which has brought more marriages at a much younger age* and . . . more divorces. The advent of "the pill" strained the relationship between the Catholic Church and its flock. Increased prosperity made most people fashion conscious. First mini-skirts, then maxis followed by mini-mini skirts. Girls wear them wisely not only for looks but also for their own safety – a motorist

* By 1973 there were some forty schoolgirl brides in Britain.

notices highly visible shapely legs from a long range in the same way as he does the luminous safety jackets of road workers! Mini skirts and plunging dresses are very fetching and great fun. They cut their cloth according to their age, not their means! Fashion mirrors people's desire for change. Suddenly long hair and side-burns were "in". Pet-shops with dogs, cats, budgerigars and mynas were in business cashing in on the affluence of animal lovers. Bingo took over many cinemas which felt the strain of television competition. More leisure meant more interest in cricket, football and all the other British sports exported all over the world from the major sporting nation. Camping and caravanning are popular pastimes.

This is not only a man's world — women armed with domestic tools like electric and gas cookers, dishwashers, fridges, electric cleaners, and helped by baby-sitters, find more time for leisure. Central heating dispensed with coal scuttles and washing machines with mangles. Domestic servants, mainly women, are gone, replaced by modern aids. These days, not only children but also their mums go to college. They deserve it, and they know it. The Women's Liberation Movement gains ascendancy. They have gone a long way since the feet of Chinese and Japanese ladies were maimed to please men. But they try to look their best, at work as well as at leisure. A woman can be as ambitious, deter-mined, talented, deft, diligent and dependable as any man, but un-fortunate experience has made her cautious with her counterpart. Dame Ethel Mary Smyth was a notable composer, writer and militant suffragette. When I hear of someone vivacious, charming, full of vi-tality and enthusiasm, I instinctively think of a woman. I am curious why we only talk of a "spokesman", and not of a "spokeswoman". In Calabria, the extreme southern part of Italy, women do all the work and men confine themselves to the fruits of their labour; there are other places like Calabria. They pronounce themselves bride*grooms* but only until they marry! And yet women are modest; a hard-pressed housewife who does *not go to work* usually says: "I am not working". Women are more open than men and have more common sense; they are not ashamed to shed tears and feel better for it. Girls develop a mature outlook earlier than boys and are the stronger sex; a male tole-rates pain, anaemia and elevated blood pressure much less than a female and commits suicide twice as often. Girls, on average, do better at school than boys. Margery Hurst started her own business on a tiny loan and became a multi-millionairess. She once said: "You can uti-lize failure but you must never remember it." We all know of Melina

Mercouri, a Greek singer who was dedicated to the freedom of her country. History tells us of many brave women. The Poles had Emilia Plater, the Israelis – Hannah Senesh, the French – Odette Churchill, the British – Edith Louisa Cavell, Violette Szabo* and Amy Johnson. 71 British Military Medals were awarded to women in World War I and 7 more since. A number of them were members of the First Aid Nursing Yeomanry (FANY) and went into the fighting line with great bravery. History reminds us of women's determination – of a great queen, Elizabeth I, in whose name the power of England was established, of the suffragettes and of the minor German princess by the name of Catherine the Great who succeeded in reaching the throne. Antoinette Poisson, mistress of Louis XV known as Madame Pompadour, influenced the arts and affairs of State. In 1971 Nicolette Walker, twenty-eight-year-old research psychologist, sailed from Britain across the Atlantic singlehanded in a sloop and reached America after a non-stop six week journey. She struggled bravely against howling gales and other perils. Nicolette remained cheerful in spite of her loneliness and tribulations. She expressed the opinion that a woman is less likely to crack up than a man. Today Mrs. Gandhi is the Prime Minister of India, Mrs. Bandanaraika** the Prime Minister of Sri Lanka, Mrs. Golda Meir was the Prime Minister of Israel. Mrs. Thatcher and Baroness Tweedsmuir were Ministers in the last Conservative Government, preceded and succeeded by Mrs. Barbara Castle and Mrs. Shirley Williams of the Labour Government. Two British women acceded to the post of university vice-chancellor. In 1963 Valentina Tereshkova, a Russian astronaut, achieved world fame. In recent years Kyung-Wha-Chung, a twenty-four-year-old Korean girl, became a world-famous violinist. It is said her playing is sweet and moving, yet she has a will of steel. I remember Shirley Temple from the moving pictures. She began her career at the age of three-and-a-half playing leading roles from the start, with enormous success. Later she became a television actress, a Director of National Multiple Sclerosis Society (N.Y.C.)***, a Delegate to the United Nations, the Ambassador to Ghana, the recipient of many decorations from various states and a mother of three. Magan Du Boisson touched the hearts of many. This Godalming housewife, disabled by multiple

* The first woman to receive the George Cross posthumously.

** The widow of the Prime Minister of Ceylon assassinated in 1959.

*** Her brother, George, was crippled with this disease. She herself underwent an operation for breast cancer in 1972.

sclerosis, came to terms with her condition. Armed with charm, great intelligence, courage, determination and passionate concern about injustice of others, she successfully campaigned for new legislation of the constant attendance allowance for the disabled. Thanks to her, state disability pensions came into being. She organized rallies in Trafalgar Square and travelled to Scotland for a demonstration. The warmth of her personality cheered many disabled; for them she wrote poetry and prose. She was killed in 1969 in a car accident on the way to a meeting. Magan, as she was affectionately known, was a gay person, in the knowledge that she would never grow old. "Be a man" is an incorrect saying. How many men would willingly go through childbirth with its pain and dangers again and again? Women are the wiser sex, and so they outlive men – there are nearly twice as many women as men over the age of seventy. Is it because they visit doctors more readily?! I think they are stronger from the start – male infants are more prone to serious infection than their opposite sex.

Women have better moral qualities. They are more faithful than men for a start. Even the lowest of them, a prostitute, may not be what men, fond of philandering, have tried to make her appear. It is men who are the coarser sex. There are prostitutes on record who took to this trade for the sake of a child or an incapacitated parent. Sixty-year-old Field Marshal von Blomberg, Hitler's Commander-in-Chief, married his much younger secretary without knowing that she had a police record as a prostitute and he was dismissed from the Army. Yet, they settled in a Bavarian village and remained loyal to each other until the Marshal's death in 1946. Nell Gwynn, the mistress of Charles II, was loved by the people for her tender heart and the founding of Chelsea Hospital – an old-soldiers home – is ascribed to her influence with the King. The French singer Edith Piaf – a nickname meaning "sparrow" in Parisian slang and given to her because of a half-starved look – scandalized people by her many love affairs which did not cease with her first marriage at thirty-six. She was capricious and intensely jealous, but also kind, generous, open and sincere, and a loyal friend – a woman par excellence. Courageously, she helped prisoners and Jews to hide and to escape from occupied France. She had to grapple with misfortunes from infancy and they never left her. Yet, she did not loose hope or belief in her fellow men. Poverty forced her to sing in the streets of Paris at a very tender age. Hardships brought ill health to her in later life and turned her into a drug addict and an alcoholic killing her at the age of forty-eight. But she had the tenacity of a bulldog. Her fragile body, anguished voice and large haunted eyes continued to enchant the audiences to the very end, and sadness – evidence of ill fate – only increased her attractiveness. The public listened to her wistful love songs which outnumbered those telling of poverty and despair. Edith Piaf's message to the world was to be happy, to love and to appreciate the blessing of being loved in return.*

Chastity is not the only virtue a woman may possess as celibacy is not the sole attribute of men, and both are of debatable value. I sometimes think that young men grow long hair and wear bracelets and pendants to appear more like their betters – the opposite sex – and on many occasions I have found it difficult to distinguish a boy from a girl. Some women resent this camouflage and retaliate by donning trousers. But in spite of all this and past chivalry which exalted ladies, husbands had a *legal* right to beat them and until recently wives had no share in the property belonging to the wage earning partner. Until recently the married women of Sark had no rights under the law and were their husbands' "chattels". They were better off though than the Arab women who have several rivals to one man and can be dismissed by him at the wave of a hand.

There is no equality between the sexes to this day. On marriage women have to change their name, even though they may not be able to pronounce it. Women's earnings remain below those of men, they are barred from many positions including the priesthood (is it God or man's will not to ordain them?), and are underprivileged in various ways in the eyes of the law (the pension scheme and unrecognized housework are such examples). Among 635 members of the British Parliament there are only 27 lady members. I was struck by the fact that on some forms, I had to fill in for women patients, only the husband's occupation was requested. Socially they are not particularly welcome in the British public institution – the "pub" – still mainly reserved for men. The 16th century King's Head public house, Harrow, had its men-only bar, a tradition dating back to Henry VIII; according to legend the King took refuge in the bar to escape from women. They had to wait until 1928 for the vote; Belgium granted it in 1948. In Switzerland only three cantons moved with the times, vacillating until 1966, and there are still two cantons where women do not have the vote.

I know of a married woman who was unable to emigrate from

* In the words of the French writer, Madame de Staël, "Love is the history of woman's life; it is an episode in man's."

266

Britain without obtaining her husband's consent; unfortunately they had not spoken to each other for a full five years while living under the same roof. "Should *he* wish to emigrate, no one would ask for my permission", she commented sadly. When a forty-year-old woman, who already had a large family became pregnant, doctors were sympathetic; not so her husband. She was told that had she no husband there wouldn't be any difficulty in carrying out the abortion.

An inquiry by a Parliamentary Select Committee concluded that sex discrimination does exist and that it was time for proper legislation. It might one day benefit men as well, as they are at present barred from midwifery,* and rarely become matrons. This is not as fanciful as it may sound, we have already male nurses, and very good they are. But women will always be favoured for some jobs and men for others which is not sex discrimination. Actions brought by jilted brides-to-be for breach of promise were stopped. Soon men could be freed from the maintenance order should a divorced woman be able to find a job. "Marriage should not be looked upon as a free meal ticket for life", commented a judge. In appropriate circumstances even husbands could claim maintenance from their wives. Some progress was certainly made even when by the end of 1973 only 40 out of 3,300 university professors in Britain were women. Women were able to enter the all-male sanctum of Students Unions and the Stock Exchange, and the 800-year-old City of London Corporation elected its first woman alderman. Those with grown-up children can go back to work should they so wish, or train for a new career. They found that more freedom can be great; they are not ageing the way they used to. Yet, it would be a pity if women decided to compete with men in every walk of life as they are different and complementary to them; I don't like to see them drinking and smoking as men do! Who would like to see them as dustmen? Spanish bull rings are opening up to women matadors: Will the Spaniards be happy to watch women's pants ripped open by bulls? Much treasured feminine grace might turn into disgrace. A woman can never be a fellow, it would be foolish of her to aspire to it anyway. For the sake of both sexes women should be encouraged to make a home, and not to strive for outside jobs. It is a thought to give a full-time housewife of below-retiring age some allowances and make her less dependant on the husband. Be that as it may, the great possibilities already offered to modern woman deflect her interests from the only

* Midwives Act 1951.

267

outlet she had in the past – rearing of children – with important consequences.

The best of fathers cannot make a good mother. The very young, when deprived of a mother's presence and love, are likely to develop unenviable traits. This opinion was expressed to me by an elderly woman whose mother left her to relatives at a tender age; from what I knew of her she was right! I view with alarm the trend of disposing with breast feeding and leaving the baby to father and the bottle. I sometimes get nightmares fearing that women's breasts might dwindle from inactivity like the eyes of a mole. Besides robbing the suckling of mother's milk and pleasure (Freud drew attention to "oral gratification" but he may be mistaken), it would deprive the adult male of womanly curves cherished by him. Another factor is the inhibitory effect of breast milk on bacteria which protects the infant from infection. Women can no longer delegate breast feeding to wet nurses. In my babyhood I was still able to be a beneficiary of such an "institution" and even got the full treatment when suckling milk mixed with alcohol from a drunken wet nurse. I was told that she was found out by my parents and dismissed on the spot. I don't mix milk with alcohol to this day! And then there is the mother's love for the child. Mrs. Hunt devoted every minute of her life to her mongol child, Nigel, and turned him into a gay, friendly, well adjusted boy. At seven he was able to read and when he grew up he published his diary – "The World of Nigel Hunt"* – an encouragement to others like him and their families. Dame Edith Sitwell delighted us with her creative work "The Mother and other Poems". Dame Edith Summerskill, although involved in politics, found time to publish "Babies without Tears" and "Letters to my Daughter". No wonder when we wish to praise nature, we rightly talk of good *mother* nature.

Marriage is a unique voluntary institution which has survived thousands of years and does not show signs of weakening. William Booth owed a great deal to his wife Catherine for the success of the Salvation Army. Men take their partners more often for better than for worse and, in the latter event, blame bad luck rather than marriage. Even woman's naughtiness can be appealing! They get divorced only to get married again, with more wisdom and experience. Bertrand Russell, an English philosopher and author of "Marriage on Morals", had been married four times. They know when they are best off, or is it the triumph of hope? Robert Koch, the discoverer of the tubercle bacillus

* 1967. Darwen, Finlay & Son Ltd., Beaconsfield, Bucks.

and the cholera vibrio, divorced his wife Emma who had not understood his work and aspirations. Much later he married Hedwig, several
years younger than himself. It was a happy marriage but did not
contribute to Koch's scientific achievements. He hurriedly announced
that his tuberculin was an antituberculous remedy; it proved dangerous.

"Running after women never hurts anybody – it's catching 'em that
does the damage" – said an American lawyer Clarence Darrow. I dis-
agree with him. The results of a survey by the Institute of Life Insurance of New York showed that married people are healthier, more
robust and live longer than the single ones; widowed and single people
are less likely to have an adequate, regular diet. Marriage can form a
very successful team. One need only remember Queen Victoria and
Prince Albert, King George VI and Queen Elizabeth, the Roosevelts,
the Churchills, the Mountbattens, the Macmillans. It was the composer Edward Elgar's wife, Caroline, who spurred him on and to
whom he owes his fame and success; after she died Elgar wrote little. I
have known several instances in which grief on loosing a life-long companion hastened the death of the spouse. In spite of prosperity there is
restlessness, rush and competition in modern life. Men of retiring age
are additionally burdened by psychological and economic stresses and
often have to struggle. Women's companionship and realism help to
mitigate the burden. They can be very understanding. Mrs. Kinsey,
whose husband Alfred wrote a famous book on sexology, stated without reproaching him that since he became interested in sex she saw
very little of him! I read a true story* about an autistic child who was
unable to communicate with the outside world and shunned all human
contact. Twenty-one years of parental love and devotion succeeded
against all odds and their daughter gained confidence and found her
rightful place in society. The present trend of early marriage, although
bringing inevitable casualties, is to be preferred to bachelorhood extended to the late thirties in the olden days owing to economic con-
siderations. These days it is usually a marriage of love, and not of
convenience. Women are more like Gladys Aylward who rescued many
Chinese children endangered by war, like Lady Hoare, the late president of the Society for Thalidomide Children, or Lady Allen who promotes the cause of playgrounds for the handicapped and rarely like Ilse
Koch, "the Bitch of Buchenwald". Joséphine Baker, a coloured star of
Folies Bergères, Casino de Paris and la Créole in the 1920's, brought

* "For the Love of Ann." James Copeland, 1973. Arrow Books Ltd.

up eleven children of various nationalities, race and creed. This wonderful woman bought a chateau for them in Dordogne ("Le Moilande").

I don't believe that women would bring us into war – they would not wish to send their children for slaughter – for they are pacifists at heart. They have better insight than men. Like the rest of the animal kingdom it is the male who is manipulated by the female without even suspecting it. We must trust their intuition. I could be biased; I knew women who gave me much help, encouragement, comfort and pleasure, and I knew men who did just the opposite.

The youth of today give a headache to their elders and a gulf has opened up between them. The young are more independent economically than were their parents, often receiving a better education, and growing up with the technological revolution and the reality of men in space and on the moon. The universe, known to the older generation only through mythology, became an object of science.

The gap was even more pronounced among families who came here from Europe during the war; many of the parents could barely speak English, had difficulty in adjusting themselves and still lived in the past. Often the only thing they had in common with their children was their name – a foreign one which conveyed little to their young who could not speak their parents' tongue. Such names could be difficult to pronounce; when the Polish film star of the silent screen, Apolonia Chalupiec, went to the U.S.A. at the age of twenty-four, she changed her name to Pola Negri.

But most of all, there was disenchantment with the record of the older generation. Youth was fed with clichés, watched unchristian Christians, the loosening of family ties and the delegation of responsibility for grandparents to the state; when an octogenarian who lived alone developed senile confusion, her daughter refused to take my patient into her house until accommodation could be found in a residential home, telling me that legally she was not responsible for her mother. The young read of famine in countries like Bangladesh and Ethiopia – their thought for food was food for thought. They were told how the Peruvians sold fish to richer countries for feeding livestock when their own children were dying of malnutrition. They have heard of the follies of war which spilled blood in torrents and annihilated many millions. They wonder why the University of Oxford conferred an Honorary Degree on Zaharoff, "the Arms King" in World War I. They have read of Hitler, Stalin and Mussolini, and of scientific experiments and the gas-chambers. They know of Heinrich Himmler who once pronounced that "we do not ask for love, only for fear" and of others in the German ruling circles of a similar mentality. They ask why previously fair-minded governments went out of their way to appease them, ready to compound with villainy. The most punishable crimes went unpunished for years. The young are dismayed by the apathy and failure to take action by their elders. They witnessed bloody coups and political assassinations. They sometimes saw ferocious animals intoxicated with the taste of blood and compared them to man – more bestial than the beasts – the most ferocious of them all – these were not herds of wild elephants but the hordes of Atilla in the fifth and twentieth century Europe. They were told of not-too-distant times in which hatred, killings and cruelty were the very qualities sought after and well rewarded. Thanks to penicillin and other innovations more wounded people survived War II than War I leaving a greater number of invalids in its wake – this was progress . . . One would think that men would get tired of war, and yet not for a moment has there been universal peace – remember the Berlin Wall,* Korea, Algeria, Congo, Biafra, Vietnam, Cambodia, Bangladesh, Russian-Chinese confrontations, Israeli-Arab wars, Mozambique, troubles in Northern Ireland, bomb outrages and blood-thirsty nationalism. No wonder people responsible for our lives are called "big-*shots*"!

The young tried desperately to find a way which would insulate mankind from wars and nuclear threat. Staggering unaware into two wars myself and feeling it, I am regretfully conscious of their feelings. They also search for the purpose of living. Some turned to religion, some to Eastern mysticism and meditation, some to charities. New names hit the headlines – Billy Graham, Maharishi Maheshyogi, Maharaj Ji (a fifteen-year-old "Guru"), "The Children of God", Oxfam, etc. They saw through the procrastination, smugness, falsehood, personal greed and pretence of their elders. To provide legal grounds for divorce one often had to make a business deal with some lady willing to spend a short time with her client in a hotel room. Young people heard that drinking and cigarette smoking was bad but one saw them doing just that on the slightest provocation; heavy drinking became an "industrial disease" for those who had to entertain their clients, and even people as able as the British poet Dylan Thomas drank themselves to death. The cream of society could not be any better, the expression "Drunk as a lord" proves it. The youth were un-

* In the first 6 years of its existence 70 people were killed.

271

able to spot among that generation a Baden Powell, a Colonel during the 217 days siege of Mafeking in the Boer's struggle for independence who dedicated himself to noble peaceful aims of the Scout Movement, or an Alfred Nobel. They were told by their elders that they are hysterical when they were enthusiastic and exuberant. They observed mediocre, falsely shy, sex starved and repressed people who acted under the guise of lawful guardians vested with status and authority when not particularly qualified for high office. These were not the people the young could talk to — neither side believed each other. Their elders lost their grip on people — "sit-in" protests and marches, organized pandemoniums, industrial and subversive actions, civil disobedience, student riots, robbery and violence were on the increase. To youth they were the men of yesterday — weak-willed and narrow-minded. Even pigeons have been disrespectful to the statues of their heroes. The young became outraged by being conned. They were told to listen and to obey but this way they would never learn to speak, and they decided to express themselves. Their views had to be heard. They called for matching of words and deeds and not just to be told to be good. A brave show of words alone was not good enough for them. Youth launched a deliberate attack on society. Seeing workers going on strike for a tea-break, students went on strike for free contraceptives. They began to assail the established religious and moral tenets and debunk the old ideas. Their elders shook their heads. With skirts getting shorter and shorter faces of older people were getting longer and longer. Yet, youth managed to stir people's conscience and mass media took their plea. A new humanism was growing. Tolerance, sympathy and understanding began to emanate towards the mentally ill, the unmarried mothers, the divorcees, the homosexuals (such relationships became legal for consenting adults over twenty-one, and recently a club was licensed for homosexuals). Youth received recognition from their elders who lowered the voting age to eighteen and enabled them to exert more influence in shaping society. Youth came into the open. Hormone loaded, they proclaimed that desire and sex are not necessarily sinful and that they ceased to be taboo for them. If there were no sex the world would cease to exist, even microbes have a sex life. Lift the ignorance which brings shame, feeling of guilt and unhappiness, they reasoned. Sex should not be left to amateurs. They spoke of a laywoman, referring not to her occasional recumbency but to her ignorance in sexual matters. "Make love, not war" was not such a bad slogan and refreshing candour. Let's face it, the mating game is

272

the game of nature observed in the whole animal kingdom. If Freud was right that suppressed sexual wishes cause certain nervous disorders which can be cured by a psychoanalyst who brings them into the patient's consciousness, there shouldn't be such patients any longer; by "do-it-yourself" they all should be cured!

The people of today are not more permissive than those in the past, even though they speak about sex more openly. When we talk of prepermissive days, we only say people had less opportunities then. Some were puritan, some pure, but many lacked both adjectives. The mythology tells us of the Greek god of herdsmen, Pan, who busied himself in pursuit of a nymph, also of lascivious satyrs. Harems had to be guarded by eunuchs, and the world has always had brothels, scandals, illegitimacy and syphilis. There are "naughty" arts and naughty jokes, and those not involved in scandals relish talking about them. If the youth of today lacks chivalry towards the opposite sex, it is yet more open and forthright. There is neither maxi-heaven-like bliss nor mini-paradise upon earth. This is an imperfect, often ruthless world and no place for saints and angels, only for sinners.

People love and hate, hope and despair, know envy, jealousy, conflicts and vengeance; if they acted differently they would be too good for this world, they would go against nature. Armies and the police made our lives just that much safer. People help each other when they are down; when they are up, they bicker, they kick, and they fight. The fellowship of suffering unites people, prosperity seems to divide them. Pure people remain poor. Boxing, a favourite "sport" of many, does cause brain damage, mutilation, even death, and in any event it is always painful. Rugby is not much better. Women's good instinct prevents them from such activities, but they are capable of sporting prowess just the same. In 1973 Wimbledon champion, Mrs. Billie-Jean King, won a decisive victory over the ex tennis champion, Bobby Riggs; the challenge came from her opponent who asserted that men are superior to women and tried to prove it. André Lwoff drew our attention to the biochemical revolution which is accompanied by gradual loss of enzymes so that higher organisms are more dependent upon the environment to provide ready-made nutrients – in short, one has to kill other species to sustain oneself. Human vegetarians suffer from various deficiencies which have to be corrected. Life is a combination of fighting, suffering, working, loving and seeking pleasure, in that order. Because of the fighting and the suffering doctors are constantly in demand since time immemorial.

273

I don't believe that youth in the main is salacious or that it is dull, negative and destructive. The opposite happens to be the truth – it is vigorous, colourful, with many positive ideas – it is our hope for the future. The young are more critical than the previous generation thanks to a better education, they also show more social awareness and less selfishness. They express more anger than their predecessors not because they are more unhappy, but because they have more freedom. Youth of today lacks prudery which does the most damage. They would not destroy the life of gifted Oscar Wilde as their forefathers did. In the days of the crinoline no one dared to utter the four-letter word as it was shunned more than the real thing; people had a chastened language but not lives. Today, being able to talk about sex helps those who are vulnerable. Youth does not *dream* of it any longer, they have no need! Besides, sexual freedom is only one of many freedoms this country enjoys. And there is nothing permissive in revealing the beauty nature bestowed on a woman, it is rather selfish to hide it. A scanty dress and G-string give justice to it and satisfaction to our visual senses for which unhibited art is only the second best. It is not immoral or harmful to see lovely willowy young ladies with fresh complexion, blond hair streaming, in colourful thigh-high skirts which reveal their elegant long legs and purposeful stride. To brighten the daily-life scene, to bring happiness is positively healthy and pleasure seeking is not wrong in itself. A *little* of what you fancy does you good. "O Calcutta" could not be such an impudent revue as it never had bare seats! It is worth mentioning that flowers whose beauty we admire are nothing else but organs of reproduction. In by-gone days one had to be rich to look "pretty". Vanity prompted women to adorn their necks with pearls – old secretions of sick oysters – and to cause death to many minks. Those who could not afford furs from minks, sables or ermines, aspired to ones from foxes, squirrels or rabbits. It was such a waste of effort, primitive tribes have shown much more common sense. Was it a healthy instinct being killed by civilization? Be that as it may, youth had little in common with the older generation and to stress how different they were, they grew their hair long and wore strange clothes. Beads were the symbols worn by both sexes. I only wish they could have had someone who would comb their hair and look after their finger nails – but then they didn't believe in servants.

It was a full swing from traditional living, convention and modesty and there were bound to be casualties. Most of the old values were fast disappearing. Religion was once a science for the illiterate for it explained everything they were unable to understand – faith was their knowledge and strength; now it is knowledge which is the object of their faith and reverence. In these days when there is little illiteracy, people have stopped looking for rewards promised them in after life. They know that thunder, lightning and natural disaster are not the sign of God's displeasure. Yet they still resort to the old blackmail: "If God does not grant me what I ask Him for, I do not wish to know Him". They like to pass the buck to Him. They began to question religion. Some young people looked upon the Son of God as a revolutionary. Creed, even race, ceased to be a barrier and people intermarried irrespectively. A patient of mine, a Catholic, underwent circumcision and took the biblical name of Abraham to be married to an orthodox Jewish girl. When I visited his mother some time later, I noticed a photograph of him, wearing a skull cap, and his bride under a canopy. It was placed in a prominent position among the statue of the Virgin Mary and holy pictures. People realized that ecclesiastical authorities cannot save unsatisfactory marriages, perpetuation of which can only bring unhappiness and frustration. The actress Sophia Loren knew it! Belief was replaced by cynicism, modesty by nudity, self-control by birth control, chastity by promiscuity. Youth, brought up by the Welfare State, never learned the word "denial" and did not practise self-denial. A Self Denial Week was definitely not their way. Good taste did not matter so long as it tasted good. Sex was on everyones lips, in everyones ears and eyes, no one could avoid it. The dirty word "fornication" was replaced by more respectable ones: "sexual experience" and "extra marital relationship" and "unlawful wife" by "common law wife". Homosexuals changed their name to "Gay People". Sex book shops, sex shows, sex films, sex posters, sex symbols, sex education and sex crime filled the scene. Exhibitionists began running stark naked imagining themselves as athletes of ancient Greece. Some older people tried to deceive themselves that they were suffering from double vision and that the things were only half as bad . . . The young people became so noisy (with the help of pop music, microphones, loud speakers and transistors) that one wonders how soon they will become hard of hearing. In music they favour cacophony. They are helped by traffic and aircraft noise, washing machines, dishwashers and many other electric appliances. Noise conquered peace. To protect oneself from hearing loss one has to turn to "ear defenders", of which there are now many types. Such situation necessitated the new slogan: "Keep Britain quiet!" The weak, the less intelligent, the unbalanced, the corrupt became overwhelmed by the changes and were unable to adapt themselves. By discarding the old values they deprived themselves of reassurance. Such people could be both cruel and kind, disruptive and helpful. Perplexity and bewilderment were destroying them. New phenomena appeared – "Beatle mania", "Osmond mania", pop festivals and the like. Well meant social protests degenerated into aggression and began to threaten the British tradition of freedom cherished by the nation. Gatherings like those at soccer matches turned into rowdyism and hooliganism. The confused hippies resorted to violence in the name of love and fought for peace. They were quickly dubbed "beatniks". People were unable to grasp that purposeful activity and not inertia, struggle and not peace are nature's main features observed on earth, in the sea and in the air. Vandalism, fanaticism, terrorism appeared on the scene. New words were heard: "Mods and Rockers", "Skinheads", "Hell's Angels", "Black Power", "Angry Brigade", "mugging" . . . New toys sprung up – flick-knives, steel rods, cudgels, knuckle-dusters, bottles, boots and explosives. Television is one of youth's principal teachers. Those who listened and watched too much had not enough time to think for themselves, and paid the price for it. They became handicapped by poor judgement so falling victim to any propaganda that sprang up around them. Those who wished to continue to live with illusions at any price and replace reality with fantasies took to pot smoking, LSD and the like; one such drug was named Bromide STP, the last letters standing for serenity, tranquillity and peace . . . They withdrew from society which they were neither able to enrich nor destroy. Society found an appropriate name for them – the "dropouts". They were no heroes; no courage was demanded of them – they lived in a free country, unmolested, among a good-tempered race. They were lucky – in some other countries they would be taken for madmen and treated as such. Theirs was not the case of the brave Soviet dissidents asking for the basic human rights against all odds. Even in the case of the Russians one could argue that they had nothing to protest about as their country had little crime, no mugging, no hooliganism, no drug taking, but no personal freedom or happiness either. Yet, the trouble-makers were in the minority. Many of them were bedevilled by lack of hardship, having an easy life, precious little to do, easy money and easy spending. They lacked the ability to refrain from trying to satisfy all their wishes. (Elvis Presley, a Mississippi country boy, made a fortune by strumming a guitar for youth everywhere; his records have sold 250 million copies.) They were deprived of conditions which would harden their characters; this was their misfortune and the root of the trouble. When Ghenghiz Khan's father was killed, he succeeded him as tribal chief at the age of thirteen and became later a bold leader who was proclaimed Khan of all the Mongols. George Stephenson, the railway pioneer, was a cow-herd who taught himself to read and write. Johann Sebastian Bach was left an orphan at the age of ten. Michael Faraday, the famous 19th century physicist, was a blacksmith's son and an errand boy to a bookbinder in his youth. William Booth was born into an impoverished family and apprenticed to a pawnbroker; his contact with poverty and sin influenced his whole life; he became an ardent evangelist and later founded the Salvation Army. Dr. David Livingstone was born of poor parents and worked in a cotton mill for thirteen years. Dr. George Hoyt Whipple who won a Nobel prize for work on the use of liver extract in pernicious anaemia, investigated Mediterranean anaemia naming it thalassaemia, and who received many awards and honours, lost his father when he was two years old and had to be self-supporting during his student years. Lord Nuffield, a public benefactor in this century, was a farmer's son who had little time for mischief as he had to work long hours in a cycle repair shop. Hans Christian Andersen, the celebrated Danish writer of fairy tales, was the son of a sickly cobbler who died at an early age when Hans was eleven years old; the child was left to his own resources. Both Frederick Hopkins, the pioneer in the study of vitamins, and Wilhelm Einthoven, the inventor of electrocardiography, lost their fathers in early boyhood. Joseph Conrad, the novelist, was exiled at the age of twelve from his native Poland by the Tsarist régime and saw both his parents die of hardship and grief; he joined a British sailing ship in search of justice and freedom. Gracie Fields, one of the best loved English variety stars, was born of poor parents and worked in a Lancashire cotton mill in her earlier years. We must not forget Aneurin Bevan, once Minister of Health, who established the National Health Service. The son of a miner, he himself went down the mines at the age of thirteen, and watched his father dying of pneumoconiosis. I would also like to mention Benjamin Frankel, a conductor and composer of chamber works, eight symphonies and instrumental Mass Songs. As a young man he had to make his living as a watchmaker's assistant and a jazz violinist in night clubs whilst studying at the Guildhall School of Music. These people had no time for boredom and mischief. Be that as it may, the majority of youth remains idealistic in outlook and helps the old and infirm, the poor, the hungry and the unfortunate in different parts of the world.

For my part I don't like many things I see and hear but I tolerate them, for instance traffic noise and super-sonic booms. I tolerate them as temporary phenomena which will be remedied. I put my trust in the Advisory Council on Noise, the Noise Abatement Society etc. Britain leads the world in the drive to lessen aircraft noise; by 1976 all jets might be noise certificated in the effort to quieten them. There are many societies which deal with undesirable products of progress. If I mention pollution here I mean it in a wider sense. I am not a pessimist who would say: "Even Big Ben *strikes* every hour". Already the pendulum has begun to swing back from the other direction and I am convinced that it will find its equilibrium. Many young people strive to save the world but it does not need saving.

Progress is not an even process devoid of unrest. To break away from the past and to be able to sail towards the future we are bound at some time to encounter stormy weather. Progress over the ages has been happening in leaps; we are privileged to live and witness one of the longest of them. After all, the strange, often irresponsible behaviour of some youths is not a sign of decay but of childish exhibitionism at an impressionable age. They are also baffled and seek answers to puzzling questions. In short, it is a part of adolescence. Somerset Maugham described it as a stage between infancy and adultery. It will not be too long before they grow up and dispel their illusions. There is no such thing as "the free world". If they choose to talk and not listen, one day they must tire of such an exercise. Life gives them valuable experience even if they burn themselves in the process. The undeniable fact is that the lives of all of us have been affected. The change we witnessed was not an academic one confined to science alone. It is unavoidable that the old might not always be able to understand the young – I don't understand abstract art – but I wouldn't dream of condemning it.

Sometimes houses and relics have to make way for new roads. The temptation to pull down everything old, even if it is beautiful and historical, is so great that the Department of Environment had to be created as a watch dog. New approaches are made to educational, economic and social problems, and the rising status of women. We witness the sex education of children, the merger of big firms, the supermarkets and such like. Bernard Shaw's "Mrs. Warren's Profession" which dealt with prostitution was barred by the Lord Chamberlain, but it is no longer. The effect of television is more often good than bad. The picture does not appear to be too gloomy so long as we retain the zest for life. There is still love and beauty left in this world. It is not all avarice, meanness, juvenile delinquency and trouble making by perverted minds, and although boils form on the flesh, they are bound to disappear and are unlikely to leave scars; in any case an infection confined to a small area does not usually ruin the body.

Some people make money by gambling, sheer luck or dishonesty, not by hard work or skill. Money (or the lack of it) brings a lot of unhappiness and anxiety. We are told that there are "poor people" no more, only because they were given a new name – "the underprivileged". In spite of great housing shortage and many people being homeless, the 32 storey London office block, built at the cost of £5 million well over ten years ago, remains empty. Yet if our capitalistic system occasionally shows an unpleasant face, it is because of our imperfections which, sadly, we must accept, and not because of the system itself; it has proved to be better than the Communistic one. The bard of the Bolshevik revolution, Vladimir Mayakovsky, commited suicide in 1930; reality killed this idealist. He joined the Bolshevik faction of the Social Democratic Labour Party in 1908 when he was barely fourteen and after their seizure of power in 1917, put his talent at the service of the Communist Party. He was praised by Stalin as the best poet of the Soviet epoch but became disillusioned. A similar fate met Sergei Esenin – "poet laureate of the Revolution" who came from a peasant family. After marrying the dancer Isadora Duncan, he travelled widely and on return to Soviet Russia found himself out of harmony with the revolution; in 1925 he took his own life. Isaac Babel, a leading proletarian writer and a protégé of Maxim Gorky, perished in one of Stalin's concentration camps, and so did Brunon Jasienski, a Polish Communist, writer and journalist of distinction. Such were the tragedies of betrayed idealists. Like André Gide before him, Salvatore Quasimodo, an Italian poet concerned with human suffering and Nobel laureate in 1959, abandoned Communism to enjoy literary freedom, and he only knew Communism – Italian style! Mrs. Jane Degras of the Royal Institute of International Affairs who came from a poor East End family – a leading authority on the history of the Soviet Union and Soviet foreign policy – was once an ardent Communist. She went to Moscow to work in the Marx-Engels Institute, but disenchanted by what she saw, returned to Britain. "Cultural revolutions" in China and Libya reminded me of the old picture when books were burnt, shops and libraries ransacked. Communist countries treat their people like Borstal children who must be deprived of freedom. Give a Borstal boy a free hand and he will become a menace. To this day many Russian people have to enter into a marriage of convenience in order to get a residence permit in their large cities, or count on favouritism. The Communist rulers do not confine themselves to their own people but attempt to influence the rest of the world. They cannot win them over by reality or deception, only by force. In Abraham Lincoln's own words "You can fool all the people some of the time, and some of the people all of the time, but you cannot fool all the people all the time." Not a single existing Communist country established the system by peaceful democratic means; it had to be imposed on people. This system remains rigid, unchanged, backed by military might. I pray that democracy can survive and that the bleak life of the unfortunate people will not reach us. Capitalism of today is, after all, the Socialism of yesterday. In practice, there is no clear cut distinction between Capitalism and Communism. I talked to my jailers at the forced labour camps and learned that theirs was a well paid job. After accumulating enough capital they intended to return to their poorly paid unskilled occupation at home, backed by the money they have saved – capitalism of Communist Brand!

There are many signs that we are sailing towards a better future for ourselves and our children after us, and I would like to mention the decrease of deaths from illegal abortions, the decrease of illegitimate births and "shot gun" marriages, the paucity of babies for adoption* and less need for hiring a woman. The liberal attitude towards illegitimate children saved us from destroying people like Willi Brandt and Catherine Cookson. Some conquest of social life has been made. The word *"permissive"* merely states that much is *permitted*. What is wrong with this? Man continues to learn how to use his resources to the best advantage – natural gas was once a useless by-product. The strange behaviour of some youths which at one time would scandalize the world, does not shock us any more; people, being more youth-orientated than before, realize that the corner has been turned, and in their heart of hearts they know they must pin their hopes to a younger generation. It is refreshing to watch youth crowding the Proms. Their elders make contact with them, they like to show sympathy and understanding and offer their support. They learn to speak on the same wave

* In 1973 there were thirty applications to every child available for adoption.

length and listen. It has been suggested that church halls could be turned into dormitories for those most needy who sleep rough. There is a tendency to distribute some of the wealth of the churches among the poor. However, there is no real need now for the clergy to act as superior guardians of illiterate people and involve themselves in politics)* Seniors are reconciled to the fact that the taboos about sexuality are broken. They realize at last their own thoughtless, irresponsible behaviour which showed itself in unwillingness to accept the emotional nature of adolescence; they contracted out of their responsibilities. It was the fault of the older generation that the young became disturbed. "Problem family" is not an empty phrase. The young who were deprived of love and affection looked for it in promiscuity and shrugged off the sexual guilt. When treated as inferior beings, stripped of self-esteem, understanding and comradeship, they attempted to assert themselves. Some turned to football or motor racing, others to violence, sex, drinking and smoking in the erroneous belief that they were building their masculine image which would give them security; self-preservation of a kind, I suppose. Seniors tried to mend their ways. It was not a matter of rivalry between generations but one of contact, understanding and goodwill. The message got through – the young had the need and the right to express and fulfill themselves. They must, however, accept the fact that they are a part of a much larger community which cannot be geared only to their own kind.

Life is a continuous movement, a continuous change and adjustment – a process which affects a single cell as much as the whole world. Perhaps we are heading towards peace and a better life after all. Besides thinking of the present one is obliged to look to the future.

Professional people were also swept by the changes, but were not submerged by the levelling up process around them. Professions have always made an imprint on their members and continue to do so. An engineer or a surgeon is usually a practical methodical man (incidentally, surgeons *cut* themselves off from the rest of doctors and call themselves "Misters"). A dentist is self-opinionated, often financially minded; a hospital consultant – aloof; a family doctor – more human; a psychiatrist – a man (or woman) *anxious* to solve other people's problems, after having solved their own; a doctor in an administrative post – a good talker; a lawyer – concise and pragmatic; a coroner a cross between a doctor and a lawyer; an acupuncturist – prickly; a

* In August 1974 the Greek Catholic Archbishop for Jerusalem, Monsignor Capucci, was charged with aiding the Palestinian terrorists.

headmaster – dictatorial; a professional soldier – brusque; a "copper" – always a copper. But, as in any generalization, there are many exceptions. There is still another factor, I could be wrong . . .

A doctor is expected to have integrity and principles, to be courageous, knowledgeable, competent, decisive but cautious, thoughtful, dedicated, tolerant, sympathetic, selfless, impartial, trustworthy, discreet, modest, good mannered, good humoured, well dressed, sensitive and understanding, aware of the needs of his fellow men. He must never, never put aside time for meals or be ill. He is expected to be a paragon of all the virtues. *Some* doctors certainly have *some* of these qualities. Frederick Banting was awarded the Military Cross in 1918 "for heroism under fire". We saw how a number of them have shaped our lives, and we remember Werner Forssmann who, single-handed, inserted a catheter into his own heart. He had to walk some distance from the operating theatre to the X-ray department and ascend stairs with the probe lying in his heart. Professor August Bier, a burly figure as I remember him from 1931 when he was lecturing in Berlin, conceived the idea of spinal anaesthesia. Thirty-two years earlier he ordered an assistant to inject cocaine* solution into his, Bier's, spinal canal. He was helped by the insight and boldness of Heinrich Quincke, Professor for internal medicine at Kiel, who demonstrated earlier that the spinal canal can be safely punctured by a needle (it is known today as "lumber puncture"). Bier suffered from an appalling headache for several days – the penalty of being a pioneer! John Hunter, a Scottish anatomist and surgeon in the 18th century, derived his knowledge from observation and experiments, some of them on himself. Dr. Mueller, a Viennese, experimented with plague germs and they killed him. William Halsted, a celebrated Baltimore surgeon and the discoverer of local anaesthesia with cocaine, was experimenting on himself and fell victim to the drug. A number of doctors lost their lives in the course of their duties. Fifteen years ago Dr. Cutts, a colleague of mine, contracted "polio" from one of his patients and died in the prime of life. There were doctors who were courageous patients. Johann von Mikulicz-Radecki, a famous Polish surgeon and teacher who was once an assistant to Theodor Billroth, the founder of gastric surgery, diagnosed a stomach cancer on himself when he was fifty-four. He underwent surgery knowing full well that he was only postponing the inevitable for a while. Mikulicz was operated on by a Viennese Professor, von Eiselsberg, whom I remember as a lean, grey haired, dis-

* Novocaine was not discovered until 1905.

282

tinguished looking man I saw in Vienna in 1930. Like his patient he was once attached to Professor Billroth's team. Professor Eiselsberg found at the operation that the growth was inoperable and simply closed the abdomen, later telling the patient that no cancer was found. Mikulicz knew it was a well intended lie but did not say so. After his death, von Eiselsberg received a letter of thanks from him and a statement that the patient had always known the truth. Despite this knowledge he continued working for some time after his operation and later on composed his own obituary. Sigmund Freud, the father of psychoanalysis, battled with a painful condition of cancer of the jaw for sixteen years without letting it interfere with his work and remained fertile to the end, succumbing to the inevitable in 1939. Sun-Yat-Sen, a practising physician in China, was a selfless idealist. In his capacity as a doctor he realized the needs of his people for social, economic and political change. He led a successful revolution against the corrupt Emperor Manchu and his régime. Another physician-revolutionary was Jean Marat who for some time had practised in London and was given the honorary degree of Doctor of Medicine by St. Andrews University. After the fall of the Bastille he preached not only revolution but murder. During the French Revolution Dr. Guillotin suggested an instrument for execution which could bring humane death. His name is mentioned with a frown, but he was not a villain. Yet another qualified doctor, Salvador Allende, involved himself in politics. His encounter with poverty as a medical student urged him to take measures which could solve Chile's social ills. He founded his country's Socialist Party and held the post of Minister of Health for three years. Allende became Chile's President in 1970, after thirty-three years of parliamentary activities. He was not a militant revolutionary but an idealist who abhorred bloodshed and gained power through free elections. His marxism was not of a Bolshevik brand and he was not subservient to Moscow. Salvador Allende was too tame to survive; after three years of rule he died in a coup. The present Prime Minister of the newly independent African state of Malawi, Dr. Hastings Banda, was in general practice in Liverpool and London and later on in the Gold Coast. Albert Schweitzer devoted his life to the needs and happiness of his fellow men and became a doctor, theologian, philosopher, missionary and an accomplished pianist. He practised in remote Lambarene in West Africa, temporarily revisiting Europe to raise money for his hospital by concerts and lectures. When he won the Nobel peace prize in 1953, he used the money to build a leper village. Dr. Thomas Barnardo, a philanthropist, felt compassion not only for 4,000 victims of cholera in the East End of London during the epidemic in 1866, but also for hundreds of neglected children, and so he started a lodging house and school for them which grew into Dr. Barnardo's Homes. There were doctors for the rich like Axel Munthe and Aldo Castellani. The latter was reported once having three queens waiting at the same time in his Harley Street consulting rooms.

Some names became household names in medicine without particular merit. In 1916 Hans Reiter, a German hygienist, reported a single patient who had diarrhoea, urethritis, conjunctivitis and polyarthritis and lent his name to the disease. Richard Julius Petri's* main achievement was a shallow glass dish used for solid culture media and "Petri dish" is mentioned many times a day in thousands of laboratories all over the world. Many doctors made their names in spheres other than medicine, politics and philanthropy. All know of Edward Jenner's smallpox vaccination but very few of his excellent paper on the cuckoo. John Bell, a physician to the British Embassy in Russia in the second decade of the 18th century, visited China, Persia and Constantinople and returned to his native Scotland where he published his "Travels". Jean Charcot, a son of the famous 19th century neurologist, himself a physician, headed two expeditions to the Antarctic, discovered Charcot Land, naming it after his father, but drowned off Western Iceland. In recent years Philip Hugh-Jones of King's College Hospital, London, engaged in exploration of the remote Mato Grosso in Brazil and combined science with adventure. Peter Steele, the medical officer for the 1971 international Everest expedition, is the author of "In a Tibetan Tent" and other books concerned with climbing and travel. He worked in a Mission hospital in Nepal and carried out work for goitre survey in Bhutan. Thomas Phaer, a physician and lawyer who lived in the 16th century, translated Vergil's "Aeneid" into English verse. A contemporary Italian painter and writer, Carlo Levi,** was trained as a physician. Roger Bannister,*** a neurologist, was once the fastest runner in the world and is the author of "First Four Minutes" and several medical papers. A hundred years ago Britain produced a world-famous doctor-sportsman. Dr. W. G. Grace, a G.P. for nearly twenty years in a working-class area of Bristol, was the greatest cricketer in the world.

* Berlin bacteriologist (1852–1921).

** The author of "Christ stopped at Eboli" in which he described the poverty-stricken villagers of the "Basilicata" region.

*** Holder of the world record for one mile in 1954.

He must also have been a good diagnostician as he soon recognized malingering in one of his patients whom he cured instantly by fetching boxing gloves and telling him: "What you need my lad is exercise, not medicine!" Hector Berlioz gave up medicine for music and Charles Darwin – for zoology. A host of doctors became world famous writers. Miss Reita Faria won the title of Miss World when still a student.

Doctors can be severely handicapped by their own illnesses. Ferdinand Sauerbruch, a celebrated Berlin surgeon, unknown to himself, lost control of his faculties when struck by cerebral sclerosis. In spite of this he was made the head of the University Hospital "Charité" in East Berlin for political reasons, an appointment which brought inevitable casualties. Paul Enrlich was forced to give up his work for a year-and-a-half because of tuberculosis contracted in the course of his researches, and the same scourge interrupted the work of the celebrated Spanish neuro-anatomist Ramóny Cajal. I remember a venerologist who became very hard of hearing which caused him to shout – he was as handicapped as Beethoven!

Even outstanding doctors might lack in stamina. Victor Schilling, a Berlin scientist renowned for his blood studies, accepted a professorship in medicine from the Nazis at Rostock University in 1941 and became their tool; a Viennese professor, Eppinger, the successor of Professor Wenkebach and a specialist in liver diseases, must have had a guilty conscience as he committed suicide on the entry of the Allies into Vienna. To save his own skin, a Polish doctor, Wladislaw Dering, himself a Nazi prisoner in the notorious concentration camp at Auschwitz, carried out many thousands of experiments consisting of mutilating operations on Jewish men and women. There was even a common murderer among the medical profession. Hawley Harvey Crippen, an American, who studied medicine and dentistry in Michigan and London, poisoned his wife, having transferred his affections to his secretary. Remembering his student days he dissected the body and attempted to destroy the bones.

Doctors vary in health, character and temperament. Edward Jenner displayed professional jealousy of his colleagues and did not easily give credit to others.* Some medical men show warmth, modesty and understanding, others only pomposity and indifference. Some are approachable and informative, others pontificate and say little in many words with the help of medical jargon alien to the patient. They have the art of saying simple things in a complex and confusing way. Some

* . Neither did they give credit to him for quite a time.

are more vocal than others. Some are blunt. Some are considerate – if a small lie can make a patient happier and feel better that way why not try? Besides doctors dedicated to patients and showing more interest in human beings than in the material world, there are ones who dedicate themselves to both or money alone. Some doctors give moral support, some immoral. Besides a gentle kind there are those relentless fighters for whom battle is life and who would go anywhere to meet it. Besides the luminaries of the medical circle, there are those who dally in medicine; besides men (and women) of stature, there are also small creatures who force their way by bullying. Some doctors give the wrong pill and the wrong dosage at the wrong time for the wrongly diagnosed condition. It might not matter should the pill come out intact at the other end; it could even make a patient feel better if he had faith in it. On one doctor, a forbidding self-centred and cold-hearted character, there was only one way I could look, and that was down, yet I was smaller than he was. Let's call him a not-so-smart Alec. The description of Joseph Mankiewicz: "He buys his suits to fit the man he'd like to be, about three sizes too large" would fit him well. Bullying and greatness do not go together. Doctors may have various complexes; piles give them an *inferiority* complex and a bald head a *superiority* one. There are morbid anatomists and morbid doctors. It takes all sorts of people to make this venerable profession. I know, I've met them all. No wonder that some doctors are liked and respected, others disliked and disrespected. No wonder that besides crusaders like Paul de Kruif who wrote "Microbe Hunters" and "Men Against Death", Ritchie Calder, author of "Medicine and Man", and Juergen Thorwald, author of "The Century of the Surgeons" and "The Triumph of Surgery", there were also outspoken critics who satirized the medical profession of *their* time, like the harassed unhappy Molière and taunting George Bernard Shaw. I have an excuse for both of them. Molière, author of "Le docteur amoreux", "Le Médécin malgré lui" and "Le Malade imaginaire" suffered from ill health and died at the age of fifty-one in spite of his doctor's efforts – we must remember that he lived in the 17th century – and doctors were not his only target. Bernard Shaw, on the other hand, who was a vegetarian, a teetotaller and a non-smoker, lived to the age of ninety-four and could afford to spurn doctors. He would have lived longer if he hadn't fractured his leg in a fall. Doctors have improved though. They neither wear top hats, sombre cloaks, stiff white collars and cuffs with cufflinks of precious stones nor big pocket watches hanging on heavy gold chains. Their appearance, far from reassuring the patient, frightened him – they reminded him of well-to-do- undertakers. Now doctors try to look more cheerful and discard their white coats when working with the push pen in their surgeries so as not to remind the patient what he came for. They act like chefs of swank restaurants preferring French names to their own. Doctors speak of the "petit and grand mal" in epilepsy, "la belle indifférence" in hysteria, "bouton de Baghdad" in cutaneous leishmaniasis, "tic douloureux" in trigeminal neuralgia or a "crise tabetic", even when they don't know a word of French! Patients believe that doctors are clever to a point of being crafty down-to-earth people. In fact they are more often than not a romantic lot; one only has to look at the descriptions they invented: "Swan deformity", "Moon face", "Honeymoon- or Anonymous cystitis" and "Sella turcica" ("Turkish saddle" for the pituitary fossa). The label "A venerable profession" is as fallacious as the myth that they are well organized, a clique, a set apart. Doctors are one of the few bodies who did not create homes for their retired people. I can only think that they have had enough of their own company during professional life . . . Yet, in writing to each other, they always sign themselves "Yours sincerely", no matter what their feelings really are! When one gets to the very bottom of it, one finds that they are not really at the top of all the professions. Again, women come to man's rescue; they constitute one-fifth of doctors in Britain. Women bring their complimentary gifts – the interest and ability to care for children, the elderly, the mentally disturbed and the disabled requiring rehabilitation. They leave the butchery to men! It is gratifying to see how many of them are able to share medicine and motherhood. They are certainly more creative – they bring new lives into being. And they have this powerful organ – the woman's voice box!

22
GP in GB

My life changed like everyone else's, perhaps more so. I was now a free man enjoying the hospitality of my adopted country. February 6, 1952 was a sad day for all of us. The bells tolled, announcing the sudden death of King George VI aged only fifty-seven. He was beloved and held in high esteem by his subjects for the unfailing concern he showed for them. On June 2, 1953 the bells rang again and the guns in Hyde Park and The Tower of London were fired, telling the world that the twenty-six-year-old Queen Elizabeth II was crowned. People from all over Britain, and indeed the whole world, converged on London. On the Sunday before the Coronation I toured the capital admiring the decorations in Oxford Street, Regent Street, the Mall and Fleet Street on the way to St. Pauls. The red banners bore the sign "ER II". It was a sunny day and the atmosphere very convivial. One met with smiles and courtesy everywhere, everybody was cheerful and nice. We knew where the sentiment lay. The British people were one big family gathering round their monarch who symbolized a thousand year old institution which united them and to whom they gave their abiding affection. I would go further – the Queen was the British nation in the flesh. It was a happy coincidence that at this time a British party led by John Hunt conquered Mount Everest. The gay enchanted atmosphere was very infectious. A fellow countryman of mine climbed a flag pole and I laughed to see him squatting on top of it. "Pole is up the pole," he shouted. "Yes," I shouted back, "You are up the pole!" In Oxford Street it was my turn. I noticed a big ladder leaning against a lamp-post and as I had a camera with me I climbed to the top and took the best picture of Oxford Street that I have ever seen. A "Bobby" just looked on and smiled. We now headed for Trafalgar Square en route to Buckingham Palace. By now it was 11 a.m. and the approach to the square was crowded with cars. We drove, or rather crawled, in three lines. Being of an impatient nature and taking advantage of the small-ness of my car, I swerved occasionally from one line to another and passed some motorists. No one cursed me and I did not hear a single hoot — to be exact I saw beaming smiles all the way. One can imagine my consternation when I suddenly noticed that my trafficators were not functioning! Near Buckingham Palace I had to come to a stop. The Household Cavalry was passing by. Luckily, I arrived home in one piece, full of praise for the British. I spent the Coronation Day in front of a television set; I was not able to watch all the programme as it lasted seven hours. What I saw was magnificent, of a fairy tale-like quality. It was a pity we couldn't see it in colour. The occasion was a triumph for the organizers and also for Mr. Hartnell who designed the dresses for the Queen and other notables. The heralds' trumpets and the four hundred strong choir added to the splendour.

My luck held. Women say that life begins at forty, it was certainly the case with me! I met a member of the species I admired, she was a credit to it. Well in my forties we got married to fortify each other. Besides being my wife, she became my part-time receptionist, secretary, cook, housekeeper, gardener and general manager. I remember one spring day when she asked me to do some weeding. I went about it with all the zest of a student of horticulture. An hour later I proudly showed her the tidy beds. I waited for praise but got a reproachful look instead. "What's the matter?" I asked anxiously. "You've taken up all my michaelmas daisies I planted this morning", she said with exasperation. But these were only moments of frustration amid long spells of happiness.

We travelled together a great deal. My wife and I flew on a visit to Rome. It was a rush to get to the airport and catch the 'plane after a busy surgery. The departure of our BEA Viscount was delayed and while waiting in the departure lounge I snatched forty winks. I was abruptly awakened to board the 'plane, leaving my ciné-camera behind. I only realized this when we had been in the air for about ten minutes, still in range of communication with London. The stewardess contacted the airport authorities and five minutes later a message came that the camera was taken care of and would be despatched to Rome. I was rather sceptical and gave up hope of turning into a temporary photographer. When next morning the telephone rang in our hotel room, my wife, afraid that she would not understand the gibbering in Italian, prompted me to answer it. She need not have worried. It was a message from the BEA office saying my camera had arrived. Another example of British efficiency and courtesy. I left for the Vatican the same morning. In St. Peter's Square, a great open space framed by the

massive colonnades of Bernini, busy with visitors and clergy in colourful robes, I waited for Pope John XXIII to appear at the window of his
apartment after the ceremony in S. Peter's Church, to bless the crowds
below. I positioned my camera on a tripod and focussed the telephoto
lens on the Papal window on the top floor of the building. Protecting
the ready-to-shoot camera from the passing crowd I eagerly awaited
the occasion. After an hour of such an ordeal, however, I found that
His Holiness was not in the Vatican . . . but I was able to film a few
passing cardinals.

On our last day in Rome we went to Via Vittoria Veneto, a tree-lined
avenue with pavement cafés and smart shops around it. I hoped to buy
an exquisite pair of shoes. In one of the windows I saw a lavish display
of such goods and we entered the large shop full of people. We soon
found we were the only customers, but no one bothered to serve us. It
was the 6th May 1960 – the day of Princess Margaret's wedding to
Anthony Armstrong-Jones – a photographer, and people crowded
around the television set which was in view of the shop. We joined in.
For a solid hour I forgot what I had come in for. We watched with
great interest the happenings on the screen and were taken by Tony's
arrival in his mini car. No less revealing were the reactions of the Italian public. They gesticulated excitedly, they uttered shouts, they
cheered, they laughed. It was obvious they were enjoying it and one felt
they were sorry that Princess Margaret was not an Italian princess. I
had a feeling they were thinking of their own Royalty which ceased to
be in the news once Italy became a Republic in 1946. They watched
with sentiment and envy British Royalty adapted to the needs of
modern times. The British monarchy was not an anachronism but a
lively institution blending with its people whom it continued to unite.
Thirteen and a half years later, on November 14, 1973 to be exact,
the same Royalty stepped down again to identify itself with its subjects
in a true democratic tradition. The event was the ceremony of Princess
Ann's wedding to Captain Mark Phillips. Once more it was watched
throughout the world.

But to return to May 6, 1960, the guests dispersed at last and I
had the full attention of an obliging salesman happy to serve the
English. I tried on many pairs of shoes but none was comfortable. I was
on the point of leaving when the assistant stopped me saying: "Please
try one more pair, sir, they are more expensive but should fit you well."
He was right, the shoes looked elegant and were most comfortable.
"Thank you," I said, "Please wrap them up for me – home in England

your shoes will remind me of Italy." The man smiled apparently satisfied that our one-and-a-half hour stay had come to a successful conclusion. It was only when I returned home and opened the parcel that I discovered the shoes bore the mark: "Lotus, made in England." I must have acquired an English taste!

Over the next twelve years we visited various countries enjoying a tour of the Dutch Canals, the Norwegian fjords, the views from the Jungfrau, Cervinia and Mount Blanc, rugged Corsica, the fragrant lavender fields of Provence, the mimosa trees of Madeira, the charm of Rhodes, the ancient ruins of Ephesus, the Alhambra of the Moorish kings, the flowered streets of Seville, the Caves of Drach with the fairy-like Martel's lake in Majorca, the picturesque Trogir on the Adriatic coast, the spell of Fez and Meknes in the centre of Morocco, the beaches of the Algarve . . . Yet, we found that with the passage of time the unspoilt character of the places, the charm of local people and the service in the hotels began to wane; the advance of tourism and its success story brought casualties.

We stopped visiting them because we wished to remember the places as we first saw them – without the newly sprung hotels, cheap entertainment, floods of people, noisy vendors and pollution. I recollect the refreshing solitude along small empty beaches and our peaceful exploration of under water marvels with a "schnorkel" and flippers. There are only a very few lonely places left. Once a district nurse with whom I was chatting outside my surgery pointed out to me a man who was passing by in a car. "What a small world," she said, "Why?", I asked. "Fancy seeing him here; I saw him sitting at a table next to me on the Costa Brava." "Have you never seen him before?" I enquired. "No never." "Fancy that," I said in turn, "he is a local doctor . . ."

And so we discovered the British Isles. The tour of Scotland was a success. Later on we added to our memories of the grandeur of the Scottish mountains, the beauty of the Welsh falls, the serenity of the Lake District and the vividness of the heather-covered slopes of Devon. We enjoyed the remoteness of Tresco Island and the slow pace of life. The British, a practical resilient race, took the challenge. In recent years their food and service has improved beyond recognition and surpassed that of the foreign hotels which often ceased to live up to the standard expected of them by reading the glossy brochures. The new motorways enabled one to commute effectively across the country. Yet I prefer the slower roads revealing the beauty of the countryside and to be orientated by the British pubs with their quaint signs – the landmarks.

291

But the biggest rediscovery was London. I have always been intrigued by the way this huge cosmopolitan metropolis is run in such a smooth manner. Its heart is the City of Westminster, its stomach – Covent Garden, Smithfield, Billingsgate, and the many street markets; one only has to visit them in the early hours of the morning. The London fog does not worry us any more, since air pollution has been reduced it has lost its bite. In this metropolis of metropolises I was able to see Paul Muni, to hear Fritz Kreisler, to admire Maurice Chevalier, to applaud the Polish Dancing Troop "Mazowsze", to watch tennis champion Ilie Nastase . . . Here, in June 1973, I saw Marlene Dietrich after forty years. She displayed the same charm, poise, figure and deep enticing voice I once admired in Berlin. The name "Jonny" pierced my ears again and left my heart thumping. But there were two new songs which the war added to Marlene's repertoire – "Underneath the lamplight" and "Where have All the Flowers Gone?". With half closed eyes I listened intently and visualized this beautiful woman standing in front of the German public, singing: "Where have all the young men gone? Gone as soldiers everyone. Where have all the soldiers gone? Gone to graveyards everyone. When will they ever learn?" When in 1960 Marlene arrived in the country of her birth, she inevitably met with a hostile reception.

In September 1972 I visited the astonishing exhibition of the "Treasures of Tutankhamun" on loan from the Arab Republic of Egypt commemorating the 50th anniversary of the discovery of the tomb by two Englishmen. In nine months 1,600,000 people visited the exhibition. The small rooms which harboured the priceless treasures were crowded to overflowing. We filed in perfect order to see the various glass cases, many people carrying children on their shoulders. I was pushed only once; it was impossible to turn to see the offender, I only heard the Italian language. The evidence of the incredible skill of the Egyptians in the 14th century B.C., displayed here, amazed me. Later on I read that the embalming technique, used by the Chinese two thousand years ago, enabled an autopsy to be carried out after all these years, which revealed that death was due to a coronary; the woman's flesh was still soft and elastic.

London pulsates with life by day and night. One finds here knowledge, entertainment, pomp and pageantry. And further, the elite look of the "City Gent" with bowler and rolled umbrella, the Scots Guards in their red coats and black bearskin hats, the "Beefeaters" in dark blue uniforms with squashed puff-hats, bemedalled Commissionaires, the good-humoured cockney Pearly King and Queen, costermongers with their barrows . . . It is a place full of contrasts – the grey solid conventional "City" and charming, trendy, bohemian, individualistic Chelsea; the dignified Mall and whirling Piccadilly Circus; the learned Bloomsbury and cockney Stepney; the glamorous, profoundly English Belgravia and Jewish Whitechapel; the solemn, traditional Westminster and gay, daringly colourful, cosmopolitan Soho; the smart, rich, snooty Mayfair and the nitty gritty of Hackney; the sophisticated Hampstead and down-to-earth Oxford Street; the Docks and Royal Parks.

London has been the home of many famous people and has witnessed numerous historical events. Karl Marx lived and died in Highgate. Sun-Yat-Sen planned the Chinese revolution when in London and was imprisoned in the Chinese delegation after being kidnapped from his lodgings by Emperor Manchus' agents; he escaped by smuggling a letter to his former tutor, an eminent London physician, who invoked the intervention of the Foreign Office. Ophthalmologist, Sir Arthur Conan Doyle, practised in the respectable medical quarter around Harley Street before Sherlock Holmes made him famous. The area only became connected with medicine in the second half of the 19th century when Florence Nightingale, in charge of the Hospital for Invalid Gentlewomen, moved it to Harley Street. (Lord Harley, who initiated the development early in the 18th century, was the patron of artists, not doctors.) In London the eight-year-old Wolfgang Amadeus Mozart conquered the English Royal court, Dr. Samuel Johnson worked as a journalist and produced his famous "Dictionary", Lord Byron, Algernon Swinburne and Oscar Wilde delighted and scandalized their fellow-citizens. Here people were able to listen to such celebrities as Mendelssohn, Chopin, Berlioz, Paderewski, Casals, Kreisler, Rubinstein, Menuhin and many other great masters of music. Mary Lloyd, the great variety comedienne, Noel Coward and Charlie Chaplin were Londoners. William Heberden, brothers Hunter, Alexander Fleming and many other famous doctors achieved their greatness when working in London. The metropolis gave shelter and a helping hand to many people – Marat, Karl Marx, Engels, Sun-Yat-Sen, Marconi, Korda, Freud, Nureyev, exiled Kings and governments, expelled writers and scientists. A great number of Jewish people settled in the East End before the first world war, driven out of Tsarist Russia by vicious pogroms; more arrived in the Thirties, particularly in North London, escaping from the Nazis. Later came

Poles, Hungarians, Yugoslavs, Czechoslovaks, Greeks, Pakistanis, Uganda Asians . . .

Londoners proved to be a good crowd who rally in adversity and remain calm, disciplined and good humoured, as seen during the Blitz. In the time of the bleak war, when their houses were burning, their streets being filled with rubble and people were being killed or fed on powdered eggs and dried milk, they circulated jokes such as: "I am sorry, darling, I could only get you a mink coat; I know you would prefer an egg." When the enemy was at Londoners' throats, we heard of "Life as usual" and "We never close". After the war blackouts were soon forgotten and it needed the notorious power cuts of 1971 to bring the memory back. Many people were too young to experience them before. No wonder that Scotland Yard received a number of calls from younger Londoners who reported seeing strange bright objects in the sky, which were the stars they were not able to see before in that City full of lights. Samuel Johnson once said: "When a man is tired of London, he is tired of life; for there is in London all that life can afford." And there are many parks, the river Thames and the beautiful surrounding country. It is not surprising that the majority of people who work in the metropolis are in fact suburban dwellers who avail themselves of the faster travelling facilities used today. It is ironic that when Hitler's wartime Minister of Armaments, Albert Speer, visited London in 1973, he declared: "I am glad Hitler did not destroy London. It is a beautiful city." He must have been disappointed not to have seen silver barrage balloons and searchlight batteries, nor to have heard the wailing of the sirens.

My work changed beyond recognition. I now had a receptionist and the help of a nurse, a midwife and a health visitor. A doctor's wife, once the Cinderella, ceased to be flogged to death. Patients' waiting time was cut down and many routine calls with social undertones were delegated to the health visitor. Less demands were made to call on patients who began to appreciate the doctor's time and learned to visit surgeries. Night calls were few and far between. The extended social services, however, put on doctors an increased amount of form-filling and correspondence, and increased travel to all parts of the world demanded of them the up-to-date knowledge of tropical diseases. The affluence brought more business to insurance companies which lean on doctors' judgement. "Are the habits of the life proposed strictly sober and temperate and have they always been so?" is one of many questions put to the medical profession. I was tempted on more than one occasion to write back: "How the hell should I know?" To the question "How much does he smoke?" the only answer was – he does not count, neither do I. Quick, reliable routine laboratory tests and plastic syringes were time savers. Deputizing services relieve the burden of night calls and a telephone answering service and dictaphones help some doctors.

It was a great satisfaction watching the kind of patients, once considered to be incurable, thriving on new treatments.

A closer liaison developed between hospitals and general practitioners. Doctors were encouraged to visit their patients in hospitals, to add their own observations on the hospital notes and to discuss cases with consultants. Laboratories, X-ray, electrocardiographic, library and other facilities were offered. A number of post-graduate centres sprung up. Seminars, week-end courses, demonstrations, hospital rounds, scientific meetings, guest lectures, discussions, medical films, symposiums ("drinking party" in Greek!) and social evenings became routine happenings. A quarter-of-a-century old computers aid programming for medical teaching and research, and help in electrocardiogram analysis. To qualify for seniority payment doctors had to attend refresher courses regularly. Clinical assistantships were offered by hospitals to general practitioners. There is still more scope to bring the general practitioner and hospital doctor closer together. Doctors were swamped with medical journals and weekly papers. I couldn't read them all, but I counted them – there were fifty-three. The B.B.C. brought "Medicine To-Day" to the screen, a monthly programme specially designed for doctors. Medical education is a life long process.

Pharmaceutical firms competed with their goodwill and hospitality. Visits from well-informed representatives, audio-visual presentations brought to our surgeries, film-lunch meetings, gimmicky presents and travelling fellowships were at large. This was as well as the requirement under the Medical Act of 1968 that pharmaceutical companies have to send complete prescribing information of their products to medical practitioners. I once heard a representative claim that he owed his ability to play the piano to one of his firm's products, an activity he was unable to perform before. I began to wonder if his pill could dispense with teachers of pianoforte . . . Loyalty of a representative to his firm can be very real. I once visited such a man in hospital after he underwent an operation for the removal of a tumour in the brain, ten days before his death. The man was obviously dying. Yet, he was still able to raise a smile and to plead in a low halting voice: "Doctor, do remember to prescribe the tonic I was telling you about . . ."

Sometime ago the technocratic, highly specialized American medicine conceived the fallacious idea that the days of general practice were numbered and that the general practitioner was an outmoded archaic figure in this age of specialization. Patients were encouraged to choose consultants as they felt fit, but it soon became apparent that this would not work. In Britain the opposite trend took shape. In 1956 the Royal College of General Practitioners was founded, collecting reference material and information on general practice, conducting bibliographical researches and epidemiological surveys, editing its own journal. One of its early planners and honorary fellows was the outstanding surgeon Professor Ian Aird. General practice has been vindicated. This much neglected subject in the curriculum of medical schools was given greater attention and several universities created professorial chairs for such an important branch of medicine; it was becoming a speciality in its own right. M.R.C.G.P.* should be a specialist's degree comparable with M.R.C.P., M.R.C.S. or M.R.C.O.G. At long last general practice started to attract medical men. Vocational training for entrance to it began to gain momentum (general practice post-graduate training scheme was evolved), and general practitioners are being groomed as trainers which will enable them to pass their life-long experiences to the younger generation.

The scope of general practice is steadily increasing as more children with weak constitutions and people with serious injuries and chronic conditions are able to survive. Techniques for early diagnosis grow and preventive methods are sought. Besides, many become conditioned to medicines from the cradle. Lastly, as soon as the patient can be nursed at home, he is discharged from hospital to the care of the family doctor.

A number of doctors carry out studies on new drugs in their practices.** Some general practitioners have their own electrocardiographs which have become a status symbol. Yet in my student days we only had a stethoscope, a reflection mirror used with an ear funnel and an opthalmoscope whose mirror had a central aperture for observing the eye. It was a treat to see a tympanic membrane or the fundus of an eye. A normal electrocardiogram dispels patient's anxiety and often results in the disappearance of his symptoms. However, even the best machine can do harm; a tracing may remain normal for some

* M.R.C.G.P. – Member of the Royal College of General Practitioners.
** This is done with the knowledge of the General Practitioners' Ethical Committee.

time after the patient has sustained a coronary thrombosis, and it does not necessarily say who is likely to do well and who not. It might indeed give a false security to both patient and doctor alike resulting in negligence. Patient's symptoms are much more significant and they are there from the start. Doctor's own ears, eyes, judgement and experience come first. History taking, although rewarding, is time consuming. "I suffer from diarrhoea, doctor." "How often do you go?" I asked. "Once," came the answer, "Loose?" I continued my enquiry. "No," I heard, "What makes you think you have diarrhoea?" I probed. "Well, before that I was going only every third day. . . ." When I said brusquely, "You have nothing to worry about," she told me she felt reassured and, being satisfied with the visit, would soon be back. I thanked her for the trust she put in me. Far from annoying me, she amused me as much as a sailor patient who, when requested to move his leg during an examination, shot at me the question "north or south?"

My first choice of a modern equipment would not be an electrocardiagraph but a defibrillator* for resuscitation of a stopped heart. It delivers a precordial shock and is life saving. This should be administered by the first person to reach the patient as the first two minutes are vital in the rescue, and the general practitioner is usually in the front line – he is the *primary* physician engaged in primary care. I wonder why life saving devices are so expensive and not usually subsidized by the Government. Be that as it may, General Practice underwent important improvements in its quality and status showing increased efficiency and effectiveness.

Patients are no different from doctors. Both share experience of many aspects of life – learning, sports, hobbies, friendships, family life, human weaknesses and illness. As with doctors, modern thinking reached patients. They expected explanation about their diseases and treatment, and they have been getting it; for doctors it was not just solemn prescribing and handing over instruction sheets any more – the voice of the ordinary man had to be heard and complied with. The Royal Society of Medicine elects lay people with medical and scientific interests to its Fellowship. I visualize times when patients may request not only booklets but also slides and audiotapes as a part of consultation! To counteract the growing specialization they might turn into medical amateurs. Yet, despite the pseudo intellectual approach they still expect to be treated solely by the doctor's effort. A patient

* A portable battery-operated apparatus is available at the cost of . . . £1,300.

told me she was having trouble with singing in her drama group, and was also unable to shout at the children she supervised. When examination showed her to be in perfect health, I advised against voice abuse . . . Patients have to grow up with doctors and be able to join in the effort of treating their own diseases, but such an evolution takes time. Old people continued their old-fashioned ways, as the woman who wrote to me, "Please doctor, can you send me a prescription for my nose as it runs as soon as I have my cup of tea and I haven't got enough hankies."

Chemists were ordered to disclose the names of the dispensed drugs to patients and I am only sorry that common remedies known to cause harm by acting on other drugs are not indicated at the same time. But what about the price! I remember a depressed patient for whom I prescribed an expensive remedy; she returned a few days later complaining that the treatment had not done her any good. I was taken aback and said on impulse: "If an expensive drug does not work on you, I will prescribe a cheaper one." On hearing this she asked if she could try it a little longer. She came to me a fortnight later, all smiles, reporting that she was cured by the drug. I suggested to the appropriate administrative body that the dispensed drugs and medicines should be marked with the cost, but was told that it might cut both ways – the patient who is prescribed the less expensive drug could assume that it would be less effective.

What patients need first and foremost is reassurance. "Is it a drug?" they often ask. What they really mean is: "Is it harmful?" And so I invariably answer emphatically "No", but they will never be reassured until they get a firm diagnosis. Even when the embarassed doctor is in doubt he must not vacillate, instead he has to furnish a descriptive identification of the patient's symptoms like "Irritable bowels", "N.Y.D.F."* or "Essential** hypertension". A descriptive term is often better than a scientific one and no doubt better than none at all; the louder a doctor's voice is, the less sure he is about what he is saying. His sphygmomanometer is a clumsy instrument and the listening method of determining blood pressure, introduced by Nicolai Korotkoff of Moscow and adopted by doctors, is far from perfect. There is another occasion which disquiets me and that is answering on a cremation form the question: "Have you any pecuniary interest in the death of the deceased?" I answer "No" when I take a fee for it!

Not only did general practitioners pander to patients, hospitals too

* N.Y.D.F. – Not yet diagnosed fever.
** Essential – of unknown causation.

stopped treating the public as illiterate children and became more informative. But all this consumed time which has to be saved by various means. Some patients were issued with sphygmomanometers which enabled them to take their own blood pressures cutting down the number of out-patient visits. Doctors notes became more concise, without losing any of their precision and freshness. "Right little finger buggered" wrote one doctor, and a gynaecologist made the entry: "It is not a ring this patient requires in her vagina."

Extension of information to patients, their half knowledge and sophistication pose various inconveniences, even hazards to doctors. Patients often read, hear or watch on the television screen the newest developments unknown to their doctor, who has less time to spare. I had a visit from a middle aged man who requested vitamin E "as it keeps one young." I could not argue, I did not know. I asked the patient to return in a few days time, wishing to look it up. I only knew it was introduced in 1922 and found essential for reproduction in rats. Vitamin E received the name tocopherol from the Greek words "tokos" (child birth) and "phereo" (to bear). I duly learned of renewed interest in this vitamin. Someone observed that it prevents certain anaemias, another found that its deficiency leads to liver damage and lesions in heart muscle in several species; yet another noticed that it spares vitamin A and also prevents damage from naturally occurring substances which may play a role in the ageing process. "It is a misnomer to call vitamin E the reproductive vitamin," I read. Unfortunately, all these claims were not based on experience with man. When the patient returned, I advised him to eat plenty of lettuce as it proved to be beneficial to rats, and in any case is less expensive than eggs, milk, liver and the vitamin.

Being better acquainted with medical subjects, neurotics were putting on fantastically artistic displays which looked very real. Knowledgeable malingerers could also be very convincing. I received a consultant's letter which read: "A manipulative lady who uses her insignificant illness as a device to get her own way and to dominate those around her."

A more serious threat was the increasing trend of claiming compensation. Admittedly, negligence and serious incompetence of a doctor which brings suffering requires recompense, and no one objects to patients organizing themselves against possible abuse if they do not trust doctors' ethical committees and similar bodies. Unfortunately, quite often trivialities are picked up by self-righteous patients who forget that if they wish doctors to be human, they must accept that they can not be infallible. A gynaecologist had to defend himself by writing: "I deny that the difficulty Mrs. X experienced with intercourse had anything to do with me as I consider the standard of my performance entirely satisfactory." Patients and doctors alike should be reminded that confidence, goodwill and mutual respect are the basis of satisfactory relationship between them. Some patients see the consultation as a game, a ticket-free entertainment. How does a doctor feel when his patient telephones him at closing time saying, "I want to save you a call" and demanding to be seen without delay because of *a very bad back*, only to rush on his bicycle to catch the doctor in surgery! Every doctor will admit that to make good communication with someone who does not feel well could be a difficult task. A doctor should be unmoved by the storms that swirl around him, he must like his patient, accept him for what he is and be resolved to carry on the task cheerfully despite frustrations and annoyances. He must show that he is sincere, concerned and willing to take care of patient's problems. A conscientious doctor anticipates the patient's desire to confide in him and must be prepared to be a good listener. Samaritans succeed by doing just that. Patients try various avenues to find sympathetic listeners. Women often confide in their hairdressers, men – in mistresses, barmaids, even prostitutes – and both sexes use doctors and ministers of religion. Stresses cannot be resolved by medicines alone, but good listening is not always too easy a task. A "By the way" disclosure might be the very problem and a trivial bodily complaint a manifestation of an emotion – physical pain is easier to bear than a psychological one.

But the foremost circumstances which underline doctor–patient relationship are those concerning abortion. In spite of relaxed abortion laws, there is still great confusion. On this difficult and emotional subject I can speak only for myself.

Women should be able to take such a decision themselves, and it is the doctor's duty to guide them. The threat to the patient's life posed by pregnancy and genetic diseases are not the only problems. By denying an abortion in a deserving case, we encroach upon woman's right and personal freedom without the justification that we are protecting society. I have met women crippled for life from criminal abortion, and I know of a grossly disabled young man in consequence of such an unsuccessful attempt. In another case, a woman who was again expecting a child told me of the ordeal she had had some eleven years earlier. She was unmarried then and, finding herself pregnant, became frantic, anxiously wanting to loose the baby. She eventually had to seek help from a backstreet abortionist when already over three months advanced in her pregnancy. An "operation" took place in the back room of her friend's house. Ether soap was injected into her womb after £25 was handed over to the abortionist. The following day she became very ill and was rushed to hospital where she had to have a blood transfusion and injections of penicillin for persistent fever. It took a long time before she was fully recovered. I asked her if she ever met the "doctor" again. "Oh no," she replied, smiling sadly, "I heard he had landed in prison." The ordeal made her depressed for a long time and she had to be admitted to a mental hospital for a while. Should society foster unplanned and unwanted pregnancies? Should it wilfully create an atmosphere conducive to illegal abortions? Abnormality in the pattern of chromosomes will often, thank God, cause a spontaneous abortion. Should we accuse Mother Nature of being an abortionist? The use of LSD and such like increases foetal abnormalities. Heroin is a good contraceptive . . . what I mean is that most heroin addicts, like the rest, have an unsuccessful sex life, if any, often their only heroine being . . . heroin. It is all to the good though. Intervention of a conscientious doctor is not aimed against nature as he realizes that it is more clever than any of them. It is clever enough not to entrust men with child-bearing! With their humble resources doctors only wish to assist nature and enlarge on its potentialities. One must not forget the sad life of unwanted little children abandoned by their mothers or increasing the ranks of battered babies. When a woman reaches labour it should be a labour of love. Has a woman not the right to termination when she already has three or four children and no strength or money, or both, to look after them? And what about the woman approaching menopause who has not planned the pregnancy and who worries about the possibility of chromosomal abnormalities. Testing for it is not fool proof yet. A sympathetic doctor would recall that in a mother over forty the risk of having a mongol child is higher than one in a hundred. The medical profession accepts that German measles contracted in the first stages of pregnancy calls for termination. Congenital heart disease, deafness, cataract, mental deficiency – they all have been traced to this source on many occasions. Again, nature in its wisdom may bring abortion in such cases.

There is too much talk about abortions and sex generally. Curiosity and a streak of adventure are healthy features in the young with which we have to reckon and act accordingly. It is of society's making that young people become curious of what it is all about and that they take to sex at an early age. They take to alcohol, cigarettes, smoking pot and experimenting with LSD and such like often for the same reason. These people may act foolishly, but they certainly are not criminals. Our aim must be to prevent rather than condemn such happenings. We must try to understand their problems and not to cry for their blood. The youngsters in question are immature and inexperienced, and find themselves in jail easily. They also become easily pregnant. I have seen girls under sixteen, complete sexual novices, in great distress, saying in tears: "Please don't tell mummy." Would it be right to refuse help, to tell them: "It serves you right." "It is your problem." Some of them are still at school and have long years of study in front of them. Should we ruin their lives deliberately? I do not think for a moment they would make good mothers. What about the unfortunate babies? I am weary of professional and not-so-professional moralizers who have no conception of what conception means. I have only one possible excuse for many of them – they have passed their sixties and are no longer subject to passion.

One should not condemn other human beings for protecting themselves from the consequences of the sexual urge imposed on them by nature in a way of exploitation – nature is interested in preserving the species, not in suffering; about one-third of all pregnancies are unplanned and often unwanted. In human as in animal female sexual responsiveness coincides with ovulation. Maurice Chevalier, an entertainer until his late seventies, sang the meaningful words: "I'm glad I'm not young any more". The well-developed human brain has a well-developed "sex centre" which, according to Professor Karl Junkmann of Berlin, governs the secretion of pituitary gonadotrophic hormones. The brain certainly controls sexual behaviour, but hormones drive the brain!

It must be remembered that the Abortion Act halved the number of deaths from abortions. But, be that as it may, I am weary of irresponsible "regulars" coming back for the second or third time with the same problem, playing on a doctor's concern. A mother brought her fifteen-year-old daughter to me requesting abortion. "She's innocent", I was told, "She does not know life and was taken advantage of". "It was her first experience and she did not enjoy it at all." I was sympathetic but I need not have been – she was enjoying sex more than her mother or I could have imagined. The girl became pregnant the next year and the year after, each time telling me that she dislikes men and does not enjoy sex! Women forget they cannot always get away with abortion scot-free, more so if it is performed on the very young who have never had a baby before, still worse if it has to be repeated. A quarter of maternal deaths are still due to abortions. It is sad to watch the ever increasing number of abortions which have reached the 150,000 mark a year – one pregnancy in seven is terminated. We should do some heart-searching as to why it all happens, since we cannot blame the pill alone for promiscuity. I personally opt for the pill and a justified abortion as opposed to treading on each other's toes with the prospect of being engulfed by a war, perhaps in the universe, which could be more formidable than the two world wars we have already experienced.

Since the beginning of this century world population has increased at an unprecedented rate. In China alone the population had increased by 300 million in the last 25 years (60 per cent). In June 1969 the 55,786,000 square miles of the global land harboured 3,552,000,000 people. Nature ravishes in abundance; to fertilize a single human egg the seminal fluid emitted by the male contains some hundred million reproductive cells, "spermatozoa", per millilitre. And so, advanced countries have a population policy and do research on such matters. In Britain the birth-rate has been decreasing since 1965, but even so it is estimated that in 40 years her population will reach at least 64 million – a 20 per cent rise on the present total of 54 million. It is the fourth densely populated country in the world. (Not everyone agrees with statistics – they show for instance that East Anglia has 7·1 flies per house today!) Family planning is becoming an integral part of the Health Service, offering free counselling and supplies on a par with other drugs. Contraception is certainly a God-sent measure in any power-cut contingency! I find it a disturbing anomaly that the under-developed countries continue to have a large birth-rate and some of their leaders have more than a dozen children.

23
The Elderly

Retirement should be through choice, not through compulsion
due to lack of employment opportunities.

John F. Kennedy

No medicine cures old age or a withered flower.

Chinese proverb

The British have shown that they were able to handle an organization
as complex as the Health Service. After 25 years of its experience it is
going from strength to strength and by and large has the confidence of
the people. Modernization is its by-word and its scope is constantly
widening. A scientific service within the National Health Service came
into existence, following the Zuckerman Report. New hospitals and
para-medical institutions have sprung up, some costing tens of million
of pounds. Organ transplants are carried out in increasing numbers; a
Cambridge professor, Roy Calne, pioneered the liver transplant.* A
fairly common condition of recurrent dislocation of the shoulder can
be successfully treated by minor bone transplantation. The life of a boy
with a rare blood disorder was saved by a bone marrow graft.

Private schemes are unable to compete with the services the egalita-
rian N.H.S. offers the chronically ill and disabled. Family planning
which promotes contraception (vasectomies included) was made a
normal part of the Service. The accent is on the community. Medical
Officers of Health were given a new name – the Community Physician
– and general practitioners are reminded of their own role in the primary medical care with the aim of prevention. Seminars are held at
which doctors get acquainted with the main features of the reorganization.

With appreciation of the problems and burdens of old age the attitude of low priority given by society to their elderly is changing. More
attention is being paid to retired people and to the part doctors have to
play in preparation for retirement and screening for possible abnormalities. Health is all important. A patient once told me: "I haven't
been to your surgery for several years, but now that I am retiring I

* He is confident that successful heart-transplantations will be introduced in
Britain in the not-too-distant future.

want to be sure that I am in good shape." The formation of a Pre-Retirement Association is a welcome event – one person in six is retired in Britain today. Loss or change of occupation, status and the people one worked with, as well as a reduced income, unavoidably bring emotional and social problems, more so as with age people become less adaptable. Retirement is the time of shattered hopes, muted ambitions and uncertainty. Conflicts arise between drive and ability on one side and opportunities on the other. One becomes a *Senior* Citizen in age only. It may lead to despondency, touchiness and strained marital relationship. People "married" only to work, without parallel hobbies, enter retirement completely unequipped and find themselves in a vacuum. Retirement is a foregone conclusion which must be anticipated and with which one has to come to terms. There are many areas of life which could bring satisfaction if one only keeps one's eyes wide open and looks for them. New skills can be built, friendships cemented, involvement with the married partner deepened, voluntary work undertaken to help others, active or creative hobbies and out-of-door activities pursued. Retirement can be turned into an interesting experience. It shouldn't be an ugly and dreaded word. There is more to do than sit and watch television, and it is not only an apple a day which keeps the doctor away! People who were unable to live within their potentials have to learn to do it now and quickly – adaptation and philosophy of life are the key words. "Many a new tune can be played on an old fiddle." But no one grows old and becomes lifeless overnight, illness apart. An abrupt retirement is not natural and can be harmful. It is a new discipline and we have only begun to scratch the surface of a very complex issue. Ideally, retirement age should be flexible, tailored more to the state of health and walk of life; it should come gradually. It is not the beginning of the end. It brings a special bonus – time available for old and new interests. Enjoyment does not cease with retirement – the phrase "a Dirty Old Man" proves it!

The elderly who are unable to look after themselves and for whom home-help, meals-on-wheels and adaptations in their own homes prove inadequate, find new residential homes geared to their needs, with nurses and a doctor in attendance, not forgetting the important catering staff. Their bad eating habits are corrected, the "sweet tooth" and overweight discouraged, smaller meals, less rich and easily digestible, are served at shorter intervals, with sufficient intake of fluids. This way diet is being adapted to the more feeble ageing bodies. Because of diminishing appetites and various states of health in the elderly, some choice of food must be available, presented in an attractive appetising way; some require it in a minced form, others will not touch it. The old people are taken out of isolation and are able to enjoy eating in company, leaving their lonely "tea and toast" habits behind. Meal times are in fact social occasions for them. The worry and irritation of daily living is taken away from these people. Dental and ophthalmic needs are looked into, and those hard of hearing are provided with small hearing aids which have replaced the old-fashioned trumpets. However, everything is not rosy. By leaving their own homes they lose the little stimulation which is still left to them. In the residential homes they don't even trouble to help make a cup of tea for each other, and can be obstreperous. They emerged from solitude and are hampered by anti-social traits. I once opened a social evening which it was hoped would stimulate the aged audience. I intended to say a few *gracious* and *warm* words. Noticing how crowded and noisy the place was, seeing some of the people dozing in their easy chairs and hearing others talking loudly, I involuntarily said: "Good *gracious* isn't it *warm* here!" How the hell can they call it a respectable age, flashed through my mind. Old folk have to be reminded that moderate physical and mental activities help to relieve tension, to retain vigour, in short – they help to prolong a happy existence. Some have to be positively pushed into human contacts, and not many have hobbies. They have radio, television and various amusements. Yet passive full-time leisure stops being leisure and becomes boredom. These people need fresh air and gentle daily exercise with helpful advice from a physiotherapist and an enthusiastic occupational therapist who could encourage what little interest was still left in them.

They should receive mental stimulation by way of participation in some activities, lectures, discussions, little "do's", outings and similar activities. Above all, they should keep up the régime they had and not give it up as soon as they enter the residential home. Their power of concentration and memory are failing and they ought to be reminded again and again that activity and not drugs is the best remedy. Rest does not make them stronger, on the contrary, it debilitates them. They experience skeletal pain more in the mornings, after a night's rest, which is eased by a day's exercise; the principal cause of osteoporosis – thinning of the skeleton – is inactivity. The elderly demand drugs instead of getting on the move; symptoms being only masked, require constant pill swallowing, a harmful pastime for the old people who often show impaired body functions. Once the drug has proved to be effective they are afraid to drop it. Perhaps the most sensible way would be to administer the wrong remedies to be sure that they won't work! Mobility and a sensible diet do better for constipation than abuse of laxatives and they obviate the consuming of binding, stomach upsetting "pain-killers." Patients request drugs to stimulate their appetites, yet the right way to help them is to drop all pills altogether. Interesting activities do more for insomnia than sleeping draughts which only lead to post-awakening confusion and depression. The number of older people is steadily increasing and money spent on uncalled-for medications could be diverted to a better, more constructive purpose. We are already heading in the right direction. Elderly patients, unlike others, require *continuous* rehabilitation to remain reasonably indpendent and geriatric day hospitals and day care centres serve such a purpose. To add contentment to fitness, social and luncheon clubs as well as work and social centres have been created. Regular events of getting together in places of past employment and meeting the old and new workmates is another exercise worth pursuing. Age is not a barring factor to a useful and happy life. Dame Sybil Thorndike remains cheerful and mentally alert at 91. Arthur (Bowden) Askey – "For ever Arthur" – started his theatrical career at 16 and is still entertaining the British public at 74. Mary Pickford, a star of the silent films, now in her 79th year, is on the National Advisory Committee on Ageing and a Director of the American Society for the Aged. Bertrand Russell retained vitality until his death at 99. Igor Stravinsky wrote his latest composition – Requiem Canticles – in 1916, when he had reached his 84th birthday. Pablo Picasso died at 90 engrossed in his work – life without it would mean nothing for him, said his friends. Leopold Stokowski, at 91, still keeps in touch with the musical world and does occasional conducting. Pablo Casals – the famous cellist who played before Queen Victoria – delighted the American audience with his cello performance at the age of 95. The occasion was the presentation of a United Nations Peace medal in 1971 for his peace crusade. He married for the third time at the age of 80 and his new bride inspired him to write love songs. Dr. George Brewster celebrated his 70th birthday with a record breaking 20 mile swim from Dover to Margate. Lord Shinwell,* affectionately called Manny, continues to show a zest for life at 90 and has just published an autobi-

* His Loyal Address in the House of Lords on October 29, 1974 in reply to the Queen's Speech met with tumultuous applause. He called for the goodwill of everyone to restore the country's prestige.

ography: "I've Lived through it All." Sir Winston Churchill became Prime Minister for the second time when he was 77 and remained in office until his resignation four years later. Lord Palmerston attained Premiership at 71 and held office for ten years, with only a year's break, dying in harness. Bernard Baruch, United States financier and advisor to three successive American Presidents, became the Chairman of the National Commission on Atomic Energy at the age of 76 and at 88 published his autobiography: "My Own Story." He expressed the opinion that "To me, old age is always fifteen years older than I am." "My Life and Times", the autobiography of the British novelist Sir Compton MacKenzie, appeared in 1963 when he was 80. Age is a most relative thing, we say that a child of 5 is *too old* for a nursery. Eamon De Valera remained in office as President of Ireland until the age of 91. Marshal Tito and General Franco are still in harness at 82, and Juan Peron reappeared on the political arena at 78. The world admired Golda Meir who continued her turbulent Premiership of Israel at 76. Of course, good health is a requisite for such activities. Besides normal ageing, one observes change due to disease. The incidence of osteoarthritis, hypertension, heart failure, diabetes, glaucoma, Parkinsonian tremor and so forth increases with age and the doctor's primary role is to improve the quality of life. For two-and-a-half years I have watched a 90-year-old whom a pacemaker* transformed from an invalid, subjected to syncopal seizures, into a reasonably active man free of discomfort. Another patient in his 91st year, treated the same way, was freed of congestive cardiac failure and fares well. Both had a complete heart block but their poor prognosis has changed.

The first artificial pacemaker was constructed in 1932; it weighed 7.2 kilos, and its spring had to be wound up every 6 minutes. Patients had to push their *external* pacemakers in front of them on a cart. In 1959 an implantable pacemaker became available but patients required repeat surgical intervention for lead repairs. The "on demand pacemakers" brought further improvement; they induce contractions, only when the heart-frequency decreases below the frequency fixed for the pacemaker. Electromechanic malfunctions are now rare, although repeated surgical efforts are unavoidable after two or three years when the waning power source has to be replaced; a nuclear powered heart is a future possibility.

* An implanted power source with leads and electrodes for continuous electric stimulation of the heart at regular intervals.

Another hope is the control of incontinence by means of electronics or other devices; it is a big problem among the elderly today.

Chairs of geriatric medicine were endowed at several Universities – a new speciality, geriatrics, was added. A modern geriatric ward is cheerful looking, not overcrowded, with the amenities required for the aged and disabled. Patients are admitted not only for treatment but also to give a break to their families and to assist them with their holidays. Geriatricians carry out studies on the causes of the ageing process, investigate functions of the thyroid gland, research in osteoporosis, examine cerebral perfusion, look into the role of fibrinogen in strokes and so forth. For instance, we do not know why when one gets older one has less bone and so fractures occur more easily, why one loses a substantial amount of the one kilogram of calcium one possessed earlier and why women should be mainly affected. The active therapy of osteoporosis remains bleak. It is only the beginning of helping people to live a good life to the end. Geriatrics is not a speciality in terminal care! People realize that one can only get older and that most of us must get old one day. It is a problem that concerns all of us. "Help the Aged" started a free-of-charge monthly magazine "Yours" which aims at better communication and brings varied and valuable information for aged citizens. This organization is helped by a number of prominent people. Much has still to be done. Housing and pensions have to be looked into. We need more homes for elderly people who are able to look after themselves provided they have purpose-built dwellings with a communal dining room, laundry facilities and a friendly warden in attendance. We need more homes for urgent social admissions on a short term basis. We will then be able to restrict the residential homes to those more disabled and to gear them to their needs.

Seeing the imposing record of the 25 year old National Health Service, I am confident we will achieve these aims. Various facets of administration, overlapping and too managerial at present – hospital management boards, regional boards, local Executive Councils and local health authorities – are giving place to a unified administration and enlarged concepts of community care. The reorganization has been under discussion for a decade and it is hoped that a more efficient structure will emerge aiming at a better service to the public. Doctors occupied by clinical duties and lacking in managerial practice are not the best source for administrators of an organization as complex as the N.H.S. Community health councils are envisaged to act as a watch dog to represent the interests of the public in the health service. The appointed day was April 1, 1974 but the reorganization is still far from completion. Existing divorce of general practice from hospital practice was certainly not in the interests of both doctors and patients. No wonder that, in spite of general affluence, private practice is far from gaining ascendancy. The best things in life are "free" . . . at the cost of £2,933 million of the National Health Bill for 1972–3, with the envisaged extra £500–£600 million annually for expanding social plans. Schemes organized by private companies, various firms, Freemasons and religious orders have difficulty in keeping pace with the most recent advances in treatment. They are certainly unable to satisfy the chronically ill and those requiring lengthy and costly treatments. There are other difficulties. How can a patient judge if the doctor's fee is fair and moderate, or excessive. No wonder that spending on private treatment comes to less than one per cent of the total N.H.S. expenditure. What the patient, however, forgets is that the N.H.S. is largely paid for by himself – the taxpayer.

Only in one medical sector does private practice continue to enjoy popularity. Appointments for patients have to be made well in advance and money does not matter so long as the sufferer is made better. Our Liz had to be put on a waiting list to have her hernia repaired; Liz is our dachshund and I am speaking of the veterinary practice. New drugs and new techniques benefit pets. I know of a doctor's wife who spent many weeks feeding a newborn puppy with a dropper as it had a harelip, until a veterinary surgeon carried out a plastic operation. The most expensive drugs are purchased and no one complains that poor cats have to buy their own contraceptive pills.

Veterinary surgeons are in an enviable position – they do not need to offer lengthy explanations to their patients and are well paid for cursory advice to a pet owner. The chiropody service is much more speedy than the one offered to our old folk. And vets are as successful as their medical colleagues. Their patients live long enough to be treated for an ageing heart, arthritis or cancer. Many an owner will spend his last penny on an animal which is his companion and trusted courageous friend. Some people receive the protection, caring, loyalty, obedience, help, love and respect from their pets – something previously denied them. One has only to see a guide dog for the blind, a St. Bernard rescue dog, huskies with their sledges, the intelligent conscientious sheep dog, a guard dog or a police dog; people have to be reminded of the animals which entertain their masters – the greyhound, the hounds, the circus performers, even film stars. I still remember "Rin-tin-tin", a

310

dog in silent films, which made a lasting impression on me. Most of the dogs take their owners for a walk! And there are cats, monkeys, rabbits, hampsters, guinea-pigs, birds . . . Lucky vets! No wonder there are scores of kennels, kennel clubs, dog shows and cemeteries for pet animals. I know of a family who had to postpone their holiday until the autumn as no boarding kennel was available for their dog during the busy season. People are justly proud of their animals who have enough sense to know not to rush to a doctor with the slightest indigestion; many pets simply eat grass to make themselves sick.

An open letter, November, 1974

FROM YOUR RELATIVE'S DOCTOR

Your relative is now in the care of a Welfare Home, away from familiar surroundings. It is important that you continue to give your support to her/him. Please consider yourself as one of the team which strives to rehabilitate the elderly resident and enhance her/his quality of life. We endeavour to provide the skill and conditions needed for the elderly, but "man does not live by bread alone". Please remember that, however good the new environment may be, it is bound to be different from the one the elderly person was accustomed to. An abrupt break must be avoided; the Elderly Resident longs for familiar faces and for talks about things and people only you know and understand. Above all she/he longs for the old love and affection. Your regular contact with her/him will do more than any medication. An ageing body does not take kindly to drugs. Your attitude, encouragement and stimulation along with our efforts could prevent depression, disturbance of sleep, poor appetite, constipation, even incontinence and aggression. Therefore, we ask you to come as often as you can to visit your relative, and also to take her/him home or to see friends from time to time. In this way you will provide your old folk with the all-important interest in life, and above all − with the essential mobility − a counter-measure against obesity, stiffness of the joints, clotting of the blood (one of the causes of strokes) and mental deterioration. Swollen legs (or feet), so often seen in the elderly, are usually caused by inactivity. Drugs which promote the secretion of urine are beneficial to the elderly mainly because they force her/him to walk frequently to the loo! Please remember that you are an important member of our team, and that we hope for your co-operation for the sake of your relative. Thank you!

24
The British and the Poles . . .
Poles Apart?

Nothing ever becomes real till it is experienced.

John Keats

By now I had been among the British for 27 years – enough time to cease to be an alien, but not long enough to become a fully fledged Britisher. I conquered, admittedly with some difficulty, the impeccable table manners of my hosts. I became less loquacious – asked "How do you do?" I answered with the same question without waiting for a reply. I also became somewhat more punctual. Yet I took mince pie and Christmas pudding as I would take medicine; it had to be taken! And I was still unable to share the British enthusiasm for their sports. Like G.B.S., I feel that "baseball has a great advantage over cricket being sooner ended . . ." But I will not say any more on this subject, trying to be on a safe wicket! How strange it is to watch adults engaged in "conker matches;" "conkers isn't only kid's stuff", they declare. Is it childish behaviour or "joie de vivre?" which an outsider is unable to understand, I wondered. As soon as I opened my mouth I have been asked "Where are you from?" What an impertinence! Their dialect was often stronger than my accent. Much of what I knew and saw puzzled me – there existed so many incongruities. Charles Lutwidge Dodgson, a renowned Oxford scholar and mathematician, is the author of several nonsense books written under the pen-name of Lewis Carroll. The serious-minded British listen with gusto to the comic operas of Gilbert and Sullivan. Practical people, they devised a most complicated tax system. Their intellectuals delight in the nonsense poetry of Edward Lear and burlesque stories of Sir William Gilbert. Sound and very proper ladies and gentlemen are interested in horoscopes, crime novels and detective stories (the popularity of Conan Doyle was passed to Agatha Christie). Saucy limericks and scandals, rape and murder are splashed in banner headlines on the front pages of reputable newspapers, the reader is left with the impression that nothing good will ever happen ("good news doesn't sell"). The Chamber of Horrors at Madame Tussauds has an assured box office. "Fanny Hill" and "My Life and Loves" were written by Englishmen. The British are honest and like fair play, yet find great attraction in gambling. For raising funds even the church depends on gambling. They are law abiding people who have been giving shelter to revolutionaries for centuries and like to demonstrate against authorities to uphold justice. The British love discipline and freedom, show tolerance and prejudices. I know a London dispensing chemist who has kept a weekly vigil for months on end in the vicinity of India House in protest about the policy of genocide against Naga tribes who live in the hills near the Assam/Burma border. They are peace loving people who coined phrases like "*fighting* fit" or "it *strikes* me". Being undemonstrative they hide their likes and dislikes and treat religion as a very private matter. Although far from bigotted, they invoke the Deity on the slightest provocation; how often one hears: "God help me," "For God's sake," "Heaven knows," "By God," "Christ," "I pray" or "To Hell." They are traditionally-minded people who have revolutionized the lives of everyone – by the dramatic art and deep thought of William Shakespeare, Newton's nature of gravity, Darwin's theory of evolution, James Watt's steam engine, George Stevenson's railway, William Cockerill's wool-carding and wool-spinning machines, Lord Rutherford's splitting of the atom, Alexander Fleming's penicillin which started the antibiotic era, to mention but a few epoch making events and discoveries. The humane British who find it necessary to have N.S.P.C.C. and R.S.P.C.A.* People fond of animals (they founded FRAME** to save much suffering in laboratory animals), and who call a good friend affectionately a pet, yet enjoy hunting, shooting and fishing. Some do not shun a cruel sport (Henry Higgins from Woking, Surrey, became a Spanish Matador of Toros), but shed tears when hearing on the radio that a budgerigar broke its neck swinging from a chain, and the most dignified of them will climb a roof to save a stranded cat. They have canine beauty salons and hospitals and homes for old animals. And further, how strange that the country of Lords (even Christ is their Lord) favours egalitarianism. How strange that her people eat porridge oats normally reserved for horses. One of the most cherished British statesmen and architects of the British Empire was an author of novels. He was of Italian/Jewish des-

* Society for the Protection of Cruelty to Children is merely National whereas that for Animals is Royal.

** Fund for Replacement of Animals in Medical Experiments.

cent and bore the symbolic name of Disraeli. The taciturn British who do cross-word puzzles to avoid conversation, claim superb orators – William Pitt, William Gladstone, Lloyd George, Winston Churchill, the lisping Aneurin Bevan . . . The British Government pays a salary to the man who leads the Opposition against it. It supports the families of strikers thus aiding them in their efforts. The same government gives money with one hand for contraception and with the other rewards mothers for having babies. The men who have been opposing sex equality do not mind being ruled by a Queen – a ruler with little power to rule. They were chivalrous enough to let an American lady take the first woman's seat in the House of Commons. She was Nancy Langhorn of Virginia who married Viscount Waldorf Astor; she remained an M.P. for 26 years. The English, the Scots and the Welsh stress their separatism yet they display loyalty to the same Monarch and unflinching unity in their adversity; this is why the Island is called the *United* Kingdom. How strange that the figure of the Greek God of Love associated with sensual passion stands not in Paris but in the centre of London. The statue of Eros which dominates Piccadilly Circus was designed by Sir Alfred Gilbert in 1893. He did not blindfold the winged boy armed with bow and arrows. He must have thought that love which the piercing arrow brings is not a haphazard meaningless affair. 43 years later Edward VIII gave up the Kingdom and Empire for the woman he loved. St. Valentine's Day on which a secret lover declares his affections to his beloved was not chosen out of religious ardour, but because of the medieval belief that birds start to mate on this particular day. Who can say that the "cold" and realistic British are unromantic! But then these logical people can be illogical. One hears them saying "Slow *up*" when their advice is to slow *down* and "*Damned* decent" for a praise. I heard a doctor saying, after having received a fee for his report, "It is a bit much, it is too little." Yes, the British are shy, yet conscious of their superiority, show common sense and . . . superstition, favour individualism, but spurn conformity. I had better stop at that – there are endless incongruities – or are there?

It could be that there are more eccentrics among the British than among other nations. They say things they do not mean, like "I am sorry" when they are not or "I am not too clever" when one knows that if this were the case they would never admit it. If by bad luck pretence is met, there is an equal chance of finding it among other nations. The French have the word "facade" for it. Others have their own words.

"Nuance" and "ambiguity" came from the French. "Hypocrite" sounds more French than English. Only "humbug" is unmistakably English; one hears a commentator saying: "How magnificently he *lost*." Yet there are so many good points in which the British score – tact, politeness, self possession, discipline, modesty, honesty, justice and tolerance. They show consideration for others, a sense of humour, a love for peace and animals and an aversion to compulsion. Both sexes are usually sporting, good looking, cheery and nice. I like their descriptions – a strapping lad or a buxom wench. They are in tune with the kind of life I cherish and it should not surprise anyone that I succeeded in the attempt to live amongst them. It is perfectly true, I was helped by the war . . . In my school days I heard a great deal of the curiously British "splendid isolation", their distrust of foreigners and their ignorance about them. They were pictured as a stiff lipped public school type, often with a hyphenated name, as snobbish colonial servants or eccentric loners. (Women were kept out of it!) The war experiences changed all that. The notion that every Englishman is an island is gone.

My contact with them proved fruitful and besides being grateful I developed admiration for much I saw – the courage and "sang froid" attitude, compassion and public spirit. In their darkest hour of 1941, when the situation appeared hopeless to all friends of Britain, when the Nazis had already prepared a list of people on these Isles they wished to eliminate, the British Command planned for the offensive and the people sang with Vera Lynn: "We'll meet again . . . some sunny day." At the height of the Battle of Britain the determined RAF raided Berlin. Douglas Bader became a legend. He lost both legs in a flying accident in 1931 but overcame his disability and returned to the R.A.F. at the outbreak of war. As a commander of the 1st R.A.F. Canadian Fighter Squadron until his capture in August 1941, he contributed to victory in the Battle of Britain. Frederick Delius, an English composer in the early 20th century, became paralyzed and totally blind at the age of 62 but with the assistance of his friend, Eric Fenby, he was able to complete some old compositions and create a number of new ones. Richard Gom, a spastic, deprived of speech, learned to type and wrote a book of poems. Roger Mallinson and Roger Chapman who sank to the bottom of the Atlantic, 1,575 feet down for 76 hours in their mini-submarine, kept their cool: "It was very quiet and peaceful down there, just a matter of waiting. We had an easy time, everybody else did the work." A journalist and broadcaster,

James Cameron, won the 1973 Italia Prize for radio drama "The Pump" – an account of his own heart attack and life with the inserted pacemaker.

The British take an interest in people who need help. History tells us of John Howard and Jeremy Bentham, 18th century reformers, responsible for mitigation of prison life and of the terrible criminal law. The life's efforts of William Wilberforce culminated in the abolition of slave trading in the British Colonies in 1807, and slavery itself in 1883. Thanks to agitation by Britain most powers have passed similar laws. Slavery in the U.S.A. ended with the victory of the Union over the Southern Confederate States in 1865. The world-wide Organization "Amnesty" which fights for the human rights of political prisoners was born in Britain, in 1961. Britain is the first country in the world to have a Minister for the Disabled.

Leonard Cheshire V.C., the war-time leader of the Dam Busters who raided Europe one hundred times, was an official British observer at the dropping of the war's second atomic bomb, at Nagasaki. It changed his life. Three years later he founded the first Cheshire Foundation Home for the Incurably Sick and since then many such homes have sprung up in Britain, Eire, various parts of Europe, Chile, African countries and the Far East. The disabled residents are being encouraged in active participation and they edit their own quarterly magazine "Cheshire Smile" among other activities.

In 1954, soon after he left the Sanatorium where he was treated for tuberculosis Group Captain Cheshire went to India to relieve human suffering. In his book: "The Face of Victory" he recalls the event. He also mentions his wife, Sue Ryder, who had been helping the survivors of Nazi atrocities stranded in various European countries; several Homes for the Sick in Poland owe their existence to her. This remarkable couple founded the Mission For the Relief of Suffering, devoting their lives to the needs of the sick and homeless and to peace and unity of mankind which, alas, has not yet become a reality. The Missionaries of Charity founded by mother Teresa in Calcutta is part of this mission. A great number of British people have shown goodwill and have become involved in charity work.

In 1866, a then unknown man of twenty-one, John Groom, with a desire to help others, cast his eyes on the needs of severely disabled young men and women in the London area. By his efforts suitable homes and work were provided for these unfortunate people. In the Crippleage's workrooms they perfected the art of artificial flower making and it became a well-known industry. John Groom's principle was "to help the disabled to help themselves." Such work continues to expand and brings help to a wide circle of the needy. Television announcer Richard Baker, disc jockey Jimmy Saville, showman Roy Castle manifest similar concern as John Groom did 107 years ago.

Many younger people of today have the same attitude. Bob Wilson and Derek Dougan, professional footballers, and Cliff Richard, an entertainer, are such examples. Gracie Fields and many others support orphanages at home and abroad. Following the unsuccessful rebellion of the Tibetan people against the "peaceful liberation" by the Peoples' Republic of China in 1959, a number of Tibetan children have been cared for at the Pestalozzi Home near Battle, Sussex. Many Vietnamese orphans found homes in Britain. I have watched one such girl grow up happily with her British "parents" and her British "sister." With the passage of time an increasing number of homes for blind babies, disabled or mentally handicapped children, orphans, cripples, the aged, and people with terminal illnesses have been founded by private voluntary organizations showing concern for people; a great proportion of them was eventually taken over or helped by the State. The nation followed the example shown by Royalty who patronizes many charities. All this goodwill exerted each day and every hour means much more to peace in the world than any demonstration, be it Remembrance Day or a display of "doves of peace."

I began to compare my fellow citizens with my old countrymen and was happy to find some similarities. The British, like the Poles, are heroic, courageous, determined and patriotic people who are always willing to pay the price of freedom, the only difference is that the British do not say so. Not much fuss was made about the daring attack on St. Nazaire which took place on March 28, 1942. In it the French sea port on the Bay of Biscay – a strongly guarded German submarine base in the battle of the Atlantic – was devastated by British Commandos. Not many knew of Geoffrey Keyes* and his men who carried out a daring raid on Rommel's headquarters in North Africa, two hundred miles behind the enemy lines. No wonder that the English people chose Saint George – a model of Knighthood and a martyr – for their patron. When on February 7, 1920 the Tsarist Admiral Alexander Kolczak faced the Soviet firing squad with great courage and dignity, the official account of his execution recorded that he had

---

* He was awarded the Victoria Cross posthumously.

borne himself "like an Englishman." Similarity does not end here. British policies are thought-provoking, those of the Poles are provoking too. I watched both Polish and British soldiers in action; the Poles were full of passion, the British full of coolness. My countrymen approached the war with bitterness, fierceness and lust for revenge, resolved to kill the enemy or be killed, the British approached it as yet another game — with fair play and without hatred — admittedly for high stakes. But they showed an adventurous spirit, defiance, and a capacity for endurance; nothing could break their spirit. Both served their countries well and were given the name of "servicemen." The name stuck. Civilians serve their countries just as well, why then reserve such a name for soldiers only? Poles and British have a sense of humour. At Victoria Station, under the warning: "Smoking can damage your health", a Britisher added the words "Inhale and farewell!" In Poland, the following joke circulated recently: "What would happen if Communism came to one of those countries near the Sahara Desert?" "Nothing for two years, and then a shortage of sand." But then many a true word is spoken in jest! Both peoples are superstitious. The Poles cross themselves when a black cat crosses their path, the British look the other way, and neither can be enticed to walk under a ladder. Both are individualistic. The British people drive on the left to be different from everyone else. When the whole world played football, they turned to rugger; in 1823 William Webb Ellis of Rugby School did the unheard of thing — he took the ball in his arms and ran with it disregarding the rules of the game. It did not satisfy the British — they changed the round ball for an oval one — and when before the ball had to be passed forward, they made a rule that it must now be passed backwards. When other nations are using the metric system, the British prefer to keep to their yards knots and stones. Both peoples deplore demagogues; in Britain Sir Oswald Mosely and Colin Jordan failed in their efforts, a similar fate was met in Poland by Roman Dmowski and General Haller. In English as in Polish the word "love" is very much in use; I would venture to say it is even more used by the British. "I love it" is constantly heard. To be more precise, many British men love music, (one of the very few sensual pleasures without vice!) others — food or women, Poles love all three and are greater individualists — they prefer solo singing to a British choir and are good at solo dancing, leaving team dancing to the British. The Poles and the British often say the same thing but in a rather different way. A Pole would say "It is important", a Britisher only says: "It is not unimportant." When a Pole stresses: "I refuse to see his point of view", an Englishman mutters apologetically: "I *fail* to see his point of view." When a Pole exclaims, "You lie!" an Englishman quietly says, "You exaggerate." He also says "It was a pleasure" when everybody knows that it was not. When he humbly talks of quite a *few*, he means quite a *lot*.

Politeness and modesty are distinctly English failings – they do everything possible not to hurt, even at the expense of the truth. There is the obvious danger that should one tell an unpalatable truth, one might be taken for a liar. And they speak of lavatories as "loos" or "W.Cs", to take the coarseness off it. I even knew a lady who called an egg "hen's fruit." The British say "please" on the slightest provocation, Poles hardly use it. They are not so refined, often uncouth, and so they call a spade a spade and do not attempt to gloss things over, being of the opinion that the language exists for the sole purpose of communicating the truth, even if it hurts. A harmony between language and thought, I suppose. Their words conceal nothing; rightly or wrongly, they feel they have nothing to conceal. Should it be consideration and politeness or the bare truth, it is simply a question of priorities. Poles are less affected by English failings, less constipated, and have less asomniacs. If they look at the defects of others with a magnifying glass, they also use it for their own virtues, and they don't like to be unnoticed. They also prefer to do their own tooth picking instead of going to a dentist. The British like to contradict themselves – they say for instance – this is *awfully* good, the Poles like to contradict others. Poles do not watch the time when they speak, neither do the British – they have no need to! Being less communicative they find that saying things is daring; they stress "I *dare* say" much too often. It puzzles me why during the war they had to have posters: "Careless talk costs lives." When Poles quarrel they enrich their own vocabulary by abusing each other, the British drop words altogether. And so it is virtually impossible to defeat Poles in argument. Both are connoisseurs. Poles favour vodka, bigos* and kisses, the British – beer, whisky and gin besides being hard tea drinkers. Perhaps a better way to compare both nations is to point out their differences.

The chemistry of a Pole can be described as mercurial, effervescent, unstable, often fuming; that of a Britisher more stable and solid. Where the Poles boast about many things, the Britisher boasts about only one thing – that he never boasts. Poles like to be in focus, the British like to keep out of it. Poles are good at preaching and enjoy *giv-*

* Hashed meat and cabbage.

319

ing council with panache, the British prefer to *take* it and have the ability to compromise where Poles are uncompromising. Poles blunder, repent and soon forget their mistakes, the British blunder too, do not repent, yet remember the mistakes they make. The British are good losers, Poles are Poles apart if they are not winning. Where the British are predictable, the Poles are not. Poles are really slaves of their emotions, the British are masters; it does not surprise me that the Poles had better warriors than politicians. To conform and keep a good reputation is the first consideration of the British, it is last to the Poles. The British are only interested in things which interest them, Poles are interested in everything fertile in mind and body. My experience with my hosts was that they show reserved friendliness; the friendliness of the Poles is always unreserved. Yet I was better served with the half promise "I might try" by the British than with a pat on my shoulder and reassuring words "Do not worry, leave it to me" of a Pole. Where Poles are good in hypothesis, the British are good in facts. The British do not believe in miracles, Poles have witnessed them. Where the British are well-bred, the Poles are of good breeding!

Organizing ability is not the strongest point of the Poles. It is not so with the British. Even their sick people have a flair for it! There is an association of colostomy patients, those with epilepsy, diabetes,* rheumatism and arthritis, an association of mouth and foot artists, limbless ex-servicemen, the blind, the deaf and dumb, the people with phobias and more. Unlike Poles, Britons are fond of understatements. I heard an Englishman answering a reporter's questions: "How did it feel to arrive back in England from Colditz after the liberation? with a concise "Nice." And then there is the word "I". The British write it with a capital letter but hardly mention it, Poles write it with a small one and can't stop using it! The way they speak is a good indication of their different temperaments. Poles speak rapidly and give no one a chance to break in, the British have the art of speaking with their mouth practically closed. Poles shout "Bravo!!!" as a sign of approval and "Hey!" or "Hello!" when trying for a lift. The British keep silent and display two-thumbs up as an "all's well" gesture, and a single-thumb sign for a lift.

The British know their own strength; when abroad they wouldn't dream of calling themselves foreigners, they reserve such a term for their hosts.

I hope to be forgiven by both nations. I know as you do that nobody

* Founded in 1934 by H. G. Wells, who was himself a diabetic.

can be impeccably Polish, or impeccably British for that matter, and we all agree with Abraham Lincoln that "folks who have no vices have very few virtues!" Besides one cannot blame an apple tree for not bearing pears; nevertheless an apple tree justifies its existence.

There are 1,400 Poles still in psychiatric wards in British hospitals – the aftermath of war. The British and Polish people got to know and understand each other when they fought together. One side showed sympathy and understanding, the other gratitude; they became friends. Bridget Monckton of Brenchley is the President of the Association of Friends of Polish Patients. Sympathizers of Poles formed the Katyn Memorial Fund to erect a memorial in Chelsea which will remind people of the war-time massacre of 10,000 Polish officers in the Katyn Wood, in Byelorussia. They chose Chelsea, a fitting place for individualists, exhibitionists and artists. The compassionate British could not forget such an atrocity. They too have suffered. In 1973 in the French village of Esquelbecq a memorial was unveiled for a hundred unarmed British soldiers taken prisoner and massacred by the S.S. Before being herded inside a cowshed where grenades were tossed in, they were marched at the double and many stabbed with bayonets to make them go faster. But there is another reason for the understanding attitude of the British towards the Poles. After all the British Isles have been accustomed to strangers – the Normans settled in a land in which Celts, Anglo Saxons and Danes lived side by side!

25

The Future

Are not the dreams of one generation the realities of the next?
Woodrow Wilson

There are stars whose radiance is visible on earth though they have long been extinct. There are people whose brilliance continues to light the world though they are no longer among the living. These lights are particularly bright when the night is dark. They light the way for Mankind. *Hannah Senesh*

Why have I never revisited Poland? I must explain, as people might find it difficult to understand. Certainly not for political reasons despite less freedom in Poland today* and bureaucratic vexations. True, the freedom I have learnt in Britain is much greater than I ever dreamed of before. It is the people of Poland who stand in my way – not the people who are there, but the people I lost, all cut off before their time. Hence much water has passed beneath the bridges. I could not face the new people for I connect each place with my nearest and dearest who are gone for ever. I might be wrong. Possibly I would never find these places again – they are gone too. But to go back would mean to erase the past which I could not do. After loosing reality I was determined that my memories would not be taken away from me.

Towards the end of the war Warsaw was a heap of rubble, flattened by German bombs, artillery and flame throwers. Nothing to start from. The Nazi revenge for the uprising. It happened before; Warsaw was severely damaged in the 17th century by the Swedish Army under King Gustavus II Adolphus. Like the vigour of Londoners which enabled them to rebuild their city after the Great Fire of 1666 and gave Christopher Wren the chance of creating St. Paul's Cathedral and other important buildings, so the vigour of the Polish people helped to raise Warsaw again and house nearly 1,500,000 inhabitants today. They were assisted by UNRRA.** The 17th century Baroque elegance

---

* In 1974 a Polish defector to the West reported that one lives in continuous fear of being taken into custody because of little negative remarks and cannot trust one's best friend; 80 countrymen absconded with him.

** United Nations Relief and Rehabilitation Association.

of the Old Town was painstakingly reconstructed and the City is dominated by the Palace of Culture and Science of Russian design. It is a *new* Warsaw. The streets and pavements are wider, the houses taller, often of modern architecture, many of them skyscrapers. The planners pride themselves on the huge communal apartment buildings on housing estates, office blocks, department stores and supermarkets. The city is adorned with monuments symbolizing its martyrdom, struggle and heroism like that of a woman armed with a sword ready to strike,* the Unknown Warrior's Tomb or slabs and plaques bearing engraved names of martyrs for freedom. The latter attest to the places of execution. Streets bear unfamiliar names, strange slogans, posters and portraits.

Czestochowa, my birthplace, still has the Jasna Gora monastery and each August Poles from all over the country journey there to venerate the holy picture of "Our Lady of Czestochowa." It was brought to the monastery by the Polish King Ladislas Jagiello in the 17th century. The river Warta still flows at the same rate. But the town has changed. Its population has greatly increased. Monotonous blocks of flats have appeared, new factories pour filth into the air through their chimneys, competing with the town's oldest industry – the production of religious and devotional articles. The river became turbid and filthy; Czestochowa developed into an industrial town, with many steel and textile factories. The beautiful avenue lined with old chestnut trees and benches which lead to the monastery has lost its charm. I remember sitting under those trees chatting to my parents. Then came progress. Cobblestones along the avenue were removed and in the process the tree roots were damaged. The chestnut trees had to be cut down and with them went the benches. The Old Market, crowded with bearded Jews before the war, changed its look; the Nazis saw to it; 35,000 lost their lives in the Czestochowa Ghetto. My birthplace changed, which is what I do not like about it; it became a poorer place *for me*.

The country's boundaries changed too. The Polish territory in the East was taken by the USSR and some German land in the north and west was added. Poland lost nearly half of her former territory to Russia, among it my university** town of Vilna, the Lake Narocz on which I did my sailing, Druskieniki to where I paddled from Augustow and Lutsk where I found myself at the time of the collapse of the Polish campaign. Polish Wilno, Russian Vilna, Lithuanian Vilnius, once the

* It portrays Nike, the Greek goddess of victory.

** Founded 1578, abolished 1832, re-established 1919.

Lithuanian capital, went to Poland in the 17th century, became Russian in 1795, was occupied by the Germans from 1915 to 1918 when it went to Lithuania and back to Poland in 1920; from 1941 to 1944 Vilna was part of the German province of Ostland and after World War II returned to Lithuania only to be annexed by the USSR with the rest of the country. Lutsk became Lithuanian in 1336, Polish in 1569, Russian in 1791, Polish in 1919 and again Russian after World War II. Western Poland had to be repopulated by Poles – they were driven out by the Nazis who put Germans in their place. Some 200,000 Poles had fallen victim to their atrocities, and poverty and hunger caused the death of at least 150,000 more. The extermination camps at Auschwitz, where some 2,200 persons a day were murdered for four and a half years, and Majdanek, responsible for the death of another 360,000 Jews, are kept as museums and young people are encouraged to visit them. At last the Germans were expelled beyond the river Oder. The invasion had cost the country more than six million lives. The new Poland had no option but to form closer ties with the Soviet Union and mirror her policies. Such is the history of Poland . . .

The country continues to show recovery. It has become more and more industrialized. Enthusiasm arose for new ideas in architecture, town planning and design. Folk art is blooming. Modern sculptors, Dunikowski and Wittig, and the abstract artist Kantor made their names. New writers appeared – Iwaszkiewicz, Putrament, Rudnicki, Andrzejewski, Rozewicz, Brandys, Breza, Przybos, Mrozek. And further, composers Penderecki and Lutoslawski, creator of a modern experimental theatre Grotowski, philosopher Kotarbinski, physicist Groszkowski, mathematician Sierpinski. I was told that Warsaw alone has twenty-six theatres and that there are numerous provincial ones. And yet I prefer to dream of pre-war Poland, my eyes shut, listening to the sound of hooves and droshkies on cobble stones and the early morning crowing of a cock. I like to think back to pleasant Polish customs like that of a "Kulig" – a merry cavalcade of horse drawn sledges and their tinkling bells at Christmas time. I like to recall my uncontrollable laughter, brought on by Harold Lloyd, Buster Keaton, the Laurel/Hardy team and Charlie Chaplin, those giants of silent comedy. I choose to look at Canaletto's* version of 18th century Warsaw when it sparked with life and culture under the auspices of King Stanislav August. This Italian painter left behind a great number of works full of realism which helped to plan the city anew after its

* Canaletto the younger.

destruction. For me, only the Poland of the past exists, with its history, its way of life and people I knew. My only fear is that the spell will be broken. I do not mind being called a bourgeois and reactionary with ossified thinking! A friend of mine told me how he was haunted throughout his adult life by the tremendously high wall he had climbed during his childhood. At 65 he decided to see the place again and was horrified to find that "his" wall was only $3\frac{1}{2}$ feet high . . . "I should never have returned", he remarked with sadness.

The present and the reality for me is Britain, the country I have learned to love. When the time comes to lay my bones, I wish them to be laid amongst the British. And Britain is, in more than one way, nearer to Europe than Poland . . . The British people will soon be fully fledged Europeans. Being cautious they began at first to sample such a possibility. They have been holidaying in Europe for a very long time. They discovered Nice on the Cote d'Azur a century ago and left behind the fashionable "Promenade des Anglais", the "Scotch Tea Rooms" still serving excellent scones, and Charley's Bar where roast beef and Yorkshire pudding or steak and kidney pudding with English ale are served. For a hundred and seventy years the British have considered a tunnel which would link them with France. Their final reappraisal makes its opening in the 1980's highly improbable. Trains taking just over half-an-hour to pass through the 32-mile-long tunnel would have added momentum to the present cross channel traffic by ferries, hover-craft and air. Bringing Britain and Europe together for the benefit of mankind is not a half-hearted affair, and so the Metrication Board is kept busy. The time will come when doctors will be free to move to any European country they choose and continue their profession. In antici-pation an *international* classification of tumours was recently pro-duced. Britain has a natural interest in Europe and played a major role in her liberation. Many sons of Britain, Guy Gibson of Dam Busters fame among them, were buried in European soil. I visualize the bidet becoming a general British commodity but there is much more to it.

Life has always been manifestly hard and violent but need it be? Must we have wars which grow more fierce as the weaponry becomes more sophisticated, with progressively worse ravages and sinister con-notations? Even a successful outcome does not spare the victor. The American War of Independence brought – besides mutilations – a craving for opium and alcohol, and the dead could not be resurrected. I do not refute the independence, only the war. There is so much madness in every war. In the Arab–Israel conflict of 1973 scores of Israeli Arabs gave their blood for the wounded Israeli soldiers and many assisted Israel's war effort. At the time of the armament race, when wars continue to be a menace and "peace" remains an overworked phrase, when several nations have to kow-tow to Moscow's wishes, when human rights and other freedoms are denied to millions of people in various parts of the globe, European unity is very much needed. The rough Channel water is unlikely to protect the British people in the modern warfare of the future. Meeting people, learning their values and their differences, watching their reactions and so forth is a logical way towards building a larger community. New names reached our ears – Council of Europe, Common Market, European Parliament, European Community, the Nine . . . The year 1974 marked the birth of the Anglo-German-Italian multi-rôle combat aircraft. I wish to remind the critics deprecating the European Community for being influenced primarily by economic reasons that just such reasons were at the root of all the wars.

I was once European, then British, now I am becoming a British European. This is progress, even though I have not reached the stage of eating snails, oysters and frog's legs. I am in a fortunate position being a doctor – medicine is accustomed to crossing national frontiers as a bridgehead between nations and races. Our planners visualize joint research and the free movement of doctors within the European Community. They are also braced for many obstacles such a big change is bound to bring.

It is intriguing to contemplate what the future will offer us. Nuclear power, similar to the discovery of fire, is bound to change our lives enormously and like fire it carries boundless possibilities as well as great dangers. Britain with her nuclear reactors and resources under the North-Sea bed (they include oil, gas and valuable metals such as manganese, nickel, copper and cobalt), backed by deep sea drilling technology, is well equipped for a successful entry into the next century, unless the human race loses its sanity and elects to commit suicide. No one can predict the unpredictable, but personally I do not believe it could happen. As a doctor I think of a syringe which, since its use was reported by Charles Pravaz of Lyons in 1853, has not always proved to be a good thing. Despite this, are we afraid to have and use it? As time goes by more potent drugs are produced with ever greater dangers. Must we ban them?

Since I ran out of tears years ago, a smile has never left me. Life studded with hardships teaches understanding, forbearance even gentleness and serenity.

My advice to you? Establish communication with your fellow men, try to help them – it will make *you* happy. By all means offer counsel, but only if you have some to offer, and remember that opinions and facts are not always the same thing. Look after yourself to the best of your ability, it is a joy to be alive, in good health and free. Science has made our tasks easier, invented various pleasures and enhanced others, like colour television and improved sound reproduction.

Do not make heavy weather of living and remember what the ancient philosopher Seneca once said, "Time heals what reason cannot." Try not to worry about little things and aim for a fraction less of what you can attain; who wants to be a celebrity anyway, they can't even be sick without publicity. Repeat after John Ruskin "There is really no such thing as bad weather, only different kinds of good weather." Adopt this principle whenever you can. But above all have hope against all odds – devils are not as black as they are painted!

I watch the movements and aspirations of the changing world; the shape of things to come. The United Nations Organization is in its 30th year. It strives to promote peace and attain better nutrition (Freedom from Hunger Campaign) and living conditions throughout the world. There is still a great deal of poverty, hunger and disease. The United Nations Organization is involved in every field of human endeavour. The Geneva Protocol of 1925 prohibited the use of gases and bacteriological weapons. The new organization aims at ending the arms race and the control of atomic energy internationally, in this way forestalling an atomic war. It endeavours to use the atomic energy exclusively for peaceful purposes – the nuclear power in industry and agriculture and the use of radio isotopes in medicine. In 1966 the international treaty on the exploration and use of outer space, including the moon and other celestial bodies, was concluded. It bans nuclear weapons from outer space and prohibits claims of national sovereignty over it. An agreement was reached on the rescue of astronauts. Concern was given to peaceful uses of the ocean floor and other natural resources, to modern technology and industrial development. United Nations Children's Fund (UNICEF) helps children of developing countries. Refugees in and outside Europe are assisted. Social justice is fostered by paying attention to human rights without distinction of race, religion or sex for all peoples and all nations. It is the United

327

Nations' Policy that "all human beings are born free and equal in dignity and rights" — rights to work, to leisure, to an adequate standard of living and education. The Organization promotes science and culture. It advances the mutual knowledge and understanding of peoples by means of mass communications (international telecommunications which include space radiocommunications) and breaks down the obstacles of the free flow of thought. The World Health Organization (WHO) keeps health statistics, combats epidemics and encourages medical research.

All this is progress and is very exciting. Yes, life has a lot in store for us, it is far from being boring. In the words of Sigmund Freud, "It is the eternal changefulness of life that makes it so beautiful. I parted company with despondency." I do not look on life as if it were an infant's dress — short and dirty; it is right in length for most of us and clean . . . if we do not make it dirty. One should be honest with oneself and oppose villainy so that the unleashing of brutal forces may be prevented. The outcome of events, no matter how they may have been caused, depends on peoples' attitudes. There is a great deal to be expected, seen and enjoyed. But do not rot as a bachelor for ever, love improves a man. As for myself, I am anxious not to let life pass me by, I may not get another opportunity.

Should I be reproached that I portrayed a very unusual period, I must ask — was there ever a typical one?

And so I come to the end of my confessions. I bid you goodbye. It was nice to take you on this at times not-so-personal journey and to share my thoughts with you. May I be forgiven for diverting you on occasions from my Memory Lane to much wider roads?

328

Postscript

By now you may think you know me well enough to take an interest in my personal affairs. Well, November 17, 1973 became another milestone in my life. It brought a novel experience to me – the first confrontation with the National Health Service as a patient. The start was innocent enough – acute appendicitis, prompt action, straight forward operation. Pre-medication, a wave to my wife, wheeling through the long hospital corridors to the operating theatre, a smile from the pretty faced woman anaesthetist and her soft harmonious voice "I am just going to give you a prick, you will soon be asleep." It was a ritual well known to me as I assisted with anaesthetics in the very same theatre in the past. With the picture familiar to me I slipped into oblivion. A moment later (or was it?) I heard the same soft voice whispering words of comfort "Wake up, wake up, you've had your operation." Such are the wonders of modern anaesthetics!

Everything went without a hitch and I made plans to go home on the seventh day. But I forgot that complications are specially reserved for the medical profession. A day before my discharge I started to run a temperature, my good spirits left me and I soon developed an agonizing pain in the chest with difficulty in breathing. I suffered a pulmonary embolism. I was given anticoagulants, antibiotics and painkillers. "Don't let it get you down", I murmured to myself, but it did and I became a burden to the coveted hospital bed. Yet, the skill at the top and devotion to duty coupled with kindness down to the lowest personnel soon put me back on my feet again. At that point it went through my mind how much worse off I would have been financially had I lived in the U.S.A. I do not know how anyone could complain of such treatment; only tiny minds and strange attitudes would be the explanation. I can only say to everyone – have your appendix out and see for yourself. If you are lucky you might have some complications which will allow you to stay in hospital just that much longer!

329

Myself, I reflected that the saying "One is as young as one feels" is only wishful thinking. You see we just do not want to admit to ourselves that we are getting older. My surgeon told me "Embolism is not so likely to occur in a younger man." My thoughts went to Iain MacLeod, Chancellor of the Exchequer, who in 1970 suffered a fatal embolism in consequence of appendicectomy, and he was three years younger than myself.

But I turned this experience to my advantage. I was able to assess who my real friends are. The list was headed by my wife who took me for better or worse and who proved to me that "a friend in need is a friend indeed." The stay in hospital confirmed my strong beliefs in the N.H.S. The experience did not change my views on life, but enhanced interests by reminding me how unimportant various vicissitudes are and how brief one's life can be. I found the physical pain easier to bear than the mental anguish I once experienced. I resolved to keep clear of it and not to become gloomy or soured by life. I learned to accept fate with good grace. I wish to live my life as fully as possible, enjoying it when still in possession of vigour. Yet, I was gently reminded of my age which prompted me to take a keen interest in geriatrics for the benefit of my elderly patients and . . . myself. But wait – the illness gave me time to think and to take stock of my life. It helped me to know myself better.

My ambition after retirement? To learn good, wholesome and interesting cooking – an *international* cuisine.

Bibliography

Anders, W., Gen., *An Army in Exile* (Macmillan, 1949)

Ayd, Frank J., Blackwell, Barry, *Discoveries in Biological Psychiatry* (Lippincott, 1970)

Borkiewicz, A., *Powstanie Warszawskie* (Pax, 1957)

Breach, R. W., *A History of Our Times: Britain, 1900–1964* (Pergamon, 1968)

Brickfield, Paul, *Reach for the Sky* (Collins, 1954)

Brickhill, Paul, *The Dam Busters* (Evans Bros., 1951)

Burckhardt, Jacob, *The Civilization of the Renaissance* (Allen & Unwin, 1944)

Calder, Ritchie, *Medicine and Man* (Allen & Unwin, 1958)

Cheshire, Leonard, V. C., *The Face of Victory* (Hutchinson, 1961)

Clark, Brian F. C., Marcker Kjeld A., *How Proteins Start* (Scientific American, Jan. 1968, vol. 218, No. 1)

Clark, Ronald W., *The Rise of the Boffins* (Phoenix, 1962)

Clark, Ronald W., *The Life and Work of J. B. S. Haldane* (Hodder & Stoughton, 1968)

Cole, Warren H., *Chemotherapy of Cancer* (Lea & Febiger, 1971)

Crossland, James, *Revised Lewis's Pharmacology* (Livingstone, 1970)

Crowther, J. G., Whiddington, R., *Science at War* (H.M.S.O., 1947)

Fitzgibbon, Constantine, *To Kill Hitler* (Tom Stacey, 1972)

Foot, Michael, *Aneurin Bevan 1945–1960* (Davis Poynter, 1973)

Freeling, Paul, *The Future General Practitioner* (Royal College of General Practitioners, 1972)

Glatt, Max M., Pittman, D. J., Gillespie, D. G., Hills, D. R., *The Drug Scene in Great Britain* (Edward Arnold, 1967)

Gregg, Pauline, *The Welfare State* (Harrap, 1967)

Hawkins, Jack, *Anything for a Quiet Life* (Hamish Hamilton, 1973)

Hibbert, Christopher, *Benito Mussolini* (Longman, 1962)

Hill, Mavis M., Williams, Norman L., *Auschwitz in England* (MacGibbon & Kee, 1965)

Jones, Sir Francis Avery, *Richard Asher Talking Sense* (Pitman Medical, 1972)

Karol, K. S., *Visa for Poland* (MacGibbon & Kee, 1959)

Kendrew, John, *The Thread of Life* (Bell, 1966)

331

Kukiel, M., *Six Years of Struggle for Independence* (Montgomeryshire Printing Co, 1947)

Landau, R., *Paderewski* (Ivor Nicholson & Watson, 1934)

Maclean, Sir Fitzroy, *Eastern Approaches* (Cape, 1949)

Macmillan, Harold, *The Blast of War* (Macmillan, 1967)

Majdalany, F., *Cassino* (Longman, 1957)

Minney, R. J., *Carve Her Name With Pride* (Collins, 1956)

Mirski, Alfred E., *The Discovery of DNA* (Scientific American, Jan. 1968, vol. 218, No. 6)

Lord Moran, *The Struggle for Survival* (Constable, 1966)

Morgan, G., Lasocki, W. A., *Soldier Bear* (Collins, 1970)

Mosley, Leonard, *Faces from the Fire* (Weidenfeld & Nicolson, 1962)

Orgill, Douglas, *The Gothic Line* (Heinemann, 1967)

Owen, David, *Unified Health Service* (Pergamon, 1968)

Roberts, J. A. Fraser, *An Introduction to Medical Genetics*, Six edition (O.U.P., 1973)

Russek, H. I., Zohman, B. L., *Coronary Heart Disease* (Lippincott, 1971)

Sampson, Anthony, *The New Anatomy of Britain* (Hodder & Stoughton, 1971)

Senesh, Hannah, *Her Life and Diary* (Vallentine, Mitchell, 1971)

Sereny, Gitta, *Into that Darkness* (André Deutsch, 1974)

Shirer, William L., *The Rise and Fall of the Third Reich* (Secker & Warburg, 1960)

Thorwald, Juergen, *The Triumph of Surgery* (Thames & Hudson, 1960)

Thorwald, Juergen, *The Dismissal* (Thames & Hudson, 1961)

Tomaszewski, Wiktor, *The University of Edinburgh and Poland* (Aberdeen University Press, 1968)

Trevor-Roper, H. R., *The Last Days of Hitler* (Macmillan, 1962)

Waage, Johan, *The Narvik Campaign* (Harrap, 1964)

Walker, Nicolette, *When I Put Out To Sea* (Collins, 1972)

Wankowicz, Melchior, *Bitwa o Monte Cassino* (Oddz. Kultury i Prasy 2go Pol. Korp., 1945–1946)

Watson, James D., *The Double Helix* (Weidenfeld & Nicolson, 1968)

Winterbottom, F. W., *The Ultra Secret* (Weidenfeld & Nicolson, 1974)

Witz, Ignacy, *Przechadzki po Warszawskich Wystawach 1945–1968* (Panstw. Inst. Wyd., 1972)

Basic Facts about the United Nations (United Nations, New York, 1970)